Culture

& Social Psychiatry

Culture

& Social Psychiatry

Marvin K. Opler

AldineTransaction
A Division of Transaction Publishers
New Brunswick (U.S.A.) and London (U.K.)

Library of Congress Catalog Number: 2006048001
ISBN: 978-0-202-30954-5
Printed in the United States of America

Library of Congress Cataloging-in-Publication Data

Opler, Marvin K. (Marvin Kaufmann), 1914-1981.
    Culture and social psychiatry / Marvin K. Opler.—[Rev. and expanded
ed.]
        p. cm.
    "Opler's classic Culture, Psychiatry, and Human values has here been
revised and expanded to nearly twice the size of the original work"—
Intro.
    ISBN 978-0-202-30954-5 (alk. paper)
    1. Social psychiatry. I. Opler, Marvin K. (Marvin Kaufmann), 1914-
1981 Culture, psychiatry, and human values. II. Title.

RC45506 2007
616.89—dc22   2006048001

To my family,
Charlotte, Ruth, Lewis,
and more recently,
Lew Perry and Curt

Preface to the
Enlarged Edition

Ten years have passed since the publication of *Culture, Psychiatry, and Human Values*. It is eleven years since the first issue of *The International Journal of Social Psychiatry* appeared. In this decade, the sciences of human behavior—cultural, social, psychological, and medical—have joined forces both in research and in practical organization. The dream of Virchow that "once medicine is established in anthropology" or "that medicine is a social science in its very bones and marrow" was uttered in the Germany of 1849 and re-echoed in the writings of Henry Sigerist, who likewise defined medicine bluntly as "a social science" with broad ethical and social responsibilities. But before these germinal ideas could take firm root, it was necessary for research to point a clear course for practical action. The central plea, documented in *Culture, Psychiatry, and Human Values*, is for a unified behavioral science combining anthropology and sociology, as basic social sciences, with psychology and social psychiatry as basic behavioral sciences, no longer compartmentalized and artificially separated into psychological medicine, as it is called in Scotland, psychiatry as it is called in the United States, or medical psychology as it is called elsewhere.

The past decade has witnessed such varied applications of social psychiatry as community psychiatry in the United States, community clinics and home treatment services in Holland, Soviet Russia, and Eastern European nations, group psychotherapy chiefly in the United States and England, and Day Hospitals, Night Hospitals, and Walk-In Emergency Clinics, along with patient Aftercare programs, widely scattered throughout the world. All these changes in the organization of medical services, spoken of programmatically in the 1940s and 1950s are in common currency on a broad international front. Although the labels vary, the international trend presents fundamental similarities, common ideological reliance upon social psychiatry as a way of recognizing social and cultural stresses appearing in individual lives, differences in those backgrounds producing the differences in disorders which we call *diagnoses,* and a more optimistic feeling throughout the world that social psychiatry can offer more than hopeless incarceration in closed-off hospitals abounding in gloomy *prognoses.* If community or culture is the vector of our widespread disease processes of functional mental disorders, then the first principle of disease prevention is to analyze the vector. Only the type of unified behavioral science described and documented in the essay of book length, originally published in 1956, can hope to accomplish this task.

Culture, Psychiatry, and Human Values documented down to 1956 the major sources of data on the epidemiology of mental disorders for continents and island areas around the world. It differentiated types of mental disorders and the amount of disorder, where known, according to social and cultural backgrounds. To do so, it was necessary to differentiate also the various etiologies of illness, their distinctive origins and courses of development. The term *etiology,* we believe, has been unnecessarily hedged with mystical meanings, whereas it means simply a continuum in the development of a disorder in which successively more serious methods and systems of defense are sometimes used. The term *ego defense* can likewise be misleading since it suggests a hypothetical intact notion of an entity, called ego, which is rather a culturally variable than a biologically uniform concept. In general, the first edition of this volume pointed to personality and abnormality in mental functioning as both being culturally determined. Mental disorders, both in their form and in amount (or epidemiology) had changed with cultural evolution. Similarly, concepts of illness and modes of treatment had changed. With population explosion in developing nations, due to relatively young age structures, young female nubility and the rising trends of births over deaths, the human welfare dimensions of the mental health problem are increased many fold from tribal to national boundaries, from rural or primitive settings to more urban ones, and from wholly localized economies to more technologically advanced or industrialized levels. The changes in disorders, the increase in prevalence of more serious illnesses in much of the world, and the accompanying ills of undeveloped economies, unemployment in urban areas, and the problems of family breakdown, suicide, drug addiction, delinquency, and prostitution make social psychiatry, as interdisciplinary research technique and practical programing, more relevant today than ever before. For the reader who finds the essay "Cultural Definitions of Illness" (in Ghana) a comforting account of lower rates of the more serious illnesses—like paranoid schizophrenia—around Kumasi, he is warned both in the book of 1956 and in later reports of the competent team of anthropologist, Meyer Fortes, and psychiatrist, Doris Y. Fortes, that the disorders in Ghana tribes like the Tallensi approach ours in type as the culture changes in our direction.

The evolutionary changes in types of illnesses, in conceptions about them, and in modes of therapy are accompanied, of course, in modern times by the interpenetration of culture-carriers occasioned by modern rapid transportation and the relocation of peoples. In Buffalo, New York, in a few short months, it is possible to have in our county hospital a Chinese case of *koro;* a Malaysian case of running amok; an East Indian hysteria; a Puerto Rican *attaque* (hysteriform and catatonic outburst form of schizophrenia) materializing ultimately into a more classic paranoid form; an Italian schizo-affective disorder; and a Haitian voodoo bewitchment. The need for social psychiatry in these circumstances is multiplied many times by the even more rapid large-scale cultural contact of populations on every continent, by the emergence of new nations, and by the cultural evolution rapidly enveloping formerly isolated parts of the globe.

A completely social and cultural approach to modal personality is a method common to cultural anthropology. Yet, as we point out in "Cultural Evolution and the Psychology of Peoples," the doctrine of modal personality in cultures is not itself a dynamic concept. While modal personality may dignify a notion of human individual development, the latter of course depends upon culture and not merely upon a wholly psychological or biological maturation set of processes. Much of what is being written today, as well as in the psychological anthropology of the 1930s and 1940s, is couched in the terms of *individual* psychological process and evolution. In Paul Tillich's *estrangement,* in George Herbert Mead's *non-realization of the self,* in Durkheim's *anomie,* in Erich Fromm's *alienation* and "escape from" freedom we are not far, really, from the Freudian idea of the individual's "ego gratification" as a central principle of an instinctual psychology, although the social realm is invoked as the arena from which ego functioning has, more or less, departed. Frankly, despite the debates, we cannot discern much difference from Freud's *The Ego and the Id* with its definition of "superego" as being fundamentally "social feelings" which "rest on the foundation of identification with others" or on "the basis of ego-ideal in common with them." The bowing out of Oedipus, and the invocation of culture as the "heir of the Oedipus complex" representing ethical standards of mankind is a prototype, written in 1923, of Mead's *Mind, Self and Society,* Ruth Benedict's *Patterns of Culture* (both published in 1934), Erich Fromm's *Escape from Freedom* (1941), or the *Individual and His Society* by A. Kardiner and R. Linton (1939). The cultural evolutionary position stands in contrast to these first steps emphasizing man's place in culture and his individual evolvement within the cultural matrix inasmuch and insofar as it adds a focus on the evolution of culture itself. Perhaps we should go back beyond Durkheim's seminal notion of *anomie* in his study on suicide (1897) to his brilliant *Rules of Sociological Method* in 1895 with its final rule for cross-cultural psychiatry: "for just comparison's sake, compare societies in the same stage of development." To do so requires the application of cultural evolutionary principles to social psychiatry.

The themes of individualism versus alienation (the German *Entfremdung*) so well exemplified in the work of Sartre suggest that man's fate in society and culture is always bound up with the same problems of self-identification. Here, of course, we think of the individual developmental system of E. H. Erikson, an attempt to broaden self-identification processes beyond sexual identification as in Freud's work. But again, the exclusive concern with the self, as such, or its admittedly important sexual aspects, falls short of the complete concerns of social psychiatry. We have therefore added immediately after our essay on cultural evolution a paper concerned really with three nearly simultaneous identification processes, although it is called "Anthropological and Cross-Cultural Aspects of Homosexuality." The three identification processes are self-identification, sexual-identification, and social-identification. Within the first year of life, not one but all of these concomitant forces begin to take root. Nor are they finalized in some life period like adolescence, though they may be (or may not be) powerfully reinforced at puberty. The fact is that, again, now in the sense of a life history or life cycle, biological, psychological, social, and cultural factors operate together. As we have pointed out, the variations in every form of mental disorder by age-sex or class-cultural analyses indicate that self- or sexual-identification processes are essentially meaningless unless one adds social-identification as a concomitant in the life cycle. As we have stated in an essay entitled "Scientific Social Psychiatry Encounters Existentialism,"* drives and conflicts actually manifest themselves in the self, but the kinds of drives and kinds of conflicts depend on culture, society, and history. For the existentialists, the key to the encounter is that in psychotherapy they mistake compelling and sometimes even horrifying subjective experiences for the objective realities. In reducing all to cross-sectional selves—so well portrayed in the harshly drawn puppet-like symbols of Jean Genet —the unique and ontologically differentiated individual actor may be allowed to emerge, while missing the whole generalizing method of social science which seeks similarities in structure and function as well as differences, and cultural processes as well as individual regularities. Both existentialism, and subjectivist interpretations of self which have always been the trademark of the tortured sensitivities of a Kierkegaard, a Nietzsche, a Dostoevski, a Sartre, or a Genet, locate "the unstable equilibrium" or "sense of bewildered precariousness" in the psychological systems which do not analyze adequately the social and cultural *conditions of existence*. In short, *Daseins*-analysis is a most incomplete analysis, though it has a certain justification in art, where partial revelation, insight, intuition, and cross-sectional descriptions allow

* *Philosophy and Phenomenological Research*, 24:2, 1963.

the perceiver to enter into the experience of the creative artist by filling the gaps, interpreting the symbols, sharing the insights, and actively participating in rounding out the interpretation of events. In all of this subjectivism, the generalizing method and even the ethical temper of science may fall by the wayside.

A broader approach of science which aims at analyzing the individual's personality development in relation to the development of society and culture is what we called a *relational* system of behavioral analysis. The key to such a relational system in any of its evolutionary parts is always the complex of cultural conditions of existence. These conditions, carried always in any social system, affect psychological development. This means they affect or indeed produce normative or modal trends in personality, statistically considered, and quantitatively also the forms or types (the etiologies) of functional mental disorders. Two essays, written in 1964 and 1961 respectively, "Sociocultural Roots of Emotional Illness," and "Social Psychiatry—Evolutionary, Existentialist, and Transcultural Findings," are next presented to draw out the implications of the view that interpersonal relations are conditioned by repetitive and meaningful social activity, fashioned for better or for worse always by environment. If, in the first essay, the reader is appalled by the high rates of impairment we discovered as a principal investigator in the Midtown Manhattan Community Mental Health Research Study, he can read of smaller counts of mental illness by M. E. Spiro in a contrasting Micronesian culture at the end of the same paper. The fact is that Midtown Manhattan's rates are alarming as are the disclosures on persons in treatment (treated prevalence of disorder) in the Yale-New Haven Study of Hollingshead, Redlich, and Myers. Nor are these matters of city size, as is indicated by discussions in the 1956 volume of Hyde's work in Boston deflating the factor of population density, or by the Stirling County Project in thinly settled areas of Nova Scotia. These studies have by implication indicted general social conditions responsible for dislocations in cultural development and disturbances in interpersonal relations. None of them holds that such conditions are immutable, though we must concede that much real damage has occurred and that some scars are transmitted by intergenerational contact.

In a relational theory, the intervention that social psychiatry can offer depends in part on developing new and flexible cross-cultural diagnostic categories not simply to understand the origin and meanings, to patients, of symptom complexes and defensive maneuvers, but to eliminate symptoms, support healthy interpersonal assets, and decrease reliance upon isolating and self-defeating tendencies in the psychic economy. The organized group with similar purposes, whether in social psychiatric team functioning, in family or group therapy, in the full use of community resources and facilities in treatment, in home services, Day and Night Hospitals, Walk-In Emergency Clinics, or community-oriented agencies, is as much preventive as it is social psychiatry.

To round out the following section and to indicate that much of this research lies in the realm of public health and preventive medicine, we have added one conference paper, hitherto unpublished, on the epidemiology of diabetes, since psychosomatic and even certain forms of metabolic disorders may have social and interpersonal connections.

In the essays that follow, various research designs are stressed. One begins with a product of the Midtown Manhattan Study in New York City, a paper entitled "Cultural Perspectives in Research on Schizophrenias." The emphasis on schizophrenias with paranoid reaction among Midtown Manhattan Irish male samples is contrasted with schizo-affective disorders in a matched sample of Italian males. The total study involved ten parameters or variables; and in each aspect these patients of different cultural background were as different as day and night. We have reported elsewhere on single variables such as the use of fantasy by Irish (tested by ten psychological methods) versus the motility of the contrasting sample. All ten variables outlined in this essay were elaborately tested, so that this account of the variables used is the more inclusive and understandable one. The reader should be aware also that *all* the hypotheses as to cultural differences in these groups and others studied in Midtown Manhattan were derived from studies of the ongoing cultural communities and of normative (or ostensibly "well") samples of nonpatient population in New York City.

In contrast to these studies in the largest city of the United xiv

States is the essay "Cultural Definitions of Illness" focusing on rural and village Ghana in West Africa. Here the plea is for introducing cultural relativity in views of ethnopsychiatry rather than applying our diagnoses crudely and uncritically to other cultural scenes. The essay by Meyer and Doris Fortes, "Psychosis and Social Change among the Tallensi of Northern Ghana,"* reinforces this view though they had not seen my essay on Ghana, published in 1963, during their field work and the period of write-up, nor was I aware what they would publish about a northern Ghana people in 1966.

In the original volume, particularly in the full descriptions of African tribal disorders, we wrote of the catatonic or catathymic outburst forms of illness and also concerning the less serious hysterical or hysteriform acting out. We noted, after Carothers, that many of these illnesses are open to spontaneous remission. They are not, therefore, of the serious dimensions of our paranoid schizophrenias and schizo-affective disorders reported for Midtown. Defensive maneuvers in nonliterate and tribal societies are more expressive, dramatic, or mimetic of the underlying conflicts than is the case in so-called "modern societies."

Having written frequently on what are called hysteriform disorders, or even simple prototypes of schizophrenias (such as *latah, imu,* Arctic Hysteria, running amok), we believe it is important for anthropologists to start commenting pointedly on the different types of mental illness developed in other cultures. If there are repressed wishes centered in some age or sex group, one finds conversion hysterias, hysteriform acting out, and others. This is stated definitely in our chapter on the Ute Indians in *Culture and Mental Health;*† before that it was stated in *Culture, Psychiatry, and Human Values.* The interesting point is that this is not just a matter of thwarted wish-fulfillment and then acting out and safety-valves provided in a cult, but rather these folk-cultural forms additionally offer group social supports which certainly counteract or take the place of isolation and private wish-fulfillment in an active way. Psychoanalysts and family group therapists usually do not have such ready resources close at hand. It is the

* *Cahiers d'Études Africaines,* 6:1, 1966, 5–40.
† Marvin K. Opler, editor. New York: The Macmillan Co., 1959.

mission of social psychiatry, we imagine, to indicate that these restitutive community supports aimed specifically at socially produced problems are a necessity in such cultures as have problems and limitations, our own included. The therapeutic methods of nonliterate peoples do not rely upon the intellectual techniques of obtaining insight alone, but they add to such rational strategies very often the wisdom of seeking directly for group support, cultural sanctions, and the aesthetic counterparts of ritual in music, dance, and dramatic verbal interventions of the shaman or the curing priest. Therefore, depth analysis which is thought necessary for cure in our society may be interwoven in nonliterate groups with methods utilizing group support, religious beliefs, and folk feeling. Such methods have greater behavioral validity in closely knit societies, and they may be utilized quite naturally to counteract the individual narcissism of the largely hysterical and hysteriform aberrations. In our modern society and culture, of course, both psychosomatic and more heavily disguised defensive maneuvers (in depth) are substituted. Hence, psychiatrists steeped in European and American psychiatric traditions often miss the cathartic value of these dramatized purification ceremonies, or they fail to see social sanctions implicit in the tightly knit society —with its beliefs about witchcraft and sorcery—and read off the native (sic!), complaining of witchcraft, erroneously as a paranoid or a schizophrenic. Our critique of M. J. Field's work (through intermediaries largely!) is based on recognizing that nonliterate peoples are mindful of their folk beliefs and social sanctions. When they state cultural rather than idiosyncratic beliefs, they are a far cry, indeed, from our paranoid schizophrenics. The best proof besides our cultural analyses is that spontaneous remissions occur; and this is hardly to be expected in schizophrenias with paranoid reaction. Further, the catathymic outburst forms, punctuated with periods of lucidity, their hysteriform underpinnings, and their expressive symbolism likewise show what we have found to be termed in the literature "spontaneous recovery." These differences must be noted in the salvaging of ethnology and ethnopsychiatry, before the so-called primitive scene disappears forever from our view, inasmuch as urban evolution brings in its wake increasing disorders like our own.

In primitive ceremonials of the curing type, the patient is often made the center of attention, and of course an element—though not the only one—of ego-gratification occurs which runs counter to narcissistic deprivation. Often, too, the practitioner is more aggressive in his spirited attack upon the illness and its sometimes sorcerous alleged perpetrators. The time-honored emphases on "sacrifices"—that is, on giving up "something"—and the shedding of symptoms as a limited goal stand in contrast to our ego-psychology attempts to explore and change *basic* identities. In our belief, this is, for all men, a fantastically large order in any society, and it is here again that we should like to contrast the essentially short-term methods and goals of most of primitive psychotherapy with depth analysis. Actually, in our own society, the methods of short-term therapy, the ideological accommodations to the greater sense of immediacy and desire for quick relief in lower-class patients, and the psychosomatic disguises (rather than the primitives' sometimes frank and obvious conversion hysterias) all argue for more flexible and often more rapid methods than depth analysis. In these shifts, we believe, we are coming full-circle to methods of herbal remedy and placebo, group ceremony and dramatization, rapid intervention and team functioning characteristic of earlier evolutionary stages in cultural development. Nonliterate tribes have often practiced social psychiatry, in effect, for countless generations; and it may be suggested by their rates before widespread cultural contact that we have much to learn from them.

In this discussion it is necessary to set aside or exclude mental disorders which have a simple organic origin. This is done simply to clarify the discussion. Actually, there are other cultures besides our own which frequently group together illnesses having an organic origin with those which do not. In Nigeria, for example, the delirium produced by smallpox fevers is regarded among the Yoruba as a mental illness because mental functioning is modified. However, Nigerian curing priests of cults distinguish with great sophistication among four classes of mental illness in a continuum; and this is consistent with their total theory of disease. There are, they say, first of all diseases of exclusively physical and organic origin. Obvious examples would be broken bones, impairments from accidents, or the kind of wasting away which might be caused by protracted famine. Their continuum proceeds to a second variety in which a disease of major organic origin has nevertheless enough psychological overtones to be called mainly organic, but *partly* psychological. Their third category comprises illnesses of psychological types but with physical and organic consequences, and here the sophistication of a tribal society like the Yoruba would supply us even today with the right formula for an approach to what we call psychosomatic illnesses. Their fourth category in the continuum is what we would call the neuroses and functional psychoses. Even here we must remember that, long before we did, the Nigerians used tranquilizers, such as Indian Snake root (reserpine), together with psychological treatments for their patients, and with a notion of varying dosages depending on age and size.

One of my Nigerian fieldworkers, a medical student, recorded data indicating that reserpine might be used along with psychological treatments in cases where a psychotic person had an illness literally called "frightened out of one's wits," the types of cases here being catatonic or at worst schizo-affective. Catatonias are not seen in our society as frequently as they used to be seen in preindustrial settings. Our medical student who conducted this field work under supervision was from Nigerian Yoruba country. Another common functional type of case he encountered was, of course, the acute confusional state with catathymic outbursts. These possibly account for the common Nigerian practice of not only sedating the patient but also putting him initially in shackles. While shackling may seem hopelessly old-fashioned to us even in a culture which had tranquilizers long before we did, one can doubt whether we can really pride ourselves on modernity in this one instance of comparison. The acting out of an illness state in Nigeria is far more spontaneous than in our urban society, and however florid the symptoms may look, the flatness of affect of our schizophrenics is often missing. We have relatively fewer catathymic outbursts, but in our urban cultures we have, as everyone knows, a superabundance of schizophrenics called "chronic or undifferentiated" along with those with paranoid reaction. Again, it seems to me, that the Nigerians come off better because their catatonias and catathymic outburst types seem to be open to remission. In our paranoid schizophrenias, spontaneous remission is uncommon.

If one went further with this catalogue of differences between Nigerian psychiatry and our own, it would emerge that they have aftercare programs in the curing cult activities for expatients and group therapy in their cult practices. They also have modes of family involvement in therapy, in which the entire family may live near the hospital or the curer's compound, as the case may be, caring for the patient and, when he is improved sufficiently, working along with him and with the practitioner or curing priest in the same work any Nigerian does.

The above example serves to illustrate a general principle of social psychiatry, true of all societies. One must start first with the social and cultural nature of the disorders themselves; the type of illness and the amount will vary with conditions in different societies and cultures. For instance, one can observe more catatonic-like schizophrenias among first- and second-generation Polish descendants in a city like Buffalo, New York, and, at the same time, more schizophrenias with paranoid reaction among those of German descent. We have already conducted such studies in local hospitals as an extension of the studies begun in New York City, using Veterans' Administration Hospitals. In Buffalo, we have also made studies of disturbed adolescents in such groups as Irish and Italian and again the form of disturbance varies with social and cultural conditions as in the Midtown Manhattan studies in New York.

The anthropological science most germane, and in fact indispensable, to social psychiatry is cultural anthropology. While not attempting here to define cultural anthropology exhaustively, we can note that most definitions emphasize a composite understanding of man and his works, usually referring to a body of customs, beliefs, practices, and artifacts. Some sense of this broad scope is indicated when we recall that practices include infant handling, child-rearing practices, the organization of life for adolescents, for sexual conduct, or for the aged. While early anthropologists discussed such *cognitive* balances in cultures by this cognitively-oriented definition of culture itself, the pendulum has swung to include emotional contents and balances as well. As a consequence, one adds today to the usual formal definitions of culture, including customs, beliefs, practices, and artifacts (or all those things engaged in and utilized by man as a member of society), the emotionally felt and creatively or negatively understood values, whether these are overtly experienced or covertly and emotionally felt. By including these unconscious or preconscious manifestations, along with conscious experiences, the anthropologist today can deal with unconscious patterning of behavior in society. The author has phrased this expansion of the scope of anthropology as including the *total conditions of existence* meaningful to man and understandable in a science of man and culture. This links culture with the vicissitudes of personality in what he has called a relativistic relational system comprising both aspects.

While primitive forms of schizophrenias are found to be open to "spontaneous" remissions—something rare in the schizophrenias with paranoid reaction of modern societies—these forms, which the author has called, following J. C. Carother's work, simple psychotic "confusional states," connect with and are catathymic outbursts, or stereotyped forms of simple catatonic schizophrenias such as the *latah* and running amok of Malaysia, the *imu* illness of Hokkaido, the Arctic Hysterias of northeastern Asia, or being frightened out of one's wits in Nigeria. All of these disorders have been reported as open to spontaneous remission, or curable by curing priest and cult, or by shamanism. They are curable, in part, because like the conversion hysteria phenomena treated through dream analysis in Ute Indian culture, they have a hysteriform basis in socially induced conflicts, though the schizophrenic forms we have listed add to this a psychotic dissociative behavior or confusions and outbursts.*

We have expanded upon these matters of classification because there is a need, now more than ever, for new diagnostic categories in social psychiatry. Such categories are as necessary today as Bleuler's reclassification of the schizophrenias from the time-worn dementia praecox was in 1911. Indeed, a half century later,

---

* Cf. Marvin K. Opler, "Dream Analysis in Ute Indian Therapy," in *Culture and Mental Health*, New York: The Macmillan Co., 1959.

following the discovery of quite different illnesses widespread in other cultural traditions, it is fitting to develop newer classifications reflecting current knowledge of other peoples rather than insisting on the universal applicability of our extraneous terms. To move this contrast ahead is not merely to stress complete differentiation. There are indeed similar processes in human behavior, and perhaps a pan-human, if not identical, set of factors accounting for a kind of kinship in the species even where conditions of existence have promoted variation.

In the main, therefore, our account goes from theory and cross-cultural epidemiological data, through group research designs and down to individual cases. In "Culture and Chronic Illness," it is interesting to see that certain cultures, more modern and urbanized to be sure, have succumbed to what may be termed psychosomatic and metabolic disorders. As a matter of fact, this is foreshadowed in "Sociocultural Roots of Emotional Illness," in an earlier section, where the data of Butler County, Pennsylvania, are adduced to indicate higher rates in many psychosomatic categories for second-generational groups (the children of immigrants).

To set the scene adequately for the individual cases, we have utilized one wartime study of the Japanese-Americans in Relocation Centers in World War II. The themes of escapism are noted in the data of formalized poetry clubs, but where the social reaction occurs, it is healthy, incisive, and instructive. This is the center where mental health epidemiology worsened as economic depletion took its toll, where suicides were a barometer of center tensions, and yet where cultural revivalism in poetry, dance, art, and even folk medicine could be studied in its most efflorescent form. The paper represents an oasis of healthful effort in a people who were the very outcasts of the American scene, subject to three years of isolation, discrimination, and prejudice. It is my tribute to their resiliency as a group.

Finally, the case presentations that follow, the story of a Japanese youth, "Cultural Dilemma of a Kibei Youth," and the accounts of two Puerto Rican men, relate to the same theme of cultural conflict and uprooting. Let them speak for themselves.

MARVIN K. OPLER

Foreword

In the last few years we have witnessed the development of a branch of psychiatric activity and research worthy of the name of Social Psychiatry. Increasingly, as psychiatrists have met with anthropologists, sociologists, and other social scientists, a blending of knowledge from all the fields has taken place, and with this came the emergence of a common language, a point of view about personality and culture, and lately the sharp delineation of research projects which draw upon all these disciplines for their resolution.

The emergence of anthropology into the field of contemporary human behavior has brought substantial enlightenment to the problems of mankind in our own contemporary western civilization. Those of us who try to view man in his total cultural setting know that the contemporary anthropologist has much to contribute to our understanding of the inter-action of the person, his family, and his total cultural heritage.

Psychiatry and the social sciences have been in need of a critical review of what is known in this complex area. There is much that we can learn and insights that we can derive about our operating psychiatric hypotheses from the studies of cultures different from ours, as well as from a more systematic delineation of our own American cultural groups and what our specific culture does to man.

Dr. Opler is particularly fitted to prepare such a critical review for us and to synthesize the available knowledge. With years of anthropological experience behind him, he has acquired a wide knowledge of the pertinent and available studies and literature. For many years his own interest in personality functioning prepared him for his role as senior anthropologist in an interdisciplinary study of urban mental health in which he has been associated with me for three years as one of the principal investigators. This living experience in interdisciplinary thought and work has led to crystallization in this present volume.

In this volume Dr. Opler ranges widely through the whole field of cultural anthropology and psychodynamics, bringing to bear upon the reported studies a fresh and critical point of view, adhering to no particular school. He has also had the courage to scrutinize and challenge some long standing convictions and hypotheses. His own synthesis of the material is original and provocative.

Dr. Opler has given us a scholarly resume of mental illness as seen in the broad framework of cultural differences and determinants. I feel confident that this book will prove stimulating to scientists of many professional backgrounds. For psychiatrists particularly it illuminates new facets of personality development, of psychodynamics, and of some of the subtle cultural determinants of psychopathology.

I have learned much from Dr. Opler in my three years of work with him. This volume summarizes for me as a psychiatrist the salient anthropological concepts and views on mental illness which would otherwise have escaped me. I hope that it will do so for a large reading public.

THOMAS A. C. RENNIE, M.D.

Professor of Psychiatry (Social Psychiatry)
Cornell University Medical College

Acknowledgments

I take pleasure in expressing my thanks and in making acknowledgments to the following editors and publishers for permission to quote from journal articles or books as the case may be; to the authors we are distinctly grateful:

To Dr. Clarence B. Farrar (editor) and *The American Journal of Psychiatry:* Volume 111, 1954, *The Psychopathologic Basis of Psychotherapy of Schizophrenia*, by Oskar Diethelm; Volume 110, 1953, *The Implications of the Psychogenetic Hypothesis*, by Paul Lemkau, Benjamin Pasamanik, and Marcia Cooper; Volume 109, 1952, *Some Characteristics of the Psychopathology of Schizophrenic Behavior in Bahian Society*, by Edward Stainbrook.

To Dr. Sol Tax (editor) and *The American Anthropologist:* Volume 44, 1942, *Some Psychological Aspects of Measurement Among the Salteaux*, by A. Irving Hallowell.

To Dr. Emil A. Gutheil (editor) and *The American Journal of Psychotherapy:* Volume 6, 1952, *The Concept of Normality*, by F. C. Redlich.

To *The Bulletin of the Menninger Clinic* and the following authors: Volume 18, 1954, *The Contribution of Psychoanalysis to American Psychiatry*, by Karl Menninger, and *The Perception Project: Progress Report*, by George S. Klein, P. Holtzman, and D. Laskin.

To Dr. C. West Churchman (editor) and *Philosophy of Science:* Volume 20, 1954, *The Concept of Values in Contemporary Philosophical Value Theory*, by Abraham Edel.

To Dr. J. O. Brew and the *Peabody Museum of Harvard University Papers:* Volume 47, 1952, *Culture: A Critical*

To Yale University Press: *An Essay on Man,* by E. Cassirer, Copyright 1944.

To W. W. Norton and Company: *Psychosocial Medicine,* by J. L. Halliday, Copyright 1948.

To Thomas Y. Crowell Company, *Essays in the Science of Culture* (edited by G. Dole and R. Carneiro): Cultural Evolution and the Psychology of Peoples, Copyright 1960.

To Basic Books, Inc., *Sexual Inversion* (edited by Judd Marmor): Anthropological and Cross-Cultural Aspects of Homosexuality, Copyright © 1965 by Basic Books, Inc., Publishers, New York.

To Dr. Wilfred Dorfman (editor) and *Psychosomatics:* Volume 5, January-February, 1964, Sociocultural Roots of Emotional Illness; Volume 2, Number 6, November-December 1961, Social Psychiatry—Evolutionary, Existentialist and Transcultural Findings.

To *The Psychiatric Quarterly:* Volume 33, July 1959, Cultural Perspectives in Research on Schizophrenia.

To The New York Academy of Medicine and International Universities Press, *Man's Image in Medicine and Anthropology* (edited by Iago Galdston): Cultural Definitions of Illness, Copyright 1963.

To the *Journal of American Folklore:* Volume 58, Number 227, January-March 1945, Senryu Poetry as Folk and Community Expression.

To The Ronald Press Company, *Clinical Studies in Culture Conflict* (edited by Georgene Seward): Cultural Dilemma of a Kibei Youth; Dilemmas of Two Puerto Rican Men, Copyright © 1958 The Ronald Press Company.

I also wish to express my gratitude to Dr. Oskar Diethelm and the late Dr. T. A. C. Rennie who read the manuscript and offered helpful suggestions, and to Mrs. Doris Slawson who typed the final draft. Any errors, however, are of my own commission.

Last, but not least, this book has been dedicated to my family for their warm and by now perennial indulgence of what are known as scholarly pursuits.

M. K. O.

Contents

PART III.   RESEARCH DESIGNS

I
Social and Cultural Backgrounds of Mental Illness

Introduction

THE IMPACT of social and cultural environment upon the development of personalities is the central concern of social psychiatry. While this environment is in no sense a fixed form or pattern into which personality falls and is moulded, neither is it simply a mere extraneous influence added to inevitable results determined by the child-rearing practices of a culture. The attempts to exaggerate the socio-cultural setting to a global and inclusive mould effect are daily belied by the variations in personalities encountered by observers, scientific or otherwise, in any given setting. On the other hand, even the most cursory acquaintance with psychiatric case histories individually considered indicates the crudity of beginning with the Freudian basic disciplines and inferring therefrom the total contours of adult personality configurations. Both methods, the grossly cultural and the rigidly psychogenetic, are only partly useful as formulae and only partly true to individual and cultural realities.

These theoretical opposites fail in that they do not assess, beyond the one-way causal scheme either for psychiatry or anthropology, the exact relationship that environmental experiences bear *throughout* the life history to individual adjustment. As Edward Sapir once said, "The worlds in which different societies live are distinct worlds, not merely the same world with different labels attached." In connection with Princeton's Perception Demonstration Center, Hadley Cantril has shown how the nature of the individual's experience in life, even upon the perceptual level, depends on his prior assumptions, how these in turn are built from past experiences; and how attitudes, opinions and percepts change only when the individual is blocked and feels frustration. No doubt, turning to psychiatry, a building up of cognitive, attitudinal and perceptual patterns has also an organic, metabolic and hormonal basis since the organism, as such, is the reactive mechanism; however, personality is more than mechanism, and the individual is more than an autonomic system, self-propelled and self-motivated.

Ordinarily, a person's experiences are in the normal course interpreted along lines laid down by his culture, even though the channels cut by culture thread through such more familiar terrain as family structure and functioning, a system of values and beliefs, a range of social and economic statuses, certain practices and taboos, attitudes towards health and illness, and such features as the characteristic styles of interpersonal relationships. All of these features are the coin of the realm of personality formation, affecting marital, parent-child, sibling, peer, and other group relations. They vary with culture, and with degree and pace of acculturation or culture change. Among the basic orientations provided by culture, A. I. Hallowell has recently listed self- and object-orientation, spatio-temporal orientation, a motivational orientation, and a sense of normative standards and values.[1] The kinds of relationships set up within a culture and defining its age-groups, its sex behavior and attitudes, its statements of the individual position in the family and in the social group are no doubt ramifications of these basic categories. They may be seen also in what Ruth Benedict once called the continuities and discontinuities of the life history pattern.

This life span, or life cycle, is lived in a constant homeostatic relationship with this total environment, parts of which become internalized and implicit in an individual's responses and reactions as well as external and explicit. On the individual level of responses in actions and symbols, unique though these are, no life is lived alone and apart from interpersonal patterns of communication and interaction. All personality formation, or the psychodynamics of well or ill alike, rely in the last analysis upon symbolic forms of communication and self-expression in which what is human *and* cultural is shared, while that which is bizarre and autistic is closer to raw impulse or guarded illusion. A psychiatry, or a behavioral science, which credits a human being with a dynamic life biography and with conditions of existence in communicated and felt socio-cultural settings, but which ends by denying reality of the social and cultural groups, cannot move from case A to case B, or indeed fully assess the impact of other people on either A or B.[2]

In his recent posthumous work, *The Interpersonal Theory of Psychiatry*, Harry Stack Sullivan has stated that progress toward a "psychiatry of peoples" can emerge only from improved understanding of significant patterns of living in the modern world coupled with the discovery of important details in personality development by which persons of different socio-cultural background "come to manifest more or less adequate behavior in their given social settings." Each of these lines of inquiry, the first in anthropology and the second in social psychiatry, he regarded as a "necessary supplement to the other." Seen from this vantage point, not merely the often unrecallable earlier stages of childhood confusion, but any appropriate and less dereistic or painful points in the life cycle are equally important in their own right "in the unfolding of possibilities for interpersonal relations in the progression . . . toward mature competence for life in a fully human world." The importance of families, communities, socio-political entities, group cultures and sub-cultures as the settings for these progressive efforts of the individual are all alluded to by Sullivan. He also stresses the special skills in the study of interpersonal relationships, participant observation and interviewing techniques using the operational approach and field theory concepts of psychiatric and anthropological science. Finally, we learn that, ideally, the psychiatrist as "participant observer" uses concepts derived from the anthropologist's analyses of other cultures.[3]

This concordance of interests in the fields of psychiatry and anthropology in three areas, the individual personality, the cultural background, and family or social group participation is a convergence in broadly integrative behavioral science. That it should appear in the consolidating and synthesizing phases of each discipline in the Twentieth Century is not surprising. If, as has been known for some time, there are intimate connections between the organization of personality and its socio-cultural background, then the study of either is revealing of outlines, demarcations and significances of conduct in the individual.

The increasing use of projective test methodologies in the study of cultures is instructive at this juncture, since it was Rorschach himself who first studied psychotic patients from two different Swiss cantons and who reported that the results obtained seemed to indicate variation in the actual form of psychoses which could be attributed to distinct cultural backgrounds. The ease with which the Rorschach, and other projective techniques, could be administered even to nonliterate peoples, and the objective criterion of "blind analyses" by psychologists who did not know the informant, opened the way for on-the-spot ethnologists to gather reasonably unbiased personality data. It is no wonder that psychologists, interpreting such materials with scoring systems which were not even well-established in our culture, found these to fall short of adequate quantitative establishment of norms elsewhere and were consequently guided by intelligent use of the raw materials and by general principles governing the use of the total instrument.

The underlying Rorschach principles, or assumptions, that the individual had no way of knowing what was expected in terms of performance and therefore characteristically responded in the way in which he handled every life situation seemed true enough if one further assumed inherent grouping principles in the perception of form, as promulgated by Gestalt psychology, and secondly, recognized the possibility of cross-cultural differences and comparisons. Indeed, Hallowell showed that certain responses were popularly given despite strongly divergent cultural backgrounds.[4] On the other hand, Laura Thompson, in a study of three different Hopi communities with variance in economic security and social organization, demonstrated through projective material the importance of cultural background and varying social organization in the personalities of members of each group.[5] Hallowell, even earlier, found significant Rorschach differences among acculturated and unacculturated Salteaux.[6]

The techniques of separate or blind analyses, initiated by the anthropologist, Cora DuBois, and Oberholzer in DuBois' *The People of Alor*, were continued with inclusion of the Thematic Apperception Test by the anthropologist Thomas Gladwin and the clinical psychologist, Seymour B. Sarason, in their joint work, *Truk; Man in Paradise*.[7] In such blind interpretations, there is remarkable similarity in interpretations given by ethnologists and clinicians, as where, in the last example, Sarason was able to draw conclusions, similar to Gladwin, about the concentration of Trukese on rigid suppression of feelings and impulses, and on the development of conformance and concreteness of thinking in these subjects. Actually, the anthropological data on the all-important lineage relationships proved to

be of crucial significance in explaining the development
of conforming, inhibited, suppressing personalities. On
the other hand, the psychological data revealed a
dominance of women and forced an ethnological re-exami-
nation of the material wherein, though seemingly more sub-
missive, they did indeed occupy the truly pivotal position
in social organization because of their primary role in the
handling of food allocations. With these basic orientations
in mind, purely descriptive data including male and female
sexual conduct, family organization and even child-rearing
practices fall in line. Equally, records examined by Oberholzer, and revealing kinds of reaction typical of patients
suffering brain injury in our culture, were adequately
understandable only when cultural themes and organization were explicit. In the Trukese study, an important
sexual problem of women was missed in Rorschach interpretations of the psychologist by merely not knowing the
female sexual symbol.

Jules Henry has pointed out that the use of rare detail in
Rorschachs of a jungle people of South America is a function of their need to observe their surroundings in order to
survive. Similarly, Cook's finding of "overuse" of space-
responses in Samoa reflected simply the special cultural
value attached to the color white. The point is clear that
in two sciences related to social psychiatry, in cultural
anthropology and clinical psychology, there is increasing
awareness that in order to understand both culture and
personality adequately, one must ascertain how the personality of the members of a given society finds expression
within a social and cultural framework. Three-dimensional
social psychiatry, involving the techniques of social science
and psychology, would likewise require as a necessary
parameter of scientific observation the notion of a socio-
cultural frame of reference for normative and aberrant;
for gauging the intensities of affect; the types and degrees

of human expressivity in different cultures; the choice of cultural symbols used in human communication; or in short, the varying cognitive, perceptual and attitudinal interpretations of any cultural human being.

Awareness of these generalized, or cultural, symbolic functions in individual psychodynamics is not limited to psychology. The fact that human communication and expression is based on symbols to which meanings are assigned was discovered, so to speak, independently in psychiatry once the notion of an inevitable course of illness and rigid diagnostic categories, as in the classical descriptive work of Kraepelin, gave way to a more dynamic view of variables in typology, illness progression, and environmental influences as in the work of Adolf Meyer. With the gradual death of the notion of a "unit psychosis," the ideological importance of longitudinal case history grew, relying at first on relating the organic and metabolic functioning to unique symbolic functioning of personality. Gradually, the hospital as a therapeutic milieu, "push therapy," the phenomena of transference and countertransference, and explorations into symbolic content and dynamics came into purview. The movement was from hospitalized to ambulatory treatment where possible; from custodial care and descriptive analysis to devices aimed at gradual socialization and improved environment; from cross-sectional symptomatology to assessment of the longitudinal course of illness; and from random exploration and probing to carefully guided support and re-education.

Increasingly the psychosocial position required a knowledge of the cultural setting and background of each patient to the end that his world of meanings and experiences be assessed in therapy, and his organic and symbolic functioning understood in terms of the contexts or milieus of family, community, social and sub-cultural groups in which he had played a role. Independently, in the social sciences, the areas of social action and interactive process were explored in social systems and social roles. The social statuses and their functions in the social structure, and the manner in which that structure was systematized were all important ingredients in defining an individual's relationships to his fellows, and his activities, to be sure, in relation to theirs. Nevertheless, the anatomy and physiology of a social system and its functioning related ultimately to a further system of meanings, at once cultural and personal in essence. This was to say that roles were, by and large, culturally defined; that social structures varied with cultural backgrounds and identities, and that whole social systems were built on foundations supplied by what Kluckhohn called implicit (Sapir's "unconsciously patterned") and explicit (consciously followed) cultural symbols.

In the work of Adolf Meyer, the challenge to an oversimplified and rigid typology and labeling process was to construct new typologies having greater range and also greater reference to the variability of process in the adaptation, or maladaptation, to environment. In therapy, too, one of his contributions was to point to possibilities of adaptation to a milieu, or to point up positive relationships which a patient was in a position to utilize. In the same intellectual period, John Dewey in philosophy was noting that a social existence was a necessary condition for the development of normative mentation processes in any individual. Physical anthropologists like Boas were pointing out the mutational plasticity of humans under environmental changes; social biologists like Hogben were documenting environmental effects in the statistical incidence of mental deficiency; and H. S. Jennings was initiating the studies of human behavior and genetics which have led ultimately to our present knowledge that of the more than five hundred single gene substitutions for which there is good evidence, only a minor few determine behavioral resultants. The psychoanalytic movement, least "organicist" of all, was at the same time enjoying a growth of popularity in the United States while giving rise to sharply varying systems like those of Horney, of Roheim, of Rado, Kardiner and Ferenczi, which like Sullivan's were directly influenced by anthropologists such as Sapir and Linton, Kluckhohn, Benedict and Mead.

In none of this transfer of interest to total life span, to situational context or milieu, to relationships within a social system, and to cultural background, were the sacred precincts of any one science inviolable. Multidisciplinary research recognized that the pathology of a society reflects its general conditions, and conversely offered important clues to an understanding of the culture. Galen's ancient phrase, "Man is a whole with his environment," found epidemiological confirmation not in the least from carefully designed public health inquiries in which the epidemiology (*how much* illness in time periods of incidence) soon came to mean *how much* illness emerged in relation to age, sex, and finally social and cultural strata. Why these problems of incidence and prevalence mean very little for certain kinds of illness such as mental disorder, unless at the same time etiological problems of the same illness groups are attacked, is a matter which will be discussed below. Suffice it to say the scenes were set for interest in the *how and why* of mental illness by a study of the incidence or occurrences of different psychopathological states in persons of specific socio-cultural background.

Psychiatry, par excellence, is a science which specializes in a knowledge of the way human experience is utilized in the total economy of personality; psychiatrists soon realized that as a generalizing behavioral science it must press beyond individual case formulations to psychosocial typologies. Indeed, J. L. Halliday in his *Psychosocial Medicine*[8] defines illness in general as "a reaction, or mode of behavior, or vital expression of a living unit in response to those forces which he encounters as he moves and grows in time." Etiology of mental illness is studied in terms of dual, relational causes which lie both in the nature of the individual and in the nature of his environment, *but in both at the same time.* While a culture is, at any point in time, more massive and imposing than any individual participant and must be distinguished from the individual, the great danger in multidisciplinary research involving relational causal systems, is to so abstract the individual from his meaningful cultural background that he ceases to be a responsive or live subject for diagnosis, case formulation or psychotherapy. There are are simply no individuals apart from specific socio-cultural background.

By culture we then mean an imposing and conditioning variable which always becomes internalized, in one way or another, in the psychic systems of human beings. Far from being a mere matter of the artifacts and social organization of a people, culture also contains their range of expressive symbolism, whether in art, language, dance or song, or in the non-verbal communication patterns involved in gestures, interpersonal emotional contacts, and the rules governing relationships of age groups and of sexes. It:[9]

"consists of patterns, explicit and implicit, of and for behavior acquired and transmitted by symbols, constituting the distinctive achievement of human groups, including their embodiments in artifacts; the essential core of culture consists of traditional (i.e., historically derived and selected) ideas and especially their attached values; culture systems may, on the one hand, be considered as products of action, on the other as conditioning elements of further action."

More specifically, it includes the patterned family and social influences, the means of symbolic communication forged into a way of life, affirmed and reaffirmed in the common currency of custom, and most importantly, always having a significant discernible meaning and value for the individual.

That these traditional ideas, or themes of culture influencing patterns of behavior; the prevailing ethics, the child-rearing practices, the notions of social integration, the taboos, religious values, and attitudes toward health and illness; that these leitmotifs of a culture were precipitates of history or could influence history was probably not the main fact about them. Surely the dynamic interplay of factors within culture influenced history. But equally important, at least for behavioral science, was the manner in which these elements in a way of life became incorporated in individual functioning, how much or to what extent ego involvements became dependent on them, and why they had much to do, positively or negatively, with superego functioning.

The tendency, in the Freudian view, to equate culture and super-ego, as in *Totem and Taboo*, was a needless oversimplification. Not all in culture, except in Dr. Pangloss' "best of all possible worlds" is positive, sublimated, humanly helpful and real achievement. Even more serious, human impulses, perceptions, emotionalized attitudes and knowledge are dependent upon cultural circumstances. The tendency to regard "normal" or "social" behavior as the sublimated, cultural achievement, and "culture" as due to successful repression or identity of feelings with others (both formulated in *Totem and Taboo*) begs two questions. May there not be what Jahoda has called "indiscriminate adjustment through passive acceptance of environmental conditions" as distinct from inability to adjust, or different from active mastery and adjustment? Secondly, the negative, destructive experiences likewise felt by the organism and interpreted on perceptual, cognitive and attitudinal levels (Rado's destructive emotions as opposed to welfare emotions) are, no matter how far from personal self-fulfillment, still caught in the same web of cultural circumstances.

If psychosomatic responding to stress or psychic distorting reactions to frustration are found, they are nevertheless referable to felt experience within a cultural framework. It has been suggested that emotion *is* bodily change plus attitudes stemming from experience, in the cumulative work of men like W. B. Cannon, Harold Wolff, or William Grace.[10] Animal experimentation on emotional conditioning has also, even in a non-cultural setting, led to similar conclusions.[11] It remains to relate emotionally charged attitudes in humans to the cultural settings and contexts, stressful or beneficial, in which they eventuate.

Therefore, while cultures are not to be confused with unique clinical cases, or with negative clinical formulations, they do contain *stress systems* of a generalized character which are capable of differentiation, one from another, and which have considerable clinical importance. Attempts to define these in terms of social structure alone, or by rates of interaction of persons in a social structure, may be misleading. Indeed, in anthropology, whole schools or systems have been developed and abandoned, on the premise that types of social structure and interactional systems may be studied alone and apart from the psychological qualifications of the *meanings of cultural conduct for individuals*. Such a system was Radcliffe-Brown's at Chicago in the 1930's, or the Chapple and Coon equilibrium-disequilibrium theories of social interaction at Harvard in the 1940's.

But if culture, social system and personality are functional variables, they are interdependent and interrelated. As concerns the always unique and personalized systems of affect and thought in any individual, it is always the *individual* who hopes, thinks, acts, dreams and aspires. Nevertheless, each individual has a particular place in social structure of a definable sort and a particular set of cultural beliefs and conditionings in his background. There is no longer serious doubt as to the overwhelming importance of life history in mental illness, but the relevance of social and cultural background in furnishing guide lines to this personalized life cycle remains to be explored.

Beginning with Kraepelin, it has been known that psychopathological illness varies in content and in type with culture. Ziehen noted variations in Holland and in German Thuringia. Bleuler, in Switzerland, remarked upon differences in English and Irish cases, Bavarians and Saxons; speaking of his own hospital, he wrote: "Indeed, in our hospital, it is easy to note the difference between the reactions of the Bernese as compared with the Zurichois who are quite closely related racially."[12] P. M. Yap has described the Latah reaction in Malaya, Arctic Hysteria in Siberia, and Imu in Hokkaido.[13] In the same British journal of psychiatry, E. H. Hare reports on variations in the Congo, Papua and India; while J. Carothers in 1947 compared incidence data among Africans of Kenya with those of American Negroes.[14] An analysis of the possible significance of these patterns of cross-cultural variances will be given below. To date, they have largely followed a rather euphoric pattern: Faris in 1934 finding no schizophrenias in Belgian Congo; Seligman in 1929 finding no protracted mental disorders in Papua, merely brief attacks; unless acculturated to the west, Seligman and Dhunjibhoy's data (1930) locating no schizophrenias, unless like Parsees, the people were highly advanced in "Western civilization"; Carothers' Kenya colonists having low incidence of disorder and with freedom from most of our social, sexual and economic problems "in consequence" having no "obsessional neuroses"; the Okinawans, unexposed to concepts of sin and guilt, being reported as notably free of anxiety and all neuroses.

For the United States, the best known statistics are of a different order. Of all persons hospitalized, psychiatric disorder equals the number of cases for all other illnesses combined; of these mental illnesses, more than half are nonorganic schizophrenias, depressive states or severe psychoneuroses. Beyond this are those ambulatory, in private care or receiving no treatment whatsoever. The probably conservative estimate of one out of twelve infants suffering from mental disease in his later life course, or one out of sixteen Americans ill now, does not include the psychological components in psychosomatic ailments (asthma, allergies, migraine, rhinitis, urticaria, neurodermatitis, ulcerative colitis, peptic ulcer, nonglandular obesity, essential hypertension, etc.), nor does it include the 20,000 suicides per year, the accident-prone, that part of crime and delinquency described by Wertham and Redl, marital discord and divorce, and such problems as impotence and frigidity. Further, there are countless cases of minor compulsions, private phobias, and transient hysteriform simulations of certain diseases. A sardonic wit has called this The Aspirin Age of the Atomic Era in Urban America.

Before the ethical or philosophic questions that this problem raises, there are first the scientific, methodological ones. The psychosocial position has supplanted what Felix and Bowers call "the older assumptions of geographic or biological determinism of human behavior . . . the product of climate, heredity or original sin."[15] In place of the solitary individual governed by such somewhat fateful and extraneous forces, Jahoda speaks of a human need for "active adjustment," "attempts at mastery of environment", "the ability to perceive correctly the world and himself," and mental health as a dynamic concept, not simply a state of being.

Human energies which utilize symbolic human constructs in interpersonal communication may do so for better or worse, but they will not act solely on behalf of a biological unit, or emotionalized *id* impulses except in the most poorly integrated personalities. What Freud interpreted as raw impulse, basic need and earliest cathected orientations are better seen in the continuum of adaptive adjustment in which impulse, need and cathexis are always modified, early in life to be sure, in the area of interpersonal communication. That integration of "mental" and emotional functions, or even cognitive adequacy, or personal insight, may be won or lost in discrete personal histories should not blind us to the fact that real, interpersonal contacts in a common, workaday world always help to define the limits of the normative and the aberrant. Within this framework, the nonintegration or the thought disturbance, or lack of judgment implied in any disorganizing illness is not there as non-conformity in the narrow sense of majority tastes and aspirations. It is the result of communicated and felt emotionality that is destructive, that is a part of no normative group, however small, no positive social force, and no tradition of a sustaining sort. Even bohemian literary and artistic movements have been aimed accurately at lace-curtained salons of dead art. There should be no confusion of regimentation with functional movements, or with principles of positive conformance. Aberration is not innovation.

It is no longer believed in most quarters that the circumstances which lead the individual inexorably into some tortured world "of his own making" are really of his making. Nor is the determinism of today one which stresses such isolated events as nursing or weaning, or the various swaddling or swathing practices of Czech, Slovak, Italians, Russians, or Polish to be read off as modal personality determinants. The individual as a psychosocial unit, capable of tremendous emotional expression, is subject to adaptive adjustment in such a way that while his experience, to be sure, is always felt and motivated, ordinarily that pattern of experience has itself context and meaning, integration, and considerable reaffirmation before it may achieve any emotional hue. If psychological field theory and anthropological behavior studies have proved anything, they have taught that while it is always the individual who functions adequately, (or who may otherwise despair, hallucinate, hate, compensate, fear, or withdraw) he is nevertheless one, in either case, whose experiences are largely imposed from without, become immediately involved in an integration of sorts, are felt within and interpreted along lines laid down by a whole series of social and cultural events. Before styles of interpersonal relationship reach individual "minds and hearts," they are subject to the greater statistical weight and frequency of socio-cultural group phenomena.

As Benedict, Horney, and Redlich have noted, each in separate ways,[16] the cultural norms and standards are present to help define both normal and aberrant. While psychiatry has noted a certain patterning, or typology, in certain disease processes, it remains to investigate specific cultural scenes and the pathology within them, to locate the affectively charged points in the cultural stress systems. There is no reason to feel that a culture may not be studied and diagrammed for ambiguities, conflicts, discontinuities in life course, obvious stress features, and handicaps to maturation and healthy development. Reaction formations, premised from one case to the next on typical anxieties, fears, hates, confusions and lack of positive communication within such systems may be balanced against studies of "normals" from matched circumstances within a culture to learn what readings of the cultural map develop the well and ill. When this is done, the functions (and limits) of both destructive and welfare emotions will be fully understood within the systems of human communication in which they alone have meaning.

This connection of culture and social group, not with modal personality constructs of dubious value clinically, but with statistically oriented epidemiology and psychiatrically valid studies of the etiology of health and illness, is the course suggested for social psychiatry. At this point, no other course, it is felt, can link experience with expression in human symbolic communication systems, or deal adequately in the triadic systems of culture, social group and personality, with such related patterns as values and attitudes; the same linkage exists between world outlooks and personal horizons, the social position of the sexes and actual sexual behavior, the status system and characteristic styles of interpersonal behavior, or in brief, between culture and personality. Since these relationships are already well known in anthropological monographs across the earth's surface, the obvious need is application to psychiatric phenomena. Let us therefore plot the course, theoretically, which marks the normative, usual experience in relation to that which marks out the aberrant.

Since both courses are functionally important, or operationally used, by the individual, a dynamic and graphic analogy may be apposite. It is suggested as an alternative to the individually centered (and limited) theory of id, ego and super-ego.

The normal, usual experience is the road most people, representing the creative aspects of a culture at its best, can follow. They take it, not simply as individuals but in groups, each with a life span and with certain age, sex and organic attributes. The line of persons and of families following the course are only in unusual systems, rigid and restrictive, in a tight line. Instead there are all the alternative routings, the by-passes, the room for occasional choice and the variant speeds, stops, impediments and hazards. The vehicles to such accomplishment are culturally designed and constructed. Generally, they vary in age within automotive or historical limits, in aspects of design and purpose, the truck and town sedan even in functional class reference. Beyond the "cultural" make and construction, denoted by name, and the "class" or usage functions, denoted by structure, there are the differentiated motives of drivers. (In view of the penchant for making individual motivational systems "basic" to some systems of social psychology, we shall add that the make or construction, the cultural label on any car, together with age, implies much, realistically considered, as to what pure motivation can really accomplish in the driver's seat.)

The road hazards or conditions, and the make or type of car, we prefer to think of as the different conditions of culture. The former might be called, in this metaphor, the cultural stress system; the latter, the vehicle intended for human accomplishment of purposes and goals, we mean to be the cultural modalities, or means, for such achievement. But some drivers, some motivational systems as it were, doubtlessly because of the hazards and stresses, the inadequacies of the vehicle and its continuing strain on the adjustive motivational system, abandon the trip and set off—presumably afoot and with certainly less efficiency—on the pathways and trails with no certain markings, armed only with their primitive energies and impulses, and with only remnants of their original purpose. We submit that the topography, the strains, the barriers, impediments and roadblocks have something to do, even as to their place of location in the journey, with the points that mark out the bypaths, the impractical shortcuts, and the meandering lonely trails.

Note one fact about the lonely trails, the ten percent of mental disorder. Epidemiologically considered, they are not wholly unique pathways, as clinical experience on similar cases, or statistics on given nosological entities indicate. As history changes and cultures vary, new styles of mental illness arise and are described. The phrase, "worlds of their own making," has little meaning in view of the Dancing Mania, or Tarantism, of Thirteenth Century Italy, described by Ferdinandus and Baglivi and redescribed by Sigerist. The imagined tarantula bite felt in the dull slack of hot summer seasons sent people to streets and market places to dance together in gay, almost ceremonial attire, until insensate or carried away. The Mania, which spread in Europe for a few centuries reads strangely like the Vailala Madness of New Guinea, reported by F. E. Williams for the dislocated, acculturated areas of that island; it is reminiscent also of certain aspects of the Ghost Dance of the Plains, described by Cora DuBois, or the Ute Indian Ghost Dance (M. K. Opler). Studies like Cantril's of the invasion from Mars, or the Mattoon, Illinois hysteria; the Beloi cult of the BaThonga or the Vada sorcery of the Trobiands; or Latah and Imu reactions demonstrate that there is little about mental illness which is immutable in time or hard to duplicate cross-culturally in special times and places. Yet if we are not hopelessly to chronicle the cross-cultural phenomena in separate, unrelated studies, the study of well and ill within the settings of modern, populous cultures and sub-cultures, including our own, is next in order.

Psychopathological differences may be expected in modern cultures. As Parsons and Shils have recently pointed out, *all* cultures regulate social and sexual behavior, control organized activities, and affect traditional behavior of any sort through processes of symbolic communication.[17] This means, at the very least, that all areas of perception, feeling and evaluation are culturally differentiated during the period when a child first experiences meaningful contacts with adults by the learning of language or by the development of what Piaget might call a social sense. Wayne Dennis' studies of infancy differentiation among Navajo and Hopi children in the Thirties and Forties, or those of Rene Spitz and John Bowlby showing the importance of maternal figures in early maturation, lend support. A variety of anthropological data points to a continuing process of differentiation, through life span. The full-length biography and a variety of personal documents were proposed early by Sapir and Kluckhohn as a firm way of testing the impact of culture upon personality.

In social psychiatry, and in ethnopsychiatric surveys such as J. C. Carothers' *The African Mind*, the study of individual patients, or of symptomatology and psychodynamics of individual disorders, has broadened into concern for the ambulatory patient and, finally, to consideration of the person in his community and sociocultural setting. As yet, few studies have been made in the kind of modern scene, marked by ethnic and status contrasts, which assure us that modernized urban cultural heterogeneity has been studied at all. A total stock-taking of methodological problems involved in epidemiological study in the United States and Europe is required. Below, in brief outline, some of the chief problems of such epidemiology are presented. They are then developed in reference to given studies in subsequent sections.

1

Methodological Considerations in Social Psychiatry

RELATIONSHIP OF EPIDEMIOLOGY AND ETIOLOGY IN THE STUDY OF MENTAL ILLNESS

IN ADVANCING social psychiatry beyond its present range of knowledge, the striking results in epidemiology, now limited to scattered and exotic parts of the world, must be extended to contemporary Western cultures. When Western studies of epidemiology are reviewed critically, the lack of articulation and significant connection between clinical studies on the one hand and sociocultural studies on the other is notable. At the outset, one is forced to agree with a recent statement by Felix and Bowers that the search for environmental factors has not yielded, as yet, any full understanding of their importance.[18] In only a few studies have psychiatrists and social scientists collaborated at all, in fewer still has this collaboration been aimed at the contemporary urban scene, and in only a mere handful has this collaborative effort involved fully the special techniques of each discipline.

In his discussion of *The Psychopathologic Basis of Psychotherapy of Schizophrenia*, Diethelm notes, " . . . The cultural influences have been considered in recent years, but were insufficiently emphasized because one has not studied sufficiently the development of individual schizophrenic illnesses over a period of 30 to 40 years, nor the changing psychopathology with changes in our own culture." Continuing later with an account of the influences of the original Freudian group upon such men as Bleuler, Jung and Abraham of the Burghölzli Clinic, Diethelm states:

" . . . Outstanding symptoms were those which could be best interpreted by the concept of regression to oral and anal levels of personality development. It is of interest to note that in a hospital with modern dynamic therapy in which interpersonal influences are constantly analyzed and studied, these symptoms of regression of 40 years ago have become rare or have disappeared completely. To this group belong incontinence, smearing, eating of feces, so-called fetal postures, verbigeration, echolalia, refusal to eat, frank catatonic motility disorders, vulgarity in words and in symbolic acts, stereotypies and mannerisms. These changes do not seem to relate to suppression or repression, but rather to lack of activation of oral and anal factors by the changed environmental attitudes and behavior."

In his total account of the essential aspects of the psychotherapy of schizophrenia, Diethelm lays proper stress upon the need "to be constantly guided by dynamic psychopathology, with a recognition of physical, environmental and cultural influences".[19] Scarcely any study of an *epidemiological* sort has combined these criteria in research on any given mental illness though Barrabee, Zborowski, and Diethelm have conducted etiological studies within ethnic sub-groups having a qualitative if not quantitative aim. Barrabee's study of psychotics of certain backgrounds is aided by psychiatric information and cultural inquiry, Zborowski's on pain reactions only partly fulfills the psychiatric criteria on dynamic psychopathology, and Diethelm's and Barnett's on alcoholism, containing, for example, negative findings on urban Chinese, discovers interesting relationships of this reaction to personality structure and numerous cultural relationships while insisting, no doubt rightly, that alcoholism is not, in itself, a mental illness. These studies, however, point the way to the kind of etiological information which is needed in any epidemiological inquiry.

When one turns from Diethelm's formulation on variability in illness typology, variation in course of illness, and change in symptomatology in accordance with changing cultural scene back to the usual, or basic, presentations of psychoanalytic dynamics, one is struck by the need to review these dynamic formulae in the light of external influences and a more variable typology·than is commonly used. In psychoanalytic dynamics, such typical mechanisms as regression, repression, projection and introjection, and their concomitants, displacement and substitution, rationalization and overcompensation, or identification and sublimation are applied to mankind *sub specie aeternitatis*. These mechanisms are discussed as if only the classical Viennese cases existed, with neither environmental nor cultural variations. Of course, much could be said for elaboration of the original Freudian insights under a variety of different influences, not the least of these being cultural and environmental change. However, a wholly mechanistic conception of these dynamics persists in some quarters, so much so that variable dynamics are lost in the rigidity of a single, orthodox point of view. Even worse, cultural subtleties and shadings are not, on occasion, recognized at all.

In opposition to the wholly erroneous idea that human behavior is subject to one typical course, dynamically speaking, and that mankind exists *sub specie aeternitatis*, it may be said that, culturally speaking, what is repressed varies, as does the availability of role models for identification. Further, who is or what becomes the target for projection, and what cultural channels for regression or sublimation are open to a person of a given sex, age and cultural background are all matters of considerable importance. It is not merely that the mechanisms of an individual's adjustment are culturally influenced, but that his *type* of adjustment *in the first place* may relate to cultural background factors. If, for example, there is no latency period, as is well known, in the Trobriands; if Zuni women feel little social sense of deprivation; Okinawans, no great sexual shame or guilt; or Samoans little spontaneity and personal freedom in contrast to Navajos; then not only do the mechanisms of adjustment vary, but the basic emotionality involved in a type of adjustment will vary as well.

While epidemiology in social psychiatry has meant the indications of an incidence and prevalence of psychiatric disorders in relation to variable social and cultural strata, the key term, mental illness, convinces one immediately that etiological factors bearing upon psychopathology are of primary importance. In a logical sense, etiology (how mental illness arises) determines epidemiology (the incidence of illness in given time periods). In the biosocial position as well, the impact of the sociocultural environment upon personality development, an etiological question, underlies epidemiological results. The first problem, therefore, in multidisciplinary research of this order is to indicate the socio-cultural environment *in its possible relation* to psychiatric disorder. Since no research worthy of note flies blind amid winds of doctrine and currents of interest, the formulation of hypothetical questions will be fast, accurate and relevant to basic problems only where the suppositions of contributing sciences are examined for pertinence and power of explanation relative to this kind of phenomena, psychiatric disorder. There is little point, in view of the scarcity of research in this field, to test the environment for dynamically irrelevant details. A. N. Whitehead, in *The Function of Reason*, points out that a limited conceptual framework, behaviorism for example, will be powerless to deal with dynamic issues.

In social psychiatry, the epidemiological interest was at

first not truly etiological in significance; it was restricted to searches for factors global enough to encompass social and psychological worlds, but unfortunately factors which were psychiatrically *unclear as to possible relevance.* These global determinants were, of course, the variations in socio-economic status, in urban and rural living, in cultural background, in ecological areas or neighborhoods of cities, in life-span mobility phenomena such as geographic or status mobility, etc. All such factors do, of course, influence personal *history.* Yet their adequacy in this generalized, and psychiatrically non-dynamic form remained questionable. Was economic deprivation in any sense the same as psychologically felt, conflictual deprivation? Were urbanites lonely in the sense that denizens of the "American Gothic" pattern were not? Did two-stage rises in upward mobility, as Ruesch and Bateson suggested, implement a sense of inadequacy and insecurity which was not dynamically there and operative already on grounds of personality structure? In addition to the mechanistic view of man *sub specie aeternitatis,* without cultural background, and the confusions of super-ego and sublimated cultural behavior "in the best of all possible worlds," there were failures to refine global notions of ecology in such a way that etiological and dynamic psychiatric questions could be tested and answered while attempting to draw epidemiological considerations and conclusions to the fore.

Considerations, such as Diethelm's of a variable typology, were lost in attempted intercorrelations of class with "schizophrenia" in general, "neuroses" in general, "depressive states" in general. The variable course of illness, dependent to so high a degree on neglect, or detection, proper diagnosis and treatment, could mean that high rates of schizophrenia in lower class groupings compared with high rates of neurosis in the upper classes might signify nothing more or less than variables in detection and treatment fa-

cilities and an unmitigated course of illness in the lower
levels. As Diethelm indicates, the variables in environmental and cultural factors, all making for differences in
psychopathology and change in personality expression
according to situation and background factors were not
adequately utilized in studies of this sort in epidemiological
psychiatry. In brief, a combination of qualitative and
quantitative methods was not devised in nosological nose-
counting, such as might answer significant etiological
questions.

In the social and psychological sciences likewise, loose
conceptualizations traceable largely to ignorance of medical and psychiatric literature, failed to convince psychiatry
of a rich field for study in socio-cultural backgrounds. At
one time, not too long ago, texts on social "pathology," or
social problems, ranged horrendous if well-meant statistics on economic poverty, broken homes, urban population
density, class and minority group membership, etc., side
by side with those on crime, delinquency, and psychiatric
disorder to let the chips fall, or to comment ruefully on
such unclear concepts as cultural "lag," the tempo of urban
life, or the presumed inadequacies of the poor.

Modern concepts reveal no such shadow-boxing with
remotely spaced variables like density and psychiatric
disorders, or like poverty, crime and mental illness, least of
all where mental disorder and anti-social behavior are
confused. In a striking study, Dunham has recently
indicated that the "quiet ones" of the slum area may be
the ones most vulnerable to serious psychic disturbance,
while open delinquent behavior in upper class homes may
be the more patent indicators of underlying sociopathic
trends. Again, etiology or illness process is considered
directly in the context of an epidemiological problem.
The tendency has been for involutional disorders to become
more rare in modern times, and to have little of the sin and

guilt ideology which was once so prevalent, for menopause to be less a point of depressive disorganization with changes in public attitude towards aging or towards sexual function in women and their social position. In the same way, the rarity of paranoid resultants of syphilitic infection due to anti-biotic discoveries and application; and a host of more subtle variations in mental illness course accompanying newer and more successful therapeutic methods; all point to etiological or developmental variants responsive to a whole range of environmental factors which have changed. The point that social and psychological analysis has not kept abreast of this changing scene is a reflection upon their slowness in adopting dynamic method.

As Diethelm notes in another source:[20]

"Cultural anthropologic investigations are highly indicated for obtaining a clarification of the meaning of the changes in psychopathology. Ethnic influences have often been mentioned but have never been studied adequately. The role of religion in the incidence of suicide is well recognized but not understood. Cultural attitudes have affected sexual life. However, neglect of careful study has permitted the development of far reaching theories."

It is suggested that careful study, in this area of problems, is guided or informed by data which have psychodynamic relevance and psychopathological detail.

At the same time, social and psychological concepts have, in psychiatric and social science literature, undergone certain changes. The emergence of the Sullivan-Sapir position has already been mentioned. In respect to the factor of socio-economic status, Karen Horney, in an early work, *The Neurotic Personality of Our Time*, has made some general observations which may prove important. In place of the sheer effects of poverty on personality, Horney instead speaks of a high rate of neurosis throughout the entire social structure as the price paid for continual, unrelenting striving for success and prestige. Inevitably, the competitive pace throughout the whole socio-economic continuum loaded the circuit with private guilt and anxiety, as well as public uncertainty. The distance between aspiration levels and actual accomplishment when thrown upon this larger screen of generally accepted values was felt by many, if not all, as full of reproach and covert condemnation. For Horney, the individually focussed conflicts arose less out of infantile experience, as such, than from cultural reaffirmations of these values favoring neurotic attitudes, albeit traceable to family scene and large segments of life course. While non-neurotic fears of poverty or insecurity, situationally realistic and valid, existed in lower social classes and could be reality tested, character neuroses involved disproportionate fears, deeply rooted anxieties, and basic conflicts developed in part by cultural factors in the culture of our time. In place of the social pathologist's factor of poverty, a concept difficult to substantiate in other cultures such as the Bolivian Siriono, (described by Allan Holmberg as a hand to mouth existence amid uniform conditions of want and uniform survival ideals) Horney has suggested psychologically felt inadequacy and deprivation, rejection and anxiety.

Central to Horney's theory is that avoidances of anxiety are also unconsciously or consciously according to cultural formulae; drowning oneself in work or developing inordinate desires for power, prestige and possessions were plotted as sure routes to denying, domineering, humiliating or depriving conduct. Such defenses in these reaction formations as the boundless craving for affection, approval and admiration were, for Horney, not simply the occasional defenses of essentially isolated cases, but in the main larger cultural constructs, or values systems, than are found simply in the uncertainties of economic structure. What is striking is that such cultural themes are to be found where, most often, the real uncertainties are least apparent in the reality sense. Such additional cultural principles (V. F. Calverton once called them the cultural compulsives) as the constant need to emphasize sexual desirability, to develop a need for prestige so great that self-evaluation suffers in excessive reliance upon others, or to become self-assertive and aggressive in a manner that finds victims unable to protect themselves—these larger constructs were hammer and anvil of the anxieties and disproportionate fears, the culturally induced denials of their existence, the *psychological* reassurances against helplessness, humiliation and destitution. They could be found anywhere in social structure where unreasoning, competitive, hostile impulses and the culturally automatic need to suppress and repress them operated.

The cultural corollaries in showing off, in inordinate narcissistic desires, in fantasy dream factories, in the ease of projecting hostilities to an "outer" world, in cravings for power and self-justification, Horney saw not merely as a cartoon panorama of American foibles, but as serious failures in the America of our time. In writing of the reaction formations among those who succumbed, she emphasized the hostile submission and withdrawal, the enhanced and sensitive anxieties, the sense of inadequacy or guilt, and the countless defensive mechanisms against rejection. Whether the account is epidemiologically sound should be tested; at least it knows, etiologically and dynamically, what requires testing.

Just as the effects of poverty have given way to such analysis, or have, like Kardiner's study of the American urban Negro, explored the dimensions of hostility and deprivation together, so the factor of sheer population density, which once was a vogue of studies in the 1930's and 1940's best exemplified, perhaps, by Dunham and by Hyde, has given way in turn to more valid psychiatric concepts. Current concepts of urbanism have used the famous Durkheimian notion of anomie in one form or another. It is important to know exactly what it means. In the hands of Robert K. Merton, or in David Riesman's *The Lonely Crowd*, anomie does not mean high density per square mile nor even a kind of nondescript anonymity in large groups. It has no connotations of crowded tenement, reprehensible though these may be on other grounds; nor does it mean "the crowd" or *Carnival* setting. Central to the conception is a personally felt and generally conceived sense of self-alienation from others. If the tenement or apartment house dwelling has thrown people together in greater proximity, or the *Carnival* or *Mardi Gras* preserves their anonymity, anomie separates them and imparts to anonymity a crucial sense of lack of communication, lack of indentity and lack of shared interests.

Increasingly, careful studies of urbanism have moved in the direction of such concepts. In one of the best delineated studies, that of Eshref Shevky and Marilyn Williams, *The Social Areas of Los Angeles*, a comparison of urban process in this city and in others has disclosed that the process is accompanied by increasing segregation, as of ethnic minorities, differentiation of socio-economic areas, and in fact greater homogeneity within areas or differentiation between them, as the process wears on. In relation to anomie, the relation of the self-alienation process to that of urbanism, social science concepts stressing size, cohesion and types of social integration are relevant. It is important to know whether family and neighborhood oriented cultures, as perhaps the rural Puerto Rican or Southern Italian exemplify, limit belongingness more or less to such units, or whether other substitutions from social structure can be made for these frameworks. Does the highly elaborated social structure and status system of the Hungarian find parallels in the American status system, or does it suffer attrition and lack of cohesion within the Hungarian community with little modification?

Are the ideas of Horney, or of Benedict, concerning psychological dislocations imbedded in our own Middletowns to be included in our own concepts of anomie? At any rate, the shift to anomie from population density considerations, such as characterized Hyde's work in Boston, implies nothing less than a psychological reworking of social science concepts. Instead of a populationally dense Transitional Zone, or Skid Row, being the class-linked matrix of the highest rates of schizophrenic illness, as it was considered in the early studies of Faris and Dunham, today the notion of downward mobility and selective "drift" of hitherto damaged personalities, as analyzed by Gerard and others, shows a pile-up, not an incidence rate, in this ecological area of those in whom the self-alienation course has possibly moved to full completion.[21]

In addition, minority or ethnic group membership no longer involves an insistence upon a unitary and cohesive cultural group, a fact which depends more upon the nature and reception of each specific sub-culture within the American scene. The nature of the culture, together with the pace and type of acculturation change in the new setting are all of importance. Today, before attempting to assess whether minority group members represent persons living in a hostile and alien world, as has been suggested in a brilliant manuscript on the development of paranoid personalities by J. S. Tyhurst, such factors as the psychological patterns of males and females within specific cultures, the intergeneration conflict or harmony, and the emotional climate of the typical "ethnic" home must first be known. Such data require not merely the recasting of psychiatric or anomie formulations in respect to foreign born, an important first step to be sure, but equally a careful analysis of self-alienation in separate and specific socio-cultural contexts with respect to the acculturation process and the changing scene. Until this is done, we shall not know whether we are dealing with alienation processes stressed by Horney for the entire urban American scene, or with socio-cultural factors of specific groupings in the population, or with economic hardship dimensions.

However, the step implied in the work of Tyhurst and Riesman, or of Merton or Gerard, a psychological working through of social science concepts, groups a lack of social cohesion and nonintegration together with self-alienation and depersonalization trends. As stated, such a reworking of general concepts must be tested in culturally distinct groups and patterns as indeed they were in Durkheim's original, brilliant work on contrasting backgrounds in *Le Suicide*.

In New York, for example, a content analysis of newspapers or an inspection of agency records will begin to describe a Puerto Rican family increasingly characterized by lack of cohesion, by struggles between parents (or parents and children) as to dominance role in a society in which male superiority was formerly unchallenged; the lesser subordination of the female in an urban scene of greater job opportunities for them; the resultant male and female role-conflicts; and the multiple common law marriages and separations; or in short, the central changes in family organization, child-rearing practices and intersexual conduct. The pace of this acculturation, the job instability for men, and the kinds and amount of personal insecurity and hostility are among the elements to consider.

As Leighton has suggested, interferences with satisfactions and security systems may foster psychological disorder. If this proposition is central in the study of environmental influence, and it appears to be, then specific kinds of interference may be connected with particular kinds of acculturation process. If further, in Puerto Rican cases which are known etiologically or dynamically, deprivation of maternal care, intersexual hostility, lack of masculine assertion among boys whose mothers compensate for absent father-figures or overprotect them in the formative years, are added to brittle marriages, floundering but not abandoned dual standards, and possibly infancy oral frustration, then a psychodynamic profile may emerge. While etiological, it will certainly relate to much of what is known epidemiologically to be striking in this group: the distillate of male fears of impotence, the psychosomatic stomach and digestive disorders, the high rates of homosexuality and prostitution, the frequent incest fears and male Oedipal conflicts. Consequently, a more coherent and dynamically valid pattern of explanation results than would by mere allusion to "alienation in a hostile world." The latter idea, while a clue, is really a circular explanation primarily because it does not begin with real people having, like all of us a cultural stock in trade, modified under certain conditions of acculturation and yet used under the conditions of time, place and specific circumstances.

Further on minority group phenomena, "the alien in a hostile world" represents a known quantity of decided epidemiological importance. The study of Barrabee at Boston Psychopathic Hospital has recognized this; Zborowski has re-emphasized it. In state hospitals and veterans' facilities, the numerical importance of such groups as German, Irish, Italian or Puerto Rican (depending of course on region) is striking. The number of first admissions to public psychiatric institutions has, since 1940, increased more than 28 per cent. This increase belongs to a period in which another half-billion outlay has been required for veterans' psychiatric needs. The figures, applying to native-born largely, do not argue that the problem of "hostility in an alien world" disappears with continued acculturation. Such study, as is required, cannot proceed on the basis of urban anonymity theory, but must include specific etiological and epidemiological inquiry. Only then could a causal nexus of specific group backgrounds and specific psychopathology become clear. Just as gross, or global, variables like socio-economic status, population density, and cultural background have undergone change and refinement, so the necessity of careful psychosocial studies, jointly guided by psychiatric and social science findings, demands a greater degree of specificity than is offered by such a breakdown of data into schizophrenias, psychoneuroses, and the like. Normative behavior and cultural background vary considerably from group to group. Presumably psychopathology can vary as well beyond such nosological labels as schizophrenic reaction, paranoid type.

This process of conceptual refinement must be made in psychiatry itself, if indeed, it stands to gain from social science collaboration. The readiness, in some quarters, for social sciences to dissolve concepts into those which have meaning and significance for psychiatry has already begun, even though the process has not been uniformly successful all along the line. In defining the specifics of psychopathology in relation to given conditions in social, cultural and environmental background no single science, whether social or psychiatric, has the analytic tools, or perhaps the time and inclination, to explore different modal reactions of human beings, as individuals and as members of groups, in physical, emotional and cultural dimensions. Yet the task must be begun against the background of enormous and sustained cultural forces which enter into behavior. Both in reference to epidemiology and etiology, the social scientist unaided has, to date, largely studied the non-biological homeostatic relationship of the individual with his total socio-cultural environment, the environment sometimes fragmentized for clarity in special problems.

In those elements which create disruptive or disorganizing tensions and anxieties, which block self-realization and self-consistency, the psychiatrist has his special province and unmatched competence. Where only an integration of sorts in a truly alien world remains, the psychiatrist alone has the skill to evaluate and explore, with caution and insight built up from clinical experience. To postpone or delay the psychiatrists' entry into and collaboration in this direction of critical socio-cultural *and* dynamic analysis is like saying, otherwise and all too philosophically, that because "society is the patient," to paraphrase L. K. Frank, therefore therapeutic and individualized efforts might just as well cease.

The sciences of man, like the sciences of his ills, must together investigate aspects of the human predicament if individualized therapy is to be linked with real progress in prevention, and in the alleviation of stressful situations. For the psychiatrist, as well as social scientist, this means that both individuals and their backgrounds may be studied and evaluated for strengths and weaknesses. In a truly epidemiological and preventive sense, the shattered lives of countless individuals and families require such fuller consideration. When the full force of human-related sciences attack the problems of psychiatric disorders in etiological and epidemiological research, then the results will be better, doubtlessly, for therapy and prevention.

The primary concern of psychiatry in the past, apart from typology and treatment, has been psychodynamic and etiological. In mental health research, the epidemiological approach, unfortunately, has too often been used alone. In much of this, statistics rather than individualized case analysis has meant that the distillate studied is removed many times from the original real product. In British social psychiatry, as in American, an effort has been made to recapture the reality of the individual in real situational contexts, just as this method informed the best work of Adolf Meyer and his associates. Neither method, the etiological or the epidemiological, can be used with any amount of assurance singly at any particular point. *How much* mental illness exists, or is produced in any society or culture within a time period depends on a series of conditions, among them the dynamic implications of specific ways of life.

As we shall see in the following sections on Prevalence and Incidence, and Multiple Causation *Versus* Single Factor Analysis, even more is contained in society and culture than primary way of life phenomena. Among these are the accuracy of methods for location and diagnosis of types of personality balance and imbalance. Suffice it to say here that in mental illnesses par excellence, the deeply rooted, insidious and slowly developing character of the disorders is especially noteworthy. If the schizophrenias account for a quarter of all those hospitalized, this probably means that both prevalence and incidence data may not be interpreted as in any sense final, unless early stages are capable of at least rough detection. In surveys of this sort, there is no reason why the institutional and expressive contexts of an individual, as a member of a family, community, society and culture, may not be searched provided the search remains psychiatric in essence.

THE INCIDENCE AND PREVALENCE OF PSYCHIATRIC DISORDERS

Prevalence and incidence studies, conducted in national and regional illness censuses, constitute one method of epidemiological survey. Although useless etiologically, they do have great practical importance in providing guidance of a general sort for over-all planning, public education in mental hygiene, and the assessment of mental ills in the total health and economy of the nation. When H. Emerson, at the First International Congress on Mental Hygiene in 1930, gave gross quantitative evidence of the magnitude and extent of mental disorders as a public health problem and in the same decade outlined the first inclusive epidemiological research of this type, the movement was felt as a part of a long-overdue attack on the chronic, degenerative, crippling and neoplastic processes, more challenging and by this time more widespread and baffling than the germ-specific, mechanically isolatable, and pharmacologically treatable ailments.

Freeman, first in a number of epidemiological research innovations, stimulated in 1936 the first comprehensive survey in a major population of over 50,000 persons, the Eastern Health District of Baltimore. This fieldwork was carried forward by Lemkau, Tietze and Cooper. Then, in rapid succession, in 1938, there was the Williamson County, Tennessee survey of Roth and Luton, next the work of Dunham in Chicago, later Hyde in Boston, and Stott; along with these, there were the formal programs of incidence study in New York and Massachusetts. The former were no doubt also influenced by Pollock's work in the 1920's, Nolan's in the decade before, and Malzberg's imposing surveys.

The two world wars, particularly World War II, gave decided impetus to studies of induction and rejection data, Hyde's mental rejection rates being wholly of this type. Subsequent studies of community population samples pushed beyond the frontiers established by Faris and Dunham, and the type of epidemiological team, now used, included the psychiatrist, anthropologist, sociologist, statistician, psychologist and social worker. The German studies of Brugger in Thuringia and Bavaria, in the 1930's, and a host of Scandinavian studies; Stromgren's in Danish rural and fishing communities, Sjögren's and Böök's in Swedish villages and island districts, and Odegaard's of the Norwegian hospitalized antedated though mostly in rural circumstances the American urban and state surveys.

These studies are not comparable because of methodological differences in the gathering of data. Many of those in small Scandinavian fishing, farming and island districts adopted the method, since redeveloped in Leighton's study of Stirling County, Nova Scotia, of gathering extensive psychiatric information on known cases through fieldwork methods and with interested informants. With far less intensive methods and certainly less psychodiagnostic information, Brugger found a constantly higher rate in every illness category per 1,000 persons in Bavaria, as compared with Thuringia. The Tennessee Survey with its rate of 69.4 per 1,000, although rural, was no more reassuring than Paul Lemkau's data, roughly comparable but in an urban scene, with its figure of 60.5 per 1,000. The Dunham, Stott and Hyde studies, hardly comparable, tell at least a similar story of high rates, in no case pinpointed to the end result of being etiologically useful to dynamic psychiatry or psychotherapy. A study by R. M. Counts and Peter F. Regan, on Army recruits, has both dynamic and therapeutic meaning.[22]

A detailed study by Joseph Eaton and R. J. Weil of several Hutterite communities described a variant culture of the United States and Canada possessing great stability and conservatism in social pattern, decided moral and religious emphasis, a distinct limiting of individualistic and impulsive tendencies, and considerable constriction in emotional expression. While this population had a seemingly higher than average occurrence of "manic-depressive disorders," the "lifetime prevalence rate" used in this study, and compared with the non-uniform methods and results obtained in Germany, Scandinavia and elsewhere remains open to serious question; if intended for comparison with incidence rates from other settings, it must be computed for incidence and not prevalence.   Further, a "lifetime prevalence rate" if not made age-specific by information as to probable age of onset is especially vulnerable in application to what Eaton terms "manic-depressive disorders" in view of an age-distribution for this illness generally older than schizophrenias.   In fact, no pattern of cultural etiology may be assumed until the age pattern of Hutterite communities, generally regarded as skewed in an elderly direction, is made manifest, and until a rate of incidence is computed in a time period for these communities commensurate with known information on the age distribution in this population.[23]

It is obvious that *how much* mental illness exists or is produced in any society or culture within a given time period depends upon a series of conditions implicit in that setting.   A methodology, however, by its definitions of illness, and by its means of locating, detecting, and diagnosing illness interposes a new series of conditions between the reality of prevalence or incidence and the findings of the study.   Here it must be remembered that chronic, degenerative or psychic diseases often develop slowly, and that for those ill the continuum of the illness state, like the life span itself, is in truth a lengthy continuum.   Detection and diagnosis is one problem to be sure, but it is a problem complicated by the sheer presence or absence of treatment. Facilities for treatment, or exacerbation by neglect, may go far to explain the striking findings of Redlich, Hollingshead and Myers in the New Haven Study, a survey in which lower class members showed 12 times the amount of schizophrenic illness as the upper class, for whom in turn the rates of psychoneurosis were distinctly higher.[24]   The fact that a survey, for a given day, of those known to private psychiatrists and to public hospitals and clinics forms the basis for these findings supports this interpretation.

Moreover, an incidence rate of *new cases occurring* in a time period, much less open to secondary questions of treatment or neglect, must be age and sex specified, not merely denoted as to class and culture. The age and sex patterns of illnesses are remarkably subject to change in time and correspondence with socio-cultural factors, of which more will be said later. Even an incidence rate, age and sex specified, will depend to some extent on attitudes towards illness and community or family modes of detection.

While the folklore of mental illness is hardly explored as yet, anyone knows that the Italian attitude towards expression of feelings directly, their dislike of introspection, and their great familial concern lest illness be detected in the family created a set of conditions quite unlike the English or "Yankee" attitude towards hospitals, clinics and individual therapeutic skills and facilities. These attitudes towards illness and treatment, modes of detection, and the presence or absence of facilities are present in any social grouping. Unlike the germ-specific diseases, for which incidence rates provide the most direct kinds of etiological clues, mental disorders as a life course process are less responsive to computation, inference and control group procedures such as served Semmelweis' discovery of specific etiological agents in puerperal fever.

However, since prevalence rates merely compound and add the piled up and time-bounded rates of incidence, they offer no recourse in method. Indeed, age and sex specific rates, if computed by incidence data alone, give more insight into the life course process of disease. The prevalence rates have merely the uses of administrative survey into present extent of a series of illness problems, which presumably grow and pile up under the rubrics of neglect, custodial care, or failure in treatment. Such indeed, is the value of the Faris and Dunham study of Chicago's Transitional Zone in which neglect and piling up of existing cases both occurred. Whereas, an epidemiological survey which can obtain incidence data and a measure of personal and biographical history for each individual has further uses.

The growing recognition of a gap, therefore, between "true incidence" and currently ascertainable incidence reported without a history of illness points not only to the serious import of case-finding in the community and institutionally (and possibly in the former area, preventive or "early" therapeutic methods), but it suggests again that such approximate epidemiological methods as are available in this field be linked with etiological knowledge and understanding. As we have seen, *how much* mental illness occurs in given social and cultural groups depends ultimately on processes best called etiological and answering the questions *how* and *why*. At the same time epidemiology, if careful, provides clues to how and why, baselines for research into further etiological questions, and if linked with prevalence studies in modern communities, some knowledge for the planning of mental health resources, preventive measures, educational and therapeutic programs.

From the point of view of mental hygiene and preventive psychiatry, the ambulatory ill and borderline cases (those for example with incipient schizophrenia, mild neurotic or psychosomatic symptoms) are of considerable importance both for therapy and mitigating educational programs. The National Mental Health Act appropriations for state aid are entirely for such purposes, and yet little knowledge of real needs in this area exists at present. While the occurrence of early symptoms among people is certainly not the same as the fuller study of disease processes, whatever factors have a bearing upon incidence are etiologically interesting. In this sense, there is better conformance to the actual meaning of incidence when applied to "early stages" of slowly developing and insidious disease processes. For incidence is the appearance of a disease entity in populations both as to distinct and clear prodromal symptoms, as well as the final occurrence and distribution of its ultimate states. Such distributions, graded or evaluated as to seriousness, are computed as to rates of appearance. If then, certain psychiatric disorders have an early development, as indeed they appear to have, the age specific data together with the noting of a course of illness will come closer to real incidence.

Further, new disease occurrences may be evaluated against the background of such larger distribution patterns as have implicit in them the failure to arrest the course of illness, or its continuity, exacerbation or worsening, or even partial cure and temporary remission. The discussions of Hoch, Polatin and others on the possibly dubious entity, pseudoneurotic schizophrenia, and the whole question of its distinctness as an entity *versus* its linkage or intermediacy between two processes could benefit immensely from such refined statistical analysis. Where, as in mental illness, there exist deeply significant differences between psychotic manifestations in which ego control and integration are lost, and neuroses in which they are retained with discomfort, considerable care must be exercised to distinguish these gradients and not to confuse or blur them with the still larger groupings as the mentally ill and sociopathic "in general." In the same way, psychodynamic and psychopathological information should correct the confusions common in epidemiological and incidence data now reported. Who has not pondered over reports where mere parts of larger disease processes (such as "chronic alcoholism," the neurotic, sociopathic or psychotic delinquent, and non-genetic types of mental deficiency) are grouped erroneously and stud the epidemiological surveys of Europe, America and Africa? In his study of alcoholism, Diethelm has suggested just such a correction.[25]

Felix and Bowers have therefore singled out two types of factors relevant to incidence rates, the first being the knowledge of etiology or how persons acquire the disorder, and the second, knowledge of methods to combat it plus the possibilities of their application in given communities and settings. The methods of casefinding, psychodynamic development, choices of therapeutic method, cultural "safety valves" and preventive programs therefore have immediate bearing upon incidence and all respond to socio-environmental factors.[26] In a paper on *Prognosis in the Psychoneuroses: Benign and Malignant Developments*, Rennie states, "Much depends upon the character or temperament, the nature and duration of pathological defenses, the intrinsic ego strength of the individual and the many modifiable or unmodifiable environmental realities which the patient must surmount . . ." Later he adds, "As Saul has pointed out, neuroses are not entities. They are ways of reacting which everyone has in some degree. Even the most 'normal' individual utilizes similar mechanisms, however rudimentary, whenever the conflicts of inner needs or the strains of life are heightened." Considering his twenty year follow-up study of 240 hospital-treated psychoneurotic patients, Rennie concludes in part:[27]

" . . . Psychoneurosis is not a specific disease entity but is a method of reacting. The clinical manifestations frequently overlap so that one can see the utilization of many kinds of defense mechanisms in a given individual. The defense mechanisms which give the clinical coloring to the particular reaction are ones which are common to everyone and are significant largely because of the degree and extent of their use by the psychoneurotic person. Such defenses may and often do change either as an immediate result

of therapy or as a spontaneous evolution subsequent to
therapy . . . Most cases present admixtures. The essential
task is to understand what and how the mechanisms operate
and in what kind of setting in terms of character organization. While the long term outcome for most psychoneurotic
patients following treatment is a benign one, the development of malignant states occurs in a sufficient number of
patients to call for special alertness in the diagnosis, prognosis and choice of therapy for every psychoneurotic patient."

The studies of incidence of psychiatric disorders have
been generally, of three types both here and abroad. These
are, first, the national and state surveys mentioned above.
There are next the studies of institutionalized cases as to
number, not etiology or follow-up phenomena, which have
been centered largely in public agencies, often state hospitals, and consequently deal for the most part with
psychotics. While the Scandinavian studies, the Stirling
Project in Nova Scotia, the New Haven study, or the Yorkville Community Mental Health Project broaden case-
finding to include all known ambulatory and institutional
cases under treatment, those based on admissions rates in
public institutions show decided incompleteness of data
because only obvious psychotics are selected into the study,
and, at times, even the private institutional and out-patient
clinic data are excluded. The Scandinavian method of
using informants and scattered sources of data to expand
this picture is methodologically loose and unsystematic.
Until the continuum of neurotic to psychotic manifestations is utilized and the community as well as institutional
scene probed by multidisciplinary methods, there is no
assurance that an area has been studied from a rounded
epidemiological point of view. There are no short cuts in
epidemiology which may successfully eliminate the field
survey, statistical study of mass phenomena, and institutional cases, public and private.

There is decided point, however, to the study within hospital settings of remission rates in response to modern methods of treatment, provided a full knowledge of both therapeutic handling and disease course has been attained. In ordering a jumble of data which may otherwise mean little, first admissions, age, sex, social and cultural data together with psychodynamic data comprise leading considerations against which style of therapy and remissions may be significant.

In psychiatry, there is increasing appreciation that epidemiology in mental disorders, the reaction patterns themselves, are rarely responsive to single agents, internal or external, for which specifics in prevention or in therapy singly apply. Notions of "precipitating events" are never active in isolation from the totality of a patient's patterns of reacting or the totality of the situation in terms of which he reacts; etiologically, the traumatic and precipitating factors, sometimes called predisposing, are to be referred to the basic facts of types of personality, the manner in which they develop, and the kinds of backgrounds responsible for such development.

The homeostatic and disequilibrium theories apply with special force only if one realizes that the only homeostasis, or lack of it, which can exist is contained in the total contours of personality, built from and operating within contexts. In anthropological experience, traumatic events and shamanistic cures, especially for hysterias, will stand as mere anecdote and vignette against the larger analysis of character, and temperament and reaction to situation. In psychiatric literature, the character neurosis with hysterical features often runs parallel so that grief reactions as in death of a close family member may mean not situationally realistic sorrow, but personally felt defeat and psychic illness, as both Lindemann and Volkart have recently pointed out. The searing and ghastly experiences which a healthy personality may meet, feel, and take in stride are proof enough that trauma, experienced by a number of personalities, will take no toll except in given configurations. Thus, hypotheses which postulate that categories of deprivation (death, want, class-necessitated job mobility, "traumatic" weaning or toilet training, etc.) are predisposing and relate to incidence of disorder are clinically assumptive and no amount of quantification, apart from distinctly known cases, can convince one that remote variables are not being manipulated. Sunspots are simply not correlated with economic cycle, though relation of such items has been assumed. The factors with which incidence rates are connected must be, on independent grounds, found to be dynamically important.

The world is full of cultures in which relatives and close associates die; it is full of cultures with hand-to-mouth marginality in which most frequently the poorer, unacculturated communities show the more optimum mental health; there are cultures like our own in which job instability in the blue collar range is often a matter of economic instabilities and periodicities and not a personal determination; and there are cultures which wean more abruptly than the Anglo-American, and yet do not have our problems of high incidence in the least. In the cities of Australia and New Zealand abrupt toilet-training and weaning seem to have no reflection in illness rates.

Just as single agents, "precipitating" and "traumatic" events require further clarification in the methodology of studies of the incidence of nonorganic mental illness, so new hypotheses setting more exact parameters of the problems are required in research design intending to use the interrelational concepts of social psychiatry. The precipitating event and predisposing factor has been used to illustrate the narrowest constriction of such parameters. However, the theory of the functioning psychosocial unit, now generally accepted as a frame of reference, needs further specification, particularly as to functioning, in order to escape vapid over-generalization. To prevent the scope of the problem from becoming too wide and general, the extremely stimulating Sullivan-Sapir theory of the emotional and expressive quality of human symbolic communication must be tested for limits.

This theory, to be applied at all, necessitates more than the generous attributing now prevalent of these positive and sensitizing qualities to the pan-human species without qualification. As Lasswell, who had much to do with originating and elaborating communication theory, pointed out recently at the Mass Communications Seminar of the Wenner-Gren Foundation for Anthropological Research, it is of utmost importance to note in the general theory of communication the place of this process *in* the social process.[28] One might add *within* the values systems *of* the social process. He needs only to ask *what* is being communicated, and *why?*

The psychiatrist, accustomed to study a personality as a whole in relation to interactions with others, frequently denotes the conditioned or habitualized stamping into the soma and personality of emotional voltages, circuits and blocked circuits that finally characterize the economy and balance of the expressive life. The social scientist, particularly the anthropologist, by much the same process of evaluative entering into the affective, expressive and structured activities of groups of people and their generalized patterns of interaction explores to a similar depth, though rarely organically (unless a physical anthropologist) the symbol-charged, communicative mileu into which he has entered. The total personality and total cultural approaches, in each realm, impose similar conditions in which affective dimensions in either loom large. Beyond the affectivity, the social conditions of existence are present in either case, whether material, ideological, or traditional. No matter how idiosyncratic and individualized the psychopathology may become, it links back at some point as do the lonely trails to more generalized routes.

In each realm, the similar conditions of the problems are: What, specifically, has been communicated and how? What values and attitudes determine the affect? What expressive symbolism has been utilized, and why? The organic and individual biological need basis of the one frame, and the historical or evolutionary and bio-social need basis of the second or cultural framework need not blind us, beyond noting the difference in numbers and in emphasis (the "ill" or "well") to the essential concern with *specified* communication processes. The varying and definable differences in values systems, roles, aspirations, and culturally determined strengths and weaknesses are still there. In either case there are constant and special problems of adaptation to milieu and characteristic methods of attempting to achieve homeostasis.

While conceivably too, whole culture groups and social classes function materially (feeding, clothing, housing and functioning in productive systems), or provide a modicum of recreation, relaxation or harnessing of energies, or organize social and sexual life, etc., our ability to learn about these functions, or psychotic distortions of them, is still dependent on these same processes of symbolic communication within structured systems. Terms like communication, adjustment, transmission of tradition, or emotional expressivity are meaningless without concretization, specification as to structures like culture or class as well as function, and a typology which indicates what is communicated, adjustment to what, passive transmission of which tradition, or emotional expressivity with what values and actions at stake.

In the same manner, mechanistic terms like projection,

repression, sublimation or regression require structural as well as functional referents, even as does the richly qualified and quantified world of mental illness in which raw hostility, tension, anxiety, displacement, distortion, hallucination, withdrawal and isolation, fear, panic, apprehension, or guilt may play a role. The identification or non-identification or misidentification patterns so important in establishing or losing ego controls function only in self-other configurations, as George H. Mead so cogently demonstrated. There are, in actuality, no genuine regressions and total withdrawals, nor can there be in self-other relational systems. The pertinent and differing amounts of ego-strength or reality tested self-reference can only be spelled out, as to emergence, by an individual's actual points of reference, to parents of same or opposite sex, parent surrogates, siblings, males, females, to people, toward cultural events and typical occurrences that mark a life course and are laden with meaning.

The fact that humans can learn to use systems of symbols and be conditioned to them swells the world of meaning far beyond the mere mammalian level of learning by signs, signals and concrete perceptions. But it promotes the less objectified universe, the gross irrationalities, and, with equal bestowal of the gifts of art, language, science and philosophy, the nonrational use and interpretation of environment, the uncommunicative nonsense, the scourge of war or blight of insanity. To enter into study of these differentials, ethically varying at base, the psychosocial position must qualify and quantify within the social system the strains and stresses that produce these last emergents, in the same sense and on the same levels of interest and valuation that psychiatry utilizes in determining degrees of ego loss, gain and asset.

This means, in either case, that thought and action in human and cultural dimensions may be measured qualitatively in terms of function and typology, provided specific conditions of culture, class or personality balance are understood as dynamic processes. If for example, displacements and misidentifications or recognitions and warm relationships characterize an adjustment; or to use Sullivan terminology, if "good-me," "bad-me" or "not-me" constellations, male or female, are developed within a milieu, both the milieu and the resultant constellation must be viewed as related and dealt with as "incidence" or emergents. The only point at which the connected series must be watched with utmost care, in view of the spare adjustive machinery and natural, compensatory mechanisms of all men, is in the endless safety valves of cultural systems and in the safe-guarding play of adjustive (and protective) mechanisms within the individual.

The uniqueness of events, individuals, and cultural systems may prevent complete determinacy or one-to-one correlates between cultural stress systems and personality breakdown, and mathematical precision or perfection may be statistically unwarranted. Nevertheless, indications of relationship between the cultural environment and pathology are fully as expectable from carefully guided studies of incidence, as is the endless documentation already achieved from studies of normative, cultural behavior, class variations and their ego-involvements in anthropology, sociology and social psychology.

In summary, of the three general methods of medicine about which knowledge of disease processes can be built—the clinical study of individual patients, laboratory experiment, and the epidemiological approach of field and statistical studies of disease processes in groups of people, psychiatry has achieved its major successes only in the first two areas. The potential of the last method to contribute, particularly where the knowledge gained has more general capacity to be turned to good effect in therapeutic practice, management, control, education and prevention, is incalculable at the present time. It has been used, somewhat gingerly, and in limited scope in such therapies as the group psychotherapy session where at present the consensus as to optimum number of small group relationships that can be handled hovers about the eight-person mark; it has been used, no doubt unconsciously, in occupational and other push-therapies, in mass educational media like the film, television and radio, in child guidance and community clinics, in trusteeship and privilege systems of larger institutions, and in recreational and self-government experimentation, supervised of course, in the smaller. In the English Borstal system for delinquency as reported by Healy and the social psychiatry methods of Belmont, reported by Maxwell Jones, using psycho-drama, group therapy sessions and carefully tested community methods of re-education, have the implications of an epidemiological approach gone furthest.[29]

But nowhere, to our knowledge, has the epidemiological method, involving cultural study in urban settings, been used first as a method of research and then applied with the perspective of "cultural push-therapy" in mind. In all this, the first aim must be to see how existing techniques for mass measurement of psychiatric disorder may be enlarged and adapted in biological, psychological and social dimensions, and next to consider their possible use in the more delicate and practical problems of therapy, control and prevention.

In view of the vast range and variation of individual mental disorders and the complexity or indefiniteness of symptomatic syndromes and subtypes, a further qualification must be added to the etiological usefulness of the kinds of surveys which are not guided by clinical, psychodynamic and socio-cultural inquiry. We have already stated that studies which reveal putative or apparent incidence rates, however approximate, may be estimating how much malfunction can exist or pile up within specific socio-cultural groups, but that they do not in this form answer the how and why of malfunction or adjustment. For this reason, research psychiatry has divided into two wings, unfortunately not always again brought into relationship. That which surveys and aggregates general statistical ranges is forced repeatedly to retreat from even the most general etiological questions. The other, dealing with specific cases and their psychodynamic and therapeutic involvements concerns single patients and nonsignificant series. No doubt, as we have seen, the statistics have partial usefulness, and the patient-formulations considerable practical importance.

But because the processes never link systematically with findings on a given backgrounded area, the repetition of surveys marks no adaptation to actual research needs in diagnostics, therapy or prevention. The continued analyses of patients must continue to have the clinical ring of a private office, of limited discovery and of lack of research consolidation of net gains. Science has always more general, incisive and inclusive concerns and methods. The limited scope of each monotonously disparate study, the one microscopic and particularized, the other quantified, but etiologically limited, suggests that only a combination of methods, the full battery of medical research methodology, applied to a given, known socio-cultural area can deliver any fresh results or prevent the current and scattered dissipations of effort.

In personality formation, or even in its repressive or dissociative processes (whether we are dealing primarily with parent-child, sibling, peer group, intersexual or status group relations, or with the values, attitudes, meanings and motivations associated with such relationships) these all vary with class and culture, with degree or pace of acculturation, or, in short, with the kinds of systems of human symbolic communication and activity set up in the first instance within a culture.   It is this normative pattern of meanings and activities to which the research methods called clinical and those called epidemiological must both make reference.   Without it, the psychodynamic and genetic approach of the Freudian movement and its successors has functional insights into personality without structural points of reference, whereas the various environmentalist and physiological schools, stemming from the pioneer work of Adolf Meyer, have the needed environmentalist emphases corrective of the early descriptive and experimental movements fostered by Kraepelin and Bleuler, without denoting accurately the variables in socio-cultural experience that finally account for details of both structure *and* function in personality.   It is this latter detail which Rennie suggests "should give us increasingly concrete data for preventive psychiatry and public mental health programs."[30]   In research operation, it requires an accommodation, if not a fusion, of various social, medical and psychological researches into a new form of multidisciplinary, social psychiatric research.   In research perspective, it necessitates an awareness, new to our times, that the individual and his peers may be studied in both functional-organic and functional-behavioral dimensions as a member of a family, community, neighborhood, status group and culture.   These last-mentioned structural referents of systems of personality are themselves dynamic or variable in operation so that their description, for these purposes, must again be made in terms of structures, functions, meanings and values and the impact these have, of necessity, upon the dynamics of personality.

In ethnologic studies, aside from such classics as Junod's BaThonga, the Chukchi of Bogoras and a dozen others, the older penchant for describing the cultural world under bare bones of social organization, economics, ritual and belief with material and social culture neatly pigeonholed and ordered under fragmented headings has long since passed away. The cultural anthropologist now leaves room for life span, for basic values and emotional expressivity, for social process, dynamic change or acculturation, and the newer rubrics of child care, economic process, status system and functional interpretations of religion. There are even psychological studies of political system, folklore and drama, art, music and belief. The methods now extant and involving a re-creation of life ways are precisely those usable to dynamic psychiatry.

Psychiatrists work empirically with just this type of data in reference to specific cases, but unlike social scientists, do not usually formulate general interrelations between cultures and personalities. The exceptions to this rule comprise a long and growing list including such names as Jung and Rank, Rado, Ferenczi and Róheim, Horney, Kardiner, Sullivan and Thompson, Diethelm, Rennie, Ruesch, Levy, Lin, Yap, Dhunjibhoy, Stainbrook, Morita, Carothers, Böök, Bergler, Murray, Joseph, Lindemann, Leighton, and to an extent in their day, even Kraepelin and Bleuler. In cultural anthropology, the contrasts among ethnic groups are vivid and dramatic particularly if one ranges across regional and continental boundaries without benefit of a cultural typology or historical frames of reference. Less because the contrasts were germane to the contemporary Western world and more because they documented man's emotional life, the psychoanalytic movement drew closer to anthropological materials than any other field within psychiatry to an extent of making the literature of the two fields at times indistinguishable. Among the famous historical collaborations of just the last two decades, one could mention the work of E. H. Erikson with A. L. Kroeber and Scudder Mekeel, of Harry Stack

Sullivan with Edward Sapir, of the Leightons with Clyde Kluckholn, Kardiner with Linton and DuBois, Redlich or Babcock and Caudill, Ruesch and Bateson, Joseph and Spicer, Lindemann and the Parsons group. As Kluckhohn points out in *One Hundred Years of American Psychiatry*, edited by J. K. Hall, Zilboorg and Bunker in 1944, a summary of these and other associations discloses that cultural anthropology was most usually to be found, until recently, in the modified psychoanalytic wings of psychiatry. Brill's studies among the Eskimo before 1920, Coriat's among the Yahgan, and Róheim's extensive fieldwork were merely historical forerunners of what increasingly has been the case.

Yet cultures, and the human psychological processes contained within them, vary sufficiently so that human patterns of thought, motivation, learning process, characteristic activities and emotional expression cannot be considered as uniform introjected patterns. Conversely, the adult personality dynamics of the human species, and the rough similarity if not identity of the human learning process anywhere make it unlikely that in culture and psychology "anything may happen." This means that a style of weaning or a mode of achieving sphincter control, as isolated and independent features of a culture, will not predetermine adult personality configurations. In any real sense of personality dynamics in the total life course, it is far more likely that the cultural attitudes towards infancy and childhood, its kinship setting, and the values of human individual worth will affect the infancy handling and disciplines, the parental behavior and the family functioning.

In a manner only unconsciously explored in anthropology and underwritten in its literature, the predominant ethical patterns and values, the conceptions of health, the meeting of individual needs throughout life span are prob-

ably the general determinants of kinds of personality encountered in a social scene. While such points seem logically patent, it is still a far cry and a crucial step for psychiatry to translate these into the language of emotional
health and illness, to find them operating in the economy
of personality, and to locate such profiles translatable into
incidence and prevalence.

It is, nevertheless, at this point that case sampling is
needed according to socio-cultural background to provide
life histories in known matrices, and further contrasts
through the study of the well and ill in each society. At
this point, also, both the methods of cultural anthropology
and social psychiatry must be used, now one and now
another in scientific demonstration, if an adequate social
psychiatry is to be developed. Therefore, psychological
mechanisms may be studied in relation to case situations,
and the histories of normal and ill, within a sample and in
a context of the cultural realities affecting patients and
respondents.

Secondly, the definition of a case may, for such etiological and incidence study, include any persons in the normal-
abnormal continuum. It is important, in addition, to
study sex and family role differentia, intergeneration conflict, and identification processes. In seeking out such
relationships, one may measure them against cultural
backgrounds and situations, matching the well and ill by
such factors as sex and age, family role and cultural
experience.

We are led, finally, to a series of distinct and definite
methodological conclusions by our consideration of prevalence and incidence study. While careful incidence studies
represent a vast advance over those of prevalence, they
cannot, in the research on mental disorder, take the place
of psychogenetic and psychodynamic studies. Put differently, neither the psychogenetic nor the epidemiological

approaches meet the requirements of etiological knowledge when used singly. When used together, the first to provide a rounded verification of psychiatrically valid hypotheses, and the second to test statistically the hypotheses concerning groups of people, the combined methods of research may yield the kind of data which withdraws support from competing explanations and really withstands rigorous scrutiny.

Before such studies are put into actual operation, however, a second corollary or principle must be used to provide the frame of reference for both types of inquiry just noted. In brief form, such a corollary states that the social and cultural referents of behavioral functioning, whether in those well or those ill, are the dynamically most relevant factors in socio-cultural environment. These last are not just class and cultural labels applied loosely, but the dynamically repeated, emotionally charged, typical and thematic values of a culture which become reflected, unconsciously at times, into the dynamic, behavioral processes of individuals. Cultures will, of course, vary in the degree to which they permit or promote ease, naturalness and positive development in interpersonal communication. In general, it is postulated that the greater the amount of intercommunication on this positive level, the greater the amount of functional good health.

While good mental health and good human relations are almost interchangeable terms, as Thomas Ling, in England, has pointed out, there are no doubt other elements.[31] Spontaneity (in the sense used above, of ease, naturalness and freedom in interpersonal communication), security and confidence, creativity and other terms have all been used to describe positive and beneficial mental functioning. However welcome such individually-centered definitions have been in clarifying kinds of emotional experience, they fail in not defining well and ill within known cultural frameworks.

Erich Fromm, both in *Escape From Freedom* and *Man For Himself*, has expressed the dilemma by which terms like "normal" or "healthy" may mean quite different things. From the point of view of the functioning society, fulfilling the social role or roles one takes, or participation in social productivity and social reproduction constitutes normalcy or health; whereas from the individual stand-point the optimum of individual growth and happiness marks this result. In this view, creativity, spontaneity, freedom, productivity and expression of one's highest potentialities are selected as the aims of mental hygiene. Indeed, in one sense they are. But the error of Fromm, or the dilemma he does not wholly solve, is implicit in the failure to analyze dynamic processes as parts of recogniz-able social situations or "fields" of cultural influence.[32]

In this sense, one may choose between the two great traditions which have directed man's thinking about him-self, the Artistotelian which holds that the behavior of all things is determined by their nature (and which might posit individual urges for freedom, creativity and spontaneity) and the Galilean tradition which holds that the behavior of all things is determined by the conditions under which it occurs. Dynamic processes as opposed to more static attributes or entities; or the behavior of people in response to specific situations, rather than as expressions of attri-butes "possessed by human organisms," is the course we favor. It is classical psychiatry and prescientific anthro-opology which both spoke descriptively, and rarely analy-tically, of organic attributes, excluded environmental in-fluence, denoted racial entities, delineated the "unit psychosis," described invariant typologies whether in illness or in culture, and failed to discover process or con-textual referents anywhere. If human behavior is ability to communicate on symbolic and conceptual levels, then the systems of communication, whether disordered or not, have reference to symbolic, conceptualized values systems. Freedom, creativity and spontaneity do not exist *sub specie aeternitatis* any more than does mankind. There are always the conditions of existence, modifying existence. Culture, human values and psychiatric resultants may be more closely linked in real cultural systems than the men of any one of them have ever dreamed. And of course the relativity of cultures, one to another, is always open to human modification.

2

The Dimensions of Culture
and Human Values

CULTURE AND PERSONALITY AS RELATED
SYSTEMS: MULTIPLE CAUSATION

PSYCHIATRISTS increasingly recognize that epidemiology of mental disorders is something more than public health detective work, designed to ferret out the factors responsible for specific diseases with the purpose of applying controls and preventive measures against their action. Epidemiologists, through association with medical historians, psychiatrists, social scientists and psychologists, are obtaining clearer understanding of group characteristics of mental diseases.

At one time, rural communities were held to be homogeneous, imposing codes and customs, involving neighbors in personal crises, and with less *anomie* presumptively, producing less personal maladjustment. The mechanization of agriculture, the increased means of communication and the virtual disappearance of the hinterland dividing city and farm did little to dispel the popular assumption that the tempo of city life, its alleged lack of neighborhood, community, and kinship connections exposed the individual to a weakened family and institutional support and control, and consequent instability.

On second thought, no one thought seriously that the "tempo of urban life," as such, had any psychiatric meaning, that urban Irish from rural countryman backgrounds turned secular, that upper status groups in the largest cities had any great rates of residential mobility, that urban neighbors were always more remote than rural ones, or that acculturation of American ethnic groups meant in the least a "melting pot" of nondescript, cultureless anonymity.   As Canon Michael Shannon, an Irish priest from abroad, recently remarked at a New York Irish Feis, "The Irish in the U.S. are more Irish than those in Ireland."

The studies of Lemert in Michigan, covering five years' admissions to state and private hospitals, and analyzed not only for counties and regions, urban and rural, but within individual counties for place of provenience, show the thinly populated fishing, mining and resort counties of the Upper Peninsula to have the highest mental illness rates (80.6 per year per 100,000), the southern agricultural counties to come next (67.5), the urban southern areas next (66.2) and the marginal forest and farming areas, last.[33] Not merely Lemert, and possibly Eaton and Weil's data on the Hutterites, have thrown doubt upon the claim that rural communities are havens of mental health, but the classic study of Roth and Luton in the Williamson County rural area of Tennessee based on house-to-house field survey showed a total of mental incapacitation of 69.4 per 1,000 in 1938 far larger than the Baltimore Survey of Lemkau, Tietze and Cooper (1936) with its total for active cases of 60.5.[34]   Mangus in Butler County, Ohio, found that differences in urban, village, and farm population rates of children's personality adjustment did not favor any of the three groups considered.[35] Leland Stott's research on intellectual and mental adjustments of urban and rural children in Nebraska pointed in the same direction.[36] In brief, by 1950, epidemiological psychiatry already knew something of the lack of clear differentiation in the incidence of mental illnesses as a whole in urban or rural settings.   In some cultural configurations, rural maladjustment rates far exceeded the urban.   From the point of view of the psychic economy and emotional life of these areas, little was known, anthropologically or psychologically, of the effects of the social and affective family settings, of the values, of different family structures, or of community organization in each case.

The presence, in the Baltimore study of Lemkau, Tietze and Cooper, of groupings like Czechs, Jewish and Negro, in contrast to the way of life of rural Tennesseans, was not analyzed in anthropological field survey to test for relevant differences. As concerns the process of urbanism in connection with the Baltimore survey, it can only be repeated that Shevky, Williams and others determined this process to be one in which more or less segregated cultural enclaves or communities tend to form into status-differentiated and ethnically delineated sets of units as the process wears on.

As Emerson noted in 1939, we have incidence rates "without any environmental counterparts to our information and . . . exquisite vignettes of individual cases without enough of them to paint a picture of the composite." In addition to having the "environmental counterparts" brought up to date with current social theory and epidemiological information, "the vignettes of individual cases" must be made consistent with modern psychiatric science. Emerson's "composite picture" is obtainable only when culture, social group and personality are studied in actual relationship, and when, as in control group studies in medical research, samples of well and ill are matched within a series that equalizes (or holds constant) each factor in turn. Sub-studies of demoralization, mass hysterias, delinquency, or suicide, where applicable, are possible within the same framework. Before this can be done, studies which consider background factors must locate sample populations with sufficient status and cultural contrasts in large enough quantities to determine age, sex, status and cultural difference. Determinations to analyze status, but not culture, or to study cultures and sub-cultures without status variations, or equally to fail to reach agreement on the necessity of considering only *the combined effects of both together* are all three, as methods, doomed to failure. If culture, status and personality are related systems, they are always relational and must be studied in combination. There are no statuses without cultural underpinnings. There are probably few American urban sub-cultures without status and role differentiation.

In a cogent article, "In Defense of Culture-Personality Studies," J. W. Eaton has suggested there is no Single Factor explanation of personality, that ordinarily experiences need frequent and consistent repetition to become emotionally meaningful, and that the child must experience personally or be aware of normal standards in reference to self-judgments.[37]   Even so, statistical assessments of the effects of cultural practices are rough approximations of probability extremely valuable for the psychiatrist to possess, to be sure, since his whole science in the nature of the case is founded upon the same approximate foundations of probability.

Yet only 13 years before, in the same journal, *The American Sociological Review*, and with culture-personality studies in their infancy, J. W. Woodard, in his article, "The Relation of Personality Structure to the Structure of Culture," was relating the Freudian doctrine of a super-ego to the "control culture" or Weltanschauung of a people as a whole and unfortunately drawing the analogy down, in what is now outmoded sociology and psychiatry, to fixed processes of "psychotic dissociation" always connected with that extremely nebulous concept of "social disorganization."[38]   The notion of fixed processes of "social disorganization" to accommodate similar fixed notions of psychological disintegration is today even more debatable in the light of figures, from England, on the diminution of neuroses in those areas most subject to conditions of severe air raid bombings in World War II.

However, the German Descriptive Schools of psychiatry, of Kraepelin, Ziehen and Wernicke which were dominant just after the turn of the century, and which provided the first adequate observational material for the Western world, persisted in the description of fixed entities and a fixed progression in illnesses. Zilboorg, in his historical survey of medical psychiatry, remarks upon the fateful view and organicist emphasis in Kraepelin which fore-shadowed Kretschmer's far-reaching hypotheses and in-sisted upon an inevitable course of illness within two basic psychotic entities, dementia praecox and the manic- depres-sive psychosis. It was not until Adolf Meyer applied the broad anthropological interests of his teacher in early folk, and social psychology that the patient was looked at from the standpoint of his emotional and ideological back-ground; or, as Brill says in his *Lectures on Psychoanalytic Psy-chiatry* from a "normal psychological viewpoint." Brill goes on to remark of Meyer's tutelage:[39] "We were taught to describe the patient's attitude and manner, his anthro-pological make-up; we examined all phases of his orienta-tion, memory, judgment, insight, etc." This was, of course, in relation to physical and neurological examination. It was at Bleuler's clinic at Burghölzli, in the company of such anthropologically-inclined figures as Jung, Brill and Riklin that the early association-test experiments of the 1900's were developed under the direction of Bleuler and Jung. There the word, "complex," originated to denote a past, repressed (and complex) emotional experience, and new descriptions of illness varied the earlier essentially dual and rigid nomenclature, the schizoid and syntonic categories of a later Kretschmer classification.

But even before American psychiatry became interpreta-tive rather than descriptive under the combined influence of men like Adolf Meyer and George H. Kirby, or even through the influences of Bleuler and Brill, an unintended by-product of Kraepelin's organicist and descriptive interests had taken him, following his Dorpat professorship, on a tour of various countries. His travels led to keen observations that his major psychopathological categories, and the sub-types within them, varied with culture. While widespread, they occurred in somewhat different arrangement and frequency in different cultures. In Java, for example, melancholia and mania were rare to begin with, and a clinical variant was the absence of any notion of having sinned as part of a depressive reaction. There were, further, no cases involving alcoholism among Javanese, and this category, as "alcoholic psychosis" in Kraepelin's system, showed elsewhere considerable cultural variability. His dementia praecox typology, on the other hand, was not only of frequent occurrence in Java but resembled the presenting symptoms described on the basis of European experience.

Ziehen's notations of differences in incidence and specific symptomatology in Holland and Thuringia; Bleuler's on English, Irish, Bavarians and Saxons; C. G. Seligman's paper on New Guinea in 1929[40] emphasizing confusional states rather than systematized insanities and disclaiming any cases of manic-depressive disorder in acculturated areas of Papua; and J. Dhunjibhoy's in 1930 [41] on regional aspects of India, already alluded to, represent the early pioneering to the third decade of the century roughly, in the field of cultural variation in symptomatology.

For the period from 1870 on, but preceding Kraepelin's discovery that the echolalia, echopraxia, "automatic obedience," and loss of will,—all characteristic of the Latah illness of Malays,—were indeed important elements in the presenting symptoms of schizophrenia of certain types among Europeans, the tendency to note crude variations by region or culture gathered momentum. Kraepelin first published on this disorder in 1896. *Dementia Praecox* was again published, in the Edinburgh edition, in 1919. For the period before, Edward Stainbrook has summarized the extensions of horizons in cultural psychiatry very well.[42] In those years, he notes, it was possible to read in the psychiatric literature frequent assertions that illness incidence, poverty and population density were connected phenomena. Following the economic depression of 1875, it was claimed that an excessive rate "of melancholy" was admitted to asylums of England and Wales. In Japan, it was reported, possibly with point if not with cultural explanation, that mental illness was more prevalent among the married than those unmarried. Melancholia and attempted suicide was less common among natives of British Guiana than in England.

In Parisian institutions, a British visitor could remark a difference from English asylums in that French children were more talkative and demonstrative, whereas in the American, the patients were noisier and more disorderly than in British psychiatric hospitals. With Bleuler, but much earlier, one observer stated, "No one of experience can escape the impression that the composition and behavior of asylum populations differ a good deal in different parts of Germany." Meanwhile, the impressionistic literature reported the increase in the number of all persons requiring care and of suicides in industrialized countries, the disproportion of suicides being one female to every three males; along with this, one reads of such variations in diagnosis as 5 per cent more "melancholics than maniacs" in Norway, but 24 per cent more "maniacs than melancholics" admitted in England in the same period, or the nonexistence of French hysteria in England.

From 1870 on, according to Stainbrook, an increasing number of observations were recorded on the ecological

and cultural "determinants of behavior disorders."   By
the time H. G. Van Loon in 1928[43] was announcing that
the much studied Malays whose characteristic symptomatology in running amok was probably the announcement of
dementia praecox in a form typical for them of "aggressive
confusion" through long habituation to "hostile tribes" and
"jungle villages" and headhunts of "any potential enemy,"
the scenes were well set both within descriptive and inter-
pretative psychiatry, and in more impressionistic reporting
as well, for the anthropological and psychiatric discoveries
which were to follow.   While acculturation was just beginning to be discussed in social science, Van Loon could
define the Latah reaction of Malay women in terms like
Kraepelin's, "the automatic obedience . . . principally in
those who have worked with Europeans," the imitation
and suggestibility assumed to be engendered by contact
with those "advanced."

It is the last three decades which have seen regional and
cultural variants emerge more clearly.   Between these
scattered and early references on cultural groups and several modern full-length and volume size accounts of psychoanalytic therapy in a person of distinctive cultural
background, there lies a literature now as impressive certainly as that of early epidemiological, and not culturally
backgrounded, psychiatry.   For the full-length analyses
of the last decade, one might refer to two which are popularly known.   The most recent, at this writing, is George
Devereux's *Reality and Dream*, the psychotherapy of a
Plains Indian, [44] and it followed by four years W. Sachs'
Black Hamlet, an analysis of a South African Bantu. [45]

In the United States, this interest in culturally backgrounded psychiatry did not exactly lie dormant until
the third decade of the Twentieth Century.   The expanding cultural horizons of anthropology and its importation,
as a discipline from Europe, through such diverse figures

as Morgan, Brinton and Boas, was matched in psychiatry by influences traceable to Freud and Bleuler, Ernest Southard and Adolf Meyer. Karl Menninger has recently summarized certain trends in psychiatric thought which mark progress in this direction through emphases on diagnostic and symptomatological variability, the treatment of ambulatory and community populations, the influence of cultural environment, and readjustments in theoretical research perspective. [46]

While Adolf Meyer, perhaps more than anyone else, at first gave currency to the descriptive classifications of Kraepelin in this country and these categories of diagnosis received enthusiastic reception in institutional psychiatry, he soon moved from more exclusively neuropathological work into increasing interest in "clinical psychiatry and began to deplore the Pandora's Box of Kraepelin name-calling and therapeutic nihilism." As new proposals for more systematic therapy in severe illnesses took form (Weir Mitchell's rest and isolation methods reminiscent of the later Morita-therapy in Japan might be cited), simplifications of psychiatric terminology, like Southard's in 1918, though based on greater "diagnostic definiteness," did not of themselves ease the therapeutic problem or lead to greater success. Other steps, like Southard's establishment of psychiatric outpatient department operations, Meyer's concept and diagnosis revision, and both his and Bleuler's notice of ranges or groupings of illness rather than fixed entities, opened the way more clearly to the concept of total personality study and advances in treatment based on dynamic ideology rather than static Kraepelinian classification and labels. It was Meyer, who, "influenced by Dewey's pragmatic 'functionalism'," according to Menninger, stressed "the importance of life experiences for the development of a mental illness."

At the same time, the Freudian concepts of personality

function and its assessment were being introduced to America by A. A. Brill, W. A. White and Smith Ely Jelliffe. Their enthusiastic reception, in theory and re-research, if not universally in therapy, was ensured by the support of such leaders as J. J. Putnam, Albert Barrett, A. P. Noyes, Richard Hutchings, Arthur Ruggles and W. A. White. As Menninger puts it, today "the Kraepelinian influence remains chiefly visible in psychiatric case records and in official nomenclature." Speaking of the eclectic position which has evolved in many quarters, he states: "The pseudo-conflict has thus been resolved. Historic vestiges remain; some psychiatrists emphasize adaptation and some adjustment and some repression. Some speak of the total personality and some of character structure. But regardless of how they speak, most psychiatrists now think in terms which express the combined ideology of Freud, Southard and Meyer."

The further step of describing illnesses in terms which include the impact of cultural experience on personality remains to be taken. The principle of homeostasis means little to any psychiatric theory or position if constructive, or destructive, efforts of the organism are viewed as "drives," modifiable by therapy, but not by life exper-ience. If Menninger is right that greater or more pro-longed stresses excite the ego and its regulatory devices to "increasingly energetic and expensive activity in the inter-ests of homeostatic maintenance," how much more is this the case if dominant themes in a cultural system present the individual, typically, with the same stressful situations. The kinds of emergency and regulatory devices which come into play "to control dangerous impulses," or to "prevent or retard the disintegrative process which threat-ens" may themselves be typically called forth *less* by some mystical *deus ex machina* of ego functioning *than* by notions, emotionally founded, of ideal behavior, cultural values, improper behavior, and the actual impediments to happiness, and positive homeostatic functioning, of actual human beings.

This notion is then to be translated into theory directly: what is important, now that clusters of illness and diagnostic prototypes are well established, is attention to the varying symptomatology, the cultural coloring, the actual experiential background of the case. It was to this point that cross-cultural work of the last three decades was addressed. A look at more recent literature on culture and psychopathology discloses that incidence studies and explorations of psychodynamics in various cultures have only just begun.

Let us look at one of the most recent of such studies, Stainbrook's on characteristics of the psychopathology of schizophrenias among Bahians of South America, based on work at the Juliano Moreira Hospital[47] About 80 per cent of these patients were rural Bahians of Brazil, approximately 85 per cent lower class and 15 per cent middle class. Many were from three ecological areas intensively studied by anthropologists. The Bahians, as Donald Pierson and others have observed, are multi-racial and their classes are not closed caste groups although largely identified with color. While culturally and biologically a gradual process of fusion has taken place, the lower and lower middle class hospital population was predominantly colored or mulatto, in large part illiterate, and exhibiting behavioral patterns, especially in religion, of both African and Brazilian origin.

This case is particularly instructive in that it shows relationship between a fused or acculturated social and cultural pattern and psychopathology directly, or between notions of ideal behavior, emotionally founded in cultural values and real cultural contexts, and resulting symptomatology. While of the 200 patients studied, all were diagnosed as schizophrenias, a scrutiny of hospital records, additional and occasionally serial interviews, and participant observation in the hospital life-space, plus projective testing, indicated several distinctive patterns. In the first place, the psychological distance between psychiatrist and patient, based on class, sub-cultural and hospital role differences, was striking. After the acute admission phase of illness subsided, the lower class patient generally related to the physician by almost uniformly passive-submissive attitudes. (The obedience and automatic imitation syndromes noticed in other native acculturating communities are parallel.) As in the schizophrenic behavior of most East Indian patients, overt impulsive and aggressive behavior was very little in evidence toward any official hospital personnel.

Beyond this, women patients much more commonly could verbalize their aggressive and fantasy feelings than men; this verbally impulsive behavior did not carry across, even in the most acutely disturbed women, to sexual acting out since they unfailingly retained their ingrained modesty in dress and posture even when squatting in the habitual Bahian sitting position. More open ideation and feeling by female patients related *both* to consistent variations in child-rearing differences and the severity of disciplines learned in connection with satisfying sexual and aggressive needs.

However, these patterns in training and expression related equally to the generalized cultural patterns of action for male and female behavior. As Stainbrook explains, "Bahian psychiatry nonetheless is prone to place a diagnosis of manic-depressive psychosis, manic phase, on such behavior because of the 'affective' characteristics." The resulting male-female ratio in manic-depressive disorder is 1 to 4 in Bahian epidemiology and since the lower class patient depressive-reactions are "extraordinarily rare, these figures apply almost entirely to the diagnosis of manic excitement." On the other hand, Stainbrook's restudy of these cases indicates them to be schizophrenias with characteristic affective features. Among the hospitalized lower-class patients, in a 10 year period, no suicidal attempts have been observed. Over half the cases of schizophrenia randomly selected (all under 40 years of age) suffered the loss of one or both parents by the time of admission at an average age of 24 years. Despite the high mortality rates of the general population, such a high proportion of parent-bereaved individuals in the hospital population was striking. It was again associated with aspects of Bahian family structure whereby the mother's near kin resided in the same house or nearby thus increasing the possibilities of substitute mothering and the presence of several, possibly confusing, parental figures. The change in the meaning of parental loss from the experience in the relatively isolated conjugal American family is clear, and it argues that deprivations, substitutions and discontinuities of this order may not be statistically considered apart from the total contours of social organization in ethnic groups.

Further, while avoidance and withdrawal behavior was a steady accompaniment of the life-long difficulties exhibited by these patients in the maintenance of poor object relationships, such catatonic symptoms as mutism, stupor and negativism were unusually rare and almost without exception "the schizophrenic patients entered readily into at least a momentarily responsive and meaningful relationship." In both chronic and acute symptomatology there occurred much less anxiety referable to other persons "than in similar disorders in our own culture." While Stainbrook agrees this observation is admittedly difficult to document with great validity, he illustrates for example the acutely catatonic girl who, with some food retained in her mouth, dilated pupils, great motor inhibition and other neurophysiological indices of extreme fear, nevertheless asserted her fear was of the spirits: "I am not afraid of people because they are human beings."

Other cases of catatonia in which such displaced and magnified fears inhibit motility but allow human relationships of a sort to continue have been reported for the Navajo; and the author in his experiences with Eskimo patients at the Morningside Hospital and Clinic in Portland, a federal center for Alaskan natives, found no dearth of Eskimo catatonics with severe motor inhibitions who would chat amiably and gaily until they focussed on supernatural fears. Obviously, catatonia operates differently if it emanates from different cultural backgrounds.

As Stainbrook puts it, the predominantly lower-class rural patient suffers from anxieties, threats and fears of retribution "interpreted as arising from the cultural deities, either . . . African or Catholic. So, too, for most of the lower class men and the majority of both lower and middle-class women, the delusional restitutional symptoms, either megalomanic or persecutory, were fantasied in terms of the cultural religious institutions. Middle-class men, however, much more frequently 'secularized' their restitutive narcissistic and self-esteem delusions in terms of economic and class conceptions of power," their paranoid ideation more frequently involving threat and persecution felt to arise from other men. Certainly here the difference in psychopathology between the lower and middle-class males relates to the point made, that in Bahian culture the intense mobility striving and identifications of middle with upper classes do not affect the lower-class Bahian. Nor will it involve the female (of lower class) whose involvement in religious behavior is as much greater as her economic aspirations lessen.

Equally striking was the fact that paranoid conceptions of impersonal causation (electricity, physical "waves," etc.) were found only in the relatively educated middle-class, private psychiatric hospital-patients of the Sanatorio de Bahia where the greater impersonality of aspiration and economic strivings were maintained in the normative cultural pattern. It is possible that an inverse proportion existed as between women in *Candomblé* cult organization and those who succumbed to idiosyncratic, autistic features. Those in sufficient control of autistic and impulsive behavior were able to conform to the relatively rigid, ritualistic group activity and passed from the period of probationary scrutiny into the possession dances. This "psychopathological screening" which distinguishes highly individualized hysterical dissociative behavior from the induced and nonindividualized conversion phenomena of the ceremonies argues against the common assumption that normative ceremonial behavior, such as Hindu-Balinese trance-dance states may be read off as "cultural psychopathology." The assumption of Benedict, Mead and others of a total relativity of culture and the abnormal, of cultural-clinical types, is a confusion of culture with cultural stress system and with incidence data. As Stainbrook described the content of *Candomblé* behavior, it was accompanied by considerable psychopathological screening. As a normative pattern, it "played a significant role in the thought and action of the schizophrenic lower-class patient," sometimes characterized by non-institutional meaningless "acting out of being possessed by an African god of goddess." However, a correlative observation "concerns the apparently low incidence of gross hysterical dissociative reactions among the lower-class Negroes in Bahia." This includes women who in *Candomblé* organization could not induce the socially approved conversion behavior, but who in personality characteristics were anxious, stubborn and hostile, no doubt others for whom the conversion phenomena acted as a cultural "safety valve," and still others who passed the organizational screening with flying colors.

The distinction between clinical and cultural manifestations is so brilliantly clear in Stainbrook's discussion that it resolves in a major dichotomy: "The clinical picture was definitely schizophrenic and not simply hysterical and usually occurred as a reaction to a situationally acute stress or deprivation. The major psychological goal achieved in the psychotic resolution seemed to be an identification with the omnipotent deity similar to the brief and transitory introjection and identification achieved" by the religious participants during the end processes of possession and conversion.[48] In brief, clinic is not culture, but cultural phenomena greatly affect the etiology and symptoms of psychopathology. The hysterical features in Balinese dances are probably not "schizoid."

A frequent distinction between the epidemiological and clinical approaches is that the first method is by definition extensive and the second intensive, the larger studies filled with inescapable errors, the smaller richly studied and accurate. It is stated above in respect to etiology and the question of cultural background, that all studies, epidemiological or clinical, must have necessary etiological reference or they cease to be psychiatry at all. The limited number of illness groupings, like the schizophrenias, and their almost universal extent in the reported cross-cultural literature suggest universal compensatory and repressive psychic mechanisms or defenses, at human disposal, but with different frequency and amount (or intensity) in given cultural contexts. Three limiting factors in addition to pan-human psychic processes can therefore operate: the cultural context and certain subcultural features such as socio-economic status; the specific conditions of a life course as these become operative in the particular psychodynamics of an individual case; and the stress system inherent in a culture under certain conditions of time, place and circumstance.

Before Stainbrook, in acculturated Bahian society of Brazil, made his remarkable studies of variations from Anglo-American and European forms of catatonia, C. Lopez reporting in the German literature in 1932 noted that no schizophrenias whatsoever could be found among Indians of interior Brazil although acculturated tribesmen living in coastal towns and settlements evidenced the illness in one or another form.[48] Such variations, from high to practically null incidence roughly correlative with cultural differentiation within a nation of "nations," argues for a range of psychodynamic processes and tendencies in the historically changeable modes of mental illness in Brazil. Further, the swift shifting in a generation of central tendencies in respect to the promotion of a kind of illness in each cultural milieu argues against an indiscriminate use of general terminology of the Kraepelinian sort.

When Ellsworth Faris, in the *Nature of Human Nature*, reported on culture and personality differences among the forest Bantu of Africa, his account was based on four hospitals of the more urbanized areas in which not a single case of schizophrenia or manic depressive psychosis was found. A subsequent search for the characteristic symptomatology of these illnesses in the outlying native villages of the region fared no better, the Bantu-speaking villagers being mystified by descriptions of the Western disorders. On the other hand, as is well known, the physiologist W. B. Cannon has analyzed the data on deaths due to extreme fears, wasting away and physiological dehydration stemming from a series of cultures in which the religious ideology concerning witchcraft attacks or the breaking of taboo systems may cause fundamental and lethal disturbances of autonomic functioning.[49] While "voodoo" death and voodoo erotic patterns are psychosomatic disturbances rare in Western European cultures, it must be remembered that they occur within values systems in which the pervasiveness of religious belief in the total round of economic and social life is very great. Such nonliterate peoples have no Sundays and it is impossible to extricate magical belief from the continuity of life processes.

Variations in circulatory and respiratory behavior run parallel, John Gillin's account of magical fright (*espanto*), with its "jumpiness" of pulse rate in San Carlos being just such an instance.[50] Jules Henry has reviewed the psychosomatic literature from the point of view of cultural variability and finds in one instance which he has studied first hand, the Pilagá Indians of Brazil, that somatic disorders center in areas of speech, hearing and muscle function; the same study indicates that the common psychosomatic ailments of Western cultures are completely absent.[51]

Anyone acquainted with the enormous anthropological literature on conversion hysterias and psychosomatic disorders among nonliterate peoples cannot fail to be impressed by the frequency of such directly somatized symptoms in these cultures as contrasted with the totally disorganizing illnesses of our own. Ebaugh notes that the frankly expressive (histrionic, in our culture) type of individual, with inner needs to obtain approval, attention or rapport, tends to develop the somatic manifestations of hysterias, as in paralysis, spasms, anesthesias and pains, or disturbances of such partially voluntary autonomic functions as eating, vomiting, breathing, coughing or lower bowel control. These correspond to the common ailments the shaman cures. Persons showing marked obsessional trends, including such ritualistic rules as temper control, cleanliness, punctiliousness, emotional constriction, and sado-masochistic standards of dutiful or truthful behavior tend to develop the often deeper seated vegetative neuroses and organic psychosomatic disorders. While the primitive literature, by and large, is full of the former, and our own of the latter dysfunctions, particularly in recent times, certain more specific rate variabilities are regularly found in the Western European and American literature. Ulcer of psychosomatic origin has been described as a middle class disease, but the duodenal ulcer variety and childhood asthma occur more often in males than in females. Worthy of note is the shift in sex ratio of peptic ulcer from being predominantly a female disorder in our own culture to one characteristically a disease of adult males.

While more than one psychosomatic disorder tends to appear in the same patient, no large study has been made of the fact that they occur usually at different times in the life cycle. While commonly also, the same disorder occurred in parents, relatives or siblings, such patterns of somatic identification have not been studied in any charted kinship sense nor have the comparative age studies been made in this sense despite the phasic nature of many of these ailments with their periods of crudescence, remission and recurrence. Such considerations require research on somatization of cultural strains. Exophthalmic goiter, gall bladder disease and rheumatoid arthritis afflict more females than males. Certain illnesses which occurred more often on the distaff side (as, peptic ulcer, exophthalmic goiter and perhaps essential hypertension) in the Nineteenth Century, have since appeared in increasing proportion among males during the Twentieth. Other diseases, like diabetes, which were predominantly male diseases of the last century have conversely increased among females of the present time. The fact of higher rates for the latter among both sexes and especially the males of Jewish and Italian cultural antecedents argues for studies in this area which combine sex, age and cultural criteria and which are historically oriented.

As Ebaugh states, "The phenomena of 'sex shift' probably provides a statistical indication of the changes that have taken place in the 'personality type of the sexes' as a

result of social changes that have led to 'female emancipation'." We should add that this is less a matter of blurring
of sex differences in social participation, the feminizing of
males and masculinizing of females, as he suggested, but
differences gradually developed in the social role of each
in the cultures from which they stem.[52]   Such studies
should be culture-specific. The related phenomena of an
age-shift, the fact that certain of these illnesses are increasingly appearing in younger age groups (most noticeable in
one large study of gastritis, peptic ulcer and anxiety states)
is evidence that the social position of the sexes, more likely
than biological difference, underlies these trends.   The
increasing incidence of psychosomatic afflictions on a non-
hysteriform level in the modern world argues that the
emotional lives of masses of adults, in Ebaugh's terms,
"have become increasingly disturbed, diverted, frustrated
or distorted."   Increasing frustration of creativity, the
need to achieve safety or security by obsessional mechanisms, the aimlessness, decline of firm life goals and values,
and the standardization and mass production extending
to information, entertainment, clothing and education are
some of the factors in social environment alluded to as
possibly important.

Two recent investigations into the problem of management of angina pectoris in geriatrics cases conclude that the
prevention of unpleasant emotional contacts will greatly
reduce the gravity and frequency of anginal attacks.   The
study of the personality type and psychotherapy in patients
with hypertension, pseudocyesis, pancreatic disease, Men-
iere's disease, and various dermatoses have, in separate
monographs, recently been concluded.   Portis, in his latest
work on *Diseases of the Digestive System* marshalls a lengthy
chapter and 70 selected references on the subject of emotional factors in gastrointestinal upsets.   It is possible that
both the deeply rooted somatizations as well as the most

incapacitating disorganizing illnesses are more prevalent in modern societies than in nonliterate cultures.

While no doubt the major functional psychoses occur in all cultures and psychosomatic symptoms involving virtually all somatic systems can be found throughout, there are notable differences in symptomatology and incidence recorded to date within various cultures. E. Winston, in attacking the extreme Rousseauan theory of a total absence of any mental disease among primitive groups, early aggregated the material from Margaret Mead's *Coming of Age in Samoa* (Appendix IV), extrapolated from the sample of cases cited, a mere six in all, and arrived at an incidence rate of 100 psychotics per 100,000! The fact that *Coming of Age . . .* patently describes a highly acculturated fringe of Samoa, despite popular assumptions to the contrary, and that figures derived from intensive anthropological observations in community settings are not comparable with those for admitted patients to public hospital facilities destroys this comparison based on a few cases.[53] A recent extrapolation from nine Saipanese cases, giving the astounding rate of 208 cases per 100,000, cannot be justified any better as incidence data though the psychiatric materials by A. Joseph and V. F. Murray in their volume, *Chamorros and Carolinians of Saipan: Personality Studies*, are clearly superior.[54] Most studies, ever since Vilhjalmur Stefansson's comparison of the unacculturated Greenland Eskimos with good mental health statistics, and the acculturated Alaskan Eskimos with decidedly poor rates, have distinguished carefully between the acculturated communities and those which are relatively untouched. While the Rorschach records obtained from frank psychotics among Saipanese show the same disintegrative patterns and serious decrease or loss of reality testing as do the records of psychotics in our own culture, it is debatable whether such a test of personality structure and psychodynamics offers the same opportunity as the Thematic Apperception to draw out differences in content and psychological experience. It is even a question in highly acculturated situations whether reality testing and disintegration are distinctions fine enough to do more than separate the very well from the clearly ill regardless of cultural context or the sub-types of disease groupings.

On the more solid grounds of symptomatology, there can be no doubt that psychopathology is culturally influenced. Geza Róheim in 1939 and P. M. Yap, in 1951, have published over a decade apart on the rapidly expanding literature of this type.[55] More pinpointed and richly descriptive studies like Stainbrook's among Bahians, E. S. Carpenter's among Aivilik Eskimos,[56] and the Berndts among Australians in West Arnhem territory[57] have since appeared along with one account, partly historical, by A. N. Berenberg and A. Jacobson on Japanese psychiatry and psychotherapy.[58] Both Carpenter and the Berndts document cases of psychoses in highly primitive cultures, technologically speaking, though neither adduce epidemiological incidence data. In each study, nevertheless, religious values and conceptions are ingredient in the etiology of the disorders, fear of witches being as important in Aivilik psychotic distortions as mistaken identifications with "the omnipotent diety" were in Stainbrook's Bahian cases. While the Japanese material is more concerned with Morita's methods of therapy in application to psychoneurotic character disorders and obsessive-phobic states, the reliance there in therapy of followers of Morita's Zikei University group in psychiatry upon culturally acceptable principles of Zen Buddhism merely strengthens the contention that religious values may configure prominently in the psychic economy, both as regards the illness and its treatment. In a more general sense of cultural influence, Jules Henry has suggested that the cultural milieu creates at once "the conditions for its own pathology (schizo-phrenia, for example) and its treatment (introspection and highly developed verbalization)."

In Western countries, the incidence of various kinds of mental and psychosomatic disorder has fluctuated or changed remarkably in populations where there is no evidence for connected changes in race, somatype or genetic composition. The contemporary rarity of "the French hysteria" anywhere in Europe; the increase in instances of peptic ulcer (in the Mauve Decade in New York, 1880-1890, and for a decade following, there were seven female to six male cases of perforated peptic ulcer, whereas in the Depression Period of 1932-1939, the ratio had changed dramatically to twelve males for every female case of tissue perforation);[59] or the fact that in World War I hysterical blindness and paralyses frequently afflicted American soldiers, while in World War II they suffered more from psychosomatic disorders of the digestive tract,[60] each constitutes a variation explainable only by a psychosocial analysis.

E. H. Ackerknecht has gathered comparable materials for similar short periods of time on a variety of nonliterate cultures such as the Kirghiz and finds that where reliably reported, shifts in psychopathology can be equally sudden and sweeping in the primitive scene.[61] Rate variability, in these instances, already suggests that processes of culture change and acculturation operate on psychodynamic levels as well as the cultural, and are as modifiable on the one as on the other. The idea of Adolf Meyer, that within such a generalized disease grouping as the schizophrenias, themselves containing similarities as well as differences, modifications can occur by reason of environmental factors, is suggested by rate variability in a number of other emotional illness groupings.

For those who maintain precarious contact with reality

or those who break seriously with real goal orientation, no clear picture is as yet afforded as to *what* overloading of what emotional or somatic circuits causes a particular disturbance. It is clear however, that interpersonal and human relations contexts, best called cultural, determine not merely whether fissures will occur in personality structure (a problem of indicating incidence), but more particularly in what area of personality adjustment they will appear, which is in final analysis a question of typology. The therapeutic predicament in psychiatry, one of dealing with end-products or epiphenomena of longstanding disease processes, and even more so the special danger of breaking through the psychic defenses of persons who have built them with frenetic purpose, poses problems in the analysis of schizophrenias for typological research results.

A continuance and expansion of Meyer's work requires moving beyond such designations, already over-generalized, as "the schizophrenias" to sub-varieties which relate lifelong situation-contexts to resulting personality contours. One course which has been suggested to overcome diagnostic pigeonholes is to study the longitudinal life course from infancy on out, a method which has been partly realized in studies limited to childhood by René Spitz in the United States and John Bowlby in English maternal-deprivation cases. Ordinarily, for a longer life process, such methods are costly and the shot is scattered; they are appropriate in the children's institutional settings in which they have been attempted. Follow-up studies, in remission states, are also decidedly useful since they have been made with persons whose ego functioning and innermost problems are to some extent known.

Far better, for cross-cultural analysis, is to study sociocultural factors in etiology directly, using cultural push therapy and positive cultural identifications to build upon strengths and avoid weaknesses in the precarious structure of a problematic personality. This method has been dimly apprehended in part in occupational and recreational therapy, but still utilizes all too little what meanings and attachments men have lived by in their best, and most maturing, periods. Such studies, if made in institutional settings, must build their own data beyond the existing record. Examples of religious variability which may be missed by social over-generalizations (as serious as the over-generalized schizophrenias) are "Catholic," without noting the variance among Irish, Polish or Italian Catholics, "Jewish," without distinguishing German and East European Jewish, or by jumbling under "Czechoslovakian," the patriarchial and formerly rural Catholic Slovakian family, and the more egalitarian or matriarchal, often urbanized and virtually nullifidian Bohemian Czech. The exploration of existing relationships in both the best human exemplifications of a cultural pattern and in its most dismal failures is the kind of data needed to throw the situational contexts and cultural stress systems into relief. When, on the other hand, researchers have no control over the amount or accuracy of data in record form, or study truncated samples of larger populations undifferentiated as to age or jumbled as to status, the lack of research design will limit the possibility of determining sub-varieties of generalized disease processes and their situational and cultural concomitants.

The limited number of disease groupings, and their presence cross-culturally though varying in rate and typology, suggest universal psychic mechanisms at human disposal varying in their frequency and intensity of use in different cultural scenes. The historically changeable modes of mental illness as these shift within one cultural tradition, in incidence or in type, we have called *rate variability*. However, if culture is not a mere tissue of externals, but is, as it appears to be in any living instance, an ingredient of personality, then as Parsons states, a culture must be conceived as being both institutionalized in systems of social activity and as internalized in individual but statistically groupable personality systems.[62] The recent, unprofitable controversies over whether cultures are entities heavily determining the activities of individual participants, or activities resolving into those of culture carriers, if brought down to concrete data, would soon accord statistical validity to a combined position. Certainly so long as non-idiosyncratic determinants are concerned, they must, in the nature of cases be cultural, whereas the actual lives and emotional contexts of behavior, or ego-involvements, are again in some proposed situations partly personal and partly cultural. The very meanings of normative, or characteristic, or typical, for the term cultural, determine at once that the probable proportion of cultural to idiosyncratic as among individuals will be heavily weighted with the cultural (perhaps nine to one in American subcultures, if epidemiological data are correct). At the same time, within discrete individuals, all we may say is that nine out of ten will show heavy normative and typical trends in emotional balance.

For the 10 percent of mental and behavioral deviancy, we may quote Felix and Bowers. The notion of studying culture and personality in actual, living relationships by any and all field and observational methods which locate the quality and type of emotion imbedded in the social process was founded in anthropology in the 1930's. It has since become congenial in social psychiatry and mental hygiene. The expression, the utilization, and the resultant course of the emotional life, as lived within cultural or subcultural boundaries, now has the kind of documentation which shifts psychiatry from limited diagnostic preoccupations to an awareness of cultural influence. As Felix and

Bowers put it in *Mental Hygiene and Socio-Environmental Factors:* [63]

" . . . The evidence for the cultural determination of ideational patterns and special motor patterns has, of course, long been established. No one can read the cross-cultural evidence without considerable respect for man's ingenuity in creating thought and motor patterns and for the resiliency of the organism in acquiring them and operating through them. The evidence for the group management of emotional or temperamental patterns is more recent, but already many of our supposed facts have been seriously questioned . . .

"Further evidence has pointed to the widespread presence of certain personality configurations in certain societies or societal sub-groups . . . Moreover, within the same society, patterned differences have been described for various status components, including such special categories as oldest as compared to younger sons. In all such cases the personality configuration has appeared to be consistent with the pattern of institutions through which the people lived. This has led to a consideration of the possible existence of a basic character or personality structure in each society with variations for class and other status differentials, a field in which several anthropologists and psychiatrists are now working.

"Evidence at the same time has been similarly accumulating on the relation between the societal setting and personality disorientation. Early and compelling examples of this are to be found in the impact of Western culture on primitive societies, where the proscribing or decay of key elements of the native culture led to a general demoralization, despondency, declining industriousness, increased infertility, compulsive clinging to elements of the traditional culture, etc. . . . . Demoralization is not the only direction that behavior patterns have taken under such circumstances . . . and the differential resiliency of cultures to change has been noted . . ."

To assume, however, that such processes as acculturation, or such forces as demoralization are single causal elements of massive proportion in disease incidence is a fallacy of reduction. The lack of certain vitamins in pellagra and beriberi, or the presence of definite agents in lead or barbiturate poisoning are different from disease processes like cardiac and psychoneurotic decompensation in which a complex of factors may play a role in varying combination. The same appears generally true of all psychiatric disorders, that various combinations and admixtures of emotionalized reactions are end-products of internalized or interpreted event sequences. There is, further, no advance warrant that any combination of such factors in any community or culture is an exact duplicate of any other. Nor are they unchanging (the meaning of culture change and of acculturation) so that a dead level of fixity and constancy may not be assumed without anthropological field work before and during case-finding procedures. The fact, for example, that a psychosomatic illness like diabetes was predominantly a male disease during the last century, and has occurred increasingly among females in the present is the beginning not the end of research into cultural etiology. In a useful paper on *Family Structure and the Transmission of Neurotic Behavior*, Jules Henry has provided an interesting coding and tabular system for recording interactions and attitudes, as for example intergeneration harmony and conflict. All these can be dated and developed in time and comparisons of interpersonal family systems to the nth family may be used to quantify. What makes the paper correct in emphasis is the statement that the "cultural milieu defines the limits within which certain types of family interaction can take place."[64] The idea of direct transmission of neuroses from one generation to the next is obviously to be modified by the range of diversities known to exist among intergeneration levels.

There are cultural diversities, or sub-cultural milieus, that exist on generation levels, and which often incorporate the religious difference, the geographic migrant, or those who have experienced social mobility upwards or down- wards. Even so, in the latter instances, it is important to settle in each individual situation whether such different factors as mobility aspirations, or parental conflicts and adolescent rebellions, reactivated and acted out, underlie the difficulty. The emotional balances of psychoneurotic and psychosomatic illnesses, clustering in family lines, among collateral relatives, and between married pairs are far from transmissible contagion; but complementary dis- eases exist from the psychiatric analysis of them, often revealing the emotional balances that have been struck in family structures. Within the individual, too, the phasic recurrence, or progressive substitution of one process for another may indicate either a continuance of a particular inability to cope with stress or a change in pattern. That unfinished business in the psychic economy is not rare is indicated by a recent survey of Bell telephone operatives in New York where recurrence of psychoneurotic absentee- ism regularly accounted for the same 25 per cent of the labor force, and appeared in them in high correlation with organic disorders. Corroborative is the research of Buell and associates in Minneapolis-St. Paul to the effect that approximately 25 per cent of the population regularly use 80 per cent of the available health resources.

In European and most American mental health studies, the field research process of obtaining the real texture of social and cultural backgrounds of patients has been omitted, or where included by hopeful intent, it is bound to the rock and limited by the last census tract information of federal origin with no attempt to refine the texture and quality of social living since that date. Where families and cultural communities have dwelled in an area for years and over generations, the absence of a history of the area, qualitative anthropological field work, or census work-ups over time to discern trends are inexcusable omissions.

In analysis, finally, the holding of socio-cultural variables constant to test one of their number should not be confused, by facile explanation, with their presumptively single-factor weight. Any explanation of mass diseases of this sort is not to be sought, as Gordon and associates warn, "in isolated factors, nor in series of factors each operating independently, but rather in a combination of mutually interacting variables that together form a causal system."[65] We may even add probable causal system, for neither psychiatry nor the social sciences enter the statistical scene of epidemiology with pristine innocence of either mental or cultural phenomena. Were this not so, the several multidisciplinary teams in operation could bow out in favor of sophomore guidance under statistical rule. In psychological studies, it is probable that emotion and cognition can not be studied apart from learning and motivation, since each set involves the complementary one. In socio-cultural studies relating to psychiatry, the causal and relational system does not become simpler.

These strictures are warranted in the light of regular, and in some cases recent publication emphasizing single processes and single factors in the epidemiology of mental illness. In a recent paper on Syracuse, New York, matters of high incidence in certain sections of the city, while not always correlated with low economic status in several census tracts, were found highly consistent with the presence of multiple rather than single-family dwellings.[66] In New Haven, the lower social stratum was said to have twelve times the incidence of schizophrenia as the upper.[67] In the classical study of Faris and Dunham on these matters, the story, as we have seen, was put differently: societies in transition were said to contain "natural areas," or ecological segments of an urban scene, which "favored" the development of certain abnormal traits.[68] As they said:

" . . . Normal Mentality and behavior develops over a long period of successful interaction between the person and these organized agencies of society. Defects in mentality and behavior may result from serious gaps in any part of of the process."

Yet the processes were never specified in psychiatric terms. While the New Haven study of Hollingshead and Redlich aims at more than allusion to "successful interaction," the "organized agencies of society," and "serious gaps" in the interactive process, it deals only with prevalence, the number of mentally ill persons as of a given stated day, with no consequent separation of incidence and disease duration. Thus the high prevalence rates in certain socio-economic strata may reflect an unmitigated course of illness in some persons plus the number of those becoming ill, or seeking treatment as of a given date.

The Syracuse study, on firmer grounds of first hospital admission rates, and dealing with the relatively firm psychiatric categories of cerebral arteriosclerosis and senile psychosis, notes a high mental hospital admissions rate for these and all other psychoses taken as a group in areas of "high concentrations of multiple family dwellings" and in areas marked "by high percentages of people living alone." The presence of census tracts of low socio-economic status, and low incidence rates of the two psychoses of the elderly "casts some doubt on the correlation between this index (of socio-economic status) and cerebral arteriosclerosis-senile psychosis hospitalization rates," according to Gruenberg. Yet the argument to date could be summed up with Faris and Dunham stating merely that older schizophrenics are no more heavily concentrated in central areas of the city than are younger (despite the general youthfulness of this category as a whole!), Gerard and Huston finding in Worcester, Massachusetts, that high rate areas of schizophrenias could be accounted for by the drift into certain areas of highly mobile, unattached individuals (no doubt many of them ill before arrival), and Morris S. Schwartz's substantiation that schizophrenics tend to go lower in the occupational scale prior to hospitalization.[69] If the additional evidence of Gerard, Huston and Schwartz is accepted, both the prevalence and gross ecological data of Faris and Dunham, and the prevalence data of New Haven are open to serious question. Further the single factor explanation of the Syracuse report, based on more careful incidence analysis, loses much of its mystery. The multiple dwelling, as a way point to illness, or more accurately, to hospital admission, is discussed tentatively as connoting social isolation without physical insulation. The danger again, of confusing effects with causes in such long and insidious processes as are involved in cerebral arteriosclerosis, senile psychosis, or psychoses in general, may be noted in the downward mobility, ecological-area drift, and occupational downgrading which accompany poor mental health. A second point, in psychoses of the elderly, is the inevitable age handicap which must first be culturally and environmentally assessed as cause before it is measured on the side of effect.

On the other hand, of these studies, only that of Gruenberg in Syracuse, and Gerard and Huston in Worcester, have the quality of an incidence study. The findings on human drift, even those on multiple dwellings, begin to tell us only where the mentally disordered are concentrated, a point of considerable importance for those interested in amelioration and prevention techniques. It is no doubt a fact, as even Algren's *Man With the Golden Arm* and other fictional accounts of deterioration and schizophrenia indicate, that slums and transitional zones lack the facilities and technique to brake deterioration and that preventive measures now current do not sufficiently block such zone aggregation, or send adequate scientific help within. Equally, a prevalence study such as that of New Haven, if not adequate to etiological analysis, nevertheless tells us that a continual lack of detection and treatment, and the tendency to use the term, schizophrenia, more freely in lower class contexts, certainly do not mitigate a serious social problem. Increasingly accurate studies on these fronts will aid in spelling out more clearly, however, the kinds of administrative and preventive measures needed in relation to those developing isolation tendencies, facing age with severe handicaps, or plunging into poorer occupational, status and housing levels.

While diagnostics or treatment will require more information on the course of illness in relation to more psychiatrically pertinent factors, the problem of treatment of cases, as they come, has importance side by side with that of etiological, and more basically preventive, questions and techniques. Nevertheless, studies which have been based on prevalence rates and global ecological survey with only the most generalized, quantified data on the population census, housing, socio-economic status and nationality have distinct limits which do not qualify them as cultural, personality, or etiologically speaking, as psychiatric research.

The description or definition of urban ecological areas is a first step, not a last, in the study of the actual lives of people in modern, urban communities. No doubt, the communities or urban regions must be differentiated and viewed in process. Gross statistical data of urban regions are, further, of critical importance in describing the main contours and *outward* living conditions of such areas. However, Robinson, in a brilliant paper on ecological correlations and the behavior of individuals, has for sound reasons of statistical analysis and the apparent inappropriateness of ecological methods to certain kinds of personality judgments, dismissed the method entirely *as a poor substitute for individual studies (correlations)*.[70] While his points on the final uniqueness of an individual's behavior are correctly taken (as they would be also for the uniqueness of a given illness process if considered in detail), there is no doubt, nevertheless, that gross urban data do describe in rough outline the main contours and conditions under which a culture, or a sub-culture, and the personalities in it, continually operate. The ecological approach, none the less, in order to accomplish this aim, must rid itself of a static quality not merely in terms of human drift within its framework, but in terms of substituting processual analysis (the history of an urban area) for the more static cross-sectional view used so constantly. Shevky and Williams, focussing on just such processes, have generalized the most important ones rather than merely delineating the statistical pattern of a current urban structure; and in so doing have demonstrated a continual change, marked over generations, in terms of sex ratio, socio-economic differentiation, increasing segregation of ethnic groups, and the like. This method, historical in essence, has greater application to intergeneration data even though it does not finally account for each individual personality variance. The point is that the gross data, if analyzed in process of change over time, succeed in describing the main contours and *conditions under which* a culture, sub-culture, or the personalities within it operated in the same time sequences.

The Chicago school of ecology, of Burgess and his group was able to point out that the medley, or checkerboard of residential segregation (cultural, racial, or socio-economic) patterned into a larger set of concentric zones such as transitional areas surrounding business districts. The correction of this pattern, by Maurice R. Davie, for other cities, in terms of transportation arteries and economic growth patterns of urban areas suggested that the developmental process of urbanism cannot simply be assumed, nor can the usual rubrics of the urban way of life be taken as existent within each region. Despite the alleged secularism of the city, its collapse of religious orientation, religious movements occur constantly in urban scenes and the larger faiths have there their most significant organizational strength. Despite the claim of individual or family job mobility within the segregated units, tremendous variations and even typical job and industry attachments may be discerned within certain cultural groups. In brief, while ecological mapping is desirable as a first step in any description of conditions under which actual people live, it is only the framework into which the texture of social integrational forms must fit and in which traditional family-kin systems, church and social organizations function.

In both the Stirling Project and the Yorkville Study, carried forward in Nova Scotia and New York respectively, actual inspection by anthropological field methods has preceded and guided survey tactics, carrying them beyond the usual rubrics of housing, income and educational level, or ethnic and religious labels, into the total texture of functioning social and cultural forms. The urbanism hypotheses of weakened social integration, through voluntary organization rather than traditional forms, or the platitude of weakened social control over individuals through replacement of family-kin controls by formal and distant ones may also be tested. Ogburn's White House report on the changing family, a Hoover Commission report of several decades back, suggested strongly that the affective life of the family under urbanism, though changed, is not modified in the least by diminishing patterns of affect and emotional solidarity, but quite the opposite, that lack of wider integrations forced family affective controls to the fore. Similar qualifications must be placed on terms like social disorganization (where aspects of the urban scene like crime or prostitution actually become highly organized), or ethnic disintegration (where the patterns of politics in city after city proclaim the existence of such formal entities).

In a Czech or Slovak community exemplified in culturally determined formal organizations, and a Hungarian community characteristically lacking in them, the affective backgrounds of social life are not even begun to be studied until family and kinship determinants of affective behavior are known in the normative patterns of such subcultural groups. The notion that, in urbanism, expedient ideas of morality take over where absolute, rigid codes of values leave off may be tested in German-American communities, like Yorkville, where patterns of cultural conservatism operate against resiliency to preserve the standards and values of first generation backgrounds. Beyond this, a pattern of acculturation may, depending on cultural groups and socio-economic contexts, interplay with urban settings in such a way as to affect the rate of change. The pace of acculturation varies notoriously with cultural group and from society to society, affecting upward social mobility and achieving a different degree of stability in different cultural groups. In New York, for example, the rapid pace among Puerto Ricans, which has not yet stabilized, and the notoriously slow pace among Irish point not only to different religious, political and economic values in the two groups, but to size of family-kin groupings, the points in time at which they enter into urban economic life, the stability of family forms, the status valuations, and the conditions within the host culture. The given status aspirations and economic placement of Hungarian-Americans and Puerto Ricans in a given decade may be simply not comparable without taking cultural variations into account. A hypothesis which otherwise failed to consider historical, economic, and social variations in subcultural groups in favor of ecological generalizations on the area as a whole would contain its own assumptive artifacts.

Ecological survey is the first mapped assessment of an area; but it cannot be assumed to touch the cultural and historical conditions under which a group of ethnic variables operate. The same strictures apply to psychiatric evaluations of people in an area which apply to cultural and socio-economic variation. Methods such as the Rorschach, the TAT, the Cornell Medical Index and others will simply not operate uniformly across cultural boundaries. In one study of the Cornell Index in application to a variant culture, the Okinawan, the psychiatrist L. G. Laufer reported, in the *American Journal of Psychiatry* recently, upon its inapplicability. The usefulness of these methods, however, in probing these differences *provided cultural variables are understood* is quite another matter. Similarly, in questionnaire technique, differences by cultural group in initial refusal rates, or in suspiciousness and guardedness, may be more characteristic of Germans, for reasons of cultural standards and values, than in Italians of first and subsequent generation levels. Blocking, fantasy, repression and defensive lying, or oral acting out, boastfulness, impulsivity, and crude imagination may be more characteristic of people in one group than in another. Questions of emotional constriction versus expressivity, the kinds of sexual and parental identifications, or the place of fantasy and imagination in early training are all, as with historical and cultural inquiry, prior to assessments of what is cultural and environmental and what is idiosyncratic in responses.

In much the same sense, Solby, in speaking of group

therapies (like occupational, musical, psychodrama and group psychotherapy) has said that differences in individual backgrounds make these supplementary, not individualized, treatments in which "lack of knowledge of the dynamics of the group as such . . . at present limits the extent of this new therapeutic procedure." To test these emotional voltages, one must obviously know, for example, when suspiciousness is culturally sanctioned in some rural ethnic peasant backgrounds, or when it becomes part of some individually autistic pattern of behavior. In either case, the inducement of emotional response has cultural and social patterning along the way, but in the one case these are externally sanctioned and expressed in the best of reality senses and within "normal limits." In the other, patently, the emotional economy is not really developed in patterns of communication or constriction with others, nor shared with them; but is internally produced, internally compelling, and basically threatening. No wonder then, that the most highly autistic systems are only in small measure and rarely in details culturally predictable, and the more completed in airtight, delusional compartments, the more liable to burst out in strange, noncultural systems. While etiological factors are situated back in time, the losses of realistic ego-directing capacities, of control of impulses, of sexual identification (and its displacement in autistic systems) are all situational losses in the sense of cultural backgrounds and the normative values and stresses they induce.

The interest in deepening ecological methods to include cultural background and the specifics of psychopathology is primarily in the usefulness of such expanded horizons for generating and testing hypotheses about the etiology of mental disturbance. The *how* and *why* of malfunctioning, or healthy adjustment, both products of culture at its best and at its worst, must be tested not within affectively empty frameworks, but in terms of the values, standards and actual lives of actual people. Epidemiological research, again, may be used to express the ratios of every category of illness incidence to healthy populations, but at some point it must turn away from preoccupation with amount to the study of actual cases within ecological *and* cultural frameworks. The idea of utilizing a question-naired sample for the drawing of cases of normal and aberrant for further study, can, for any area, be linked with the study of psychopathology and cultural background directly in hospitalized cases. Such findings, if applied later in preventive programs or in action settings (hospitals and community clinics) have the practical value of essentially therapeutic and etiological work in British social psychiatry under the influence of John Bowlby, Maxwell Jones,[71] Aubrey Lewis[72] and others. In American programs, few studies have left their communities better than they found them, and few demonstration areas of this sort have been linked with epidemiological research. While the work of R. A. Spitz,[73] for example, has been parallel to that of John Bowlby,[74] the exigencies of the British postwar scene have forced more practicality into the latter program.

Equally important in the sense of larger populations and etiologically pressing problems are the attempts to specify particular psychopathological differences in American cultural groups. The well-known higher incidence of alcoholism in the Irish has been noted by R. F. Bales,[75] only two years later than claims of a greater incidence of sociopathic disorder in Italians of the Boston area were remarked upon in studies of Hyde and associates of Selective Service registrants.[76] Even the different rates of suicide in western countries, or in Ceylon or Japan[77] can clearly be related to cultural, or specifically religious variations, high rates in Czechoslovakia, Germany and Switzerland being matched by low rates among the Irish (Eire and North Ireland), Ceylonese or Dutch. Writing of clinical work in the Northside Center for Child Development in New York City, Drs. Stella Chess, Kenneth B. Clark, and Alexander Thomas have discussed the importance of cultural evaluation in psychiatric diagnosis and treatment from the point of view of noting variations in cases which would otherwise be confusing.[78]

Speaking of both the British and American experience in culture and personality studies, Aubrey Lewis has this to say:[79]

"Individuals are the objects of a psychiatrist's daily concern; consequently he cannot help looking at the problem of interaction between individual and culture from the individual's standpoint. This point of view has its most extreme statement in psychoanalytic theory, which makes the individual incorporate his environment rather than interact with it. As Ernest Jones put it, human behavior is not the product of interaction between the external world and the inner urges and cravings of the individual, but 'it would appear to be nearer to the truth to describe it as the interaction of two separate sets of internal forces on the outer world . . .' He is, in short, concerned almost entirely with what man does to, and with, his environment, not with what it does to him. With this extreme position goes, of course, a corresponding emphasis on the relations between individuals, especially within the family, transcending the influence of the whole social heritage, i.e., the culture. Not every psychiatrist accepts the psychoanalytic view of this—even psychoanalysts, for example Karen Horney, desert it. . . . Consequently in studies that originate with the psychiatrist there is a strong bias. The psychiatrist moreover is so close to the problems of his patients (which are disclosed within the same culture, usually, as that the doctor lives in) that he forgets that some of these problems might cease to be problems if the culture changed . . ."

As E. M. Lemert states in his *Social Pathology*, [80] there is first of all the difficulty of quantitative and qualitative studies in mental disorders where the amount and particular varieties of the illnesses, or even their presence or absence can in certain instances become a matter of dispute, even among psychiatrists. Lewis goes on:

" . . . We are apt to say that this uncertainy of detection and diagnosis is an overrated difficulty in psychiatry, but it seems to me that it is a fundamental weakness in any studies that profess to be exact, and that it, quite as much as the number of independent uncontrolled variables, makes the study of large groups with the appropriate statistical treatment essential, rather than the minute studies of individuals which have hitherto been the psychiatrist's more usual contribution. To come back to Lemert's work. He considers the ethnic, economic and cultural characteristics of those admitted to mental hospitals, taking these characteristics as indicators of role, status and cultural conflict. He looks at the situation in which the mental disorder developed; the social context of the illness. Then he takes in turn a number of socio-personal matters: the common beliefs about mental illness . . ., the institutions developed to meet the real and supposed needs of the mentally sick person and of society in relation to him, the changing attitudes in different classes and in different cultures and countries at different periods, . . . the social structure of the mental hospital . . ."

While Lewis lists the different problems associated with age and sex arrangements in various cultures, it is obvious that throughout both he and Lemert have been speaking broadly of cultures, classes and the importance of environmental contexts. To this one might add the recent work of Stanton, Schwartz and Davies at Chestnut Lodge where aspects of psychopathology seemed to be a response to therapeutic milieu. [81] That the latter can itself be viewed as a cultural setting, of a sort, is seen in such phenomena as further withdrawals conditioned by lack of understood communication, or by soiling which vanishes in more proper environments, where lack of authoritarianism and higher social expectations in the hospital setting respectively lessen the intensity of defiant behavior.

These viewpoints place a particular obligation upon the science of psychiatry at this time, which has, moreover, much to do with individual therapeutic perspectives over and beyond the importance of environment in general disease etiology. This obligation has nowhere been put more simply and cogently than by Redlich and Bingham in their book, *The Inside Story: Psychiatry and Everyday Life.* Here the authors feel one should know about cultural backgrounds of patients consistently so that psychiatrists in actual practice can judge which of their patient's "odd seeming thoughts, feelings and actions are the result" of cultural teachings and which come from his own "unique development." According to them, it is essential that the doctor who wants to "help us relearn" should understand the cultural background and learning milieu in which behavioral reactions were formed.[82] If *stress* is what is happening in the interpersonal relations of a patient's particular case, we may be sure it is produced not merely in terms of energy and its psychobiological processes of transformation, but in terms of linked cultural and personal realities in which coded symbols as mediating agents mark the quality and quantity of these very relationships.

Neither qualitative nor quantitative assertions about hostility, fear, anxiety, displacement, or repression have much meaning without reference to the analysis of how energies are typically used or dissipated in a culture, a family, or a person. On the other hand, personality traits may be qualitatively and quantitatively discussed with far more meaning for the individual when the thoughts, feelings and actions that summarize his behavior are seen in relation to the thoughts, feelings and actions he experienced in his total life course and his total cultural milieu. The contrary theory, that symbols are merely coded signals of human energies and their processes of transformation, begs the questions: To whom and from whom? And for what socially realistic or unrealistic purposes?

Diethelm has recently summarized the same points;[83] under the heading of *Changing Psychopathology*, he wrote:

"Psychopathology, i. e., the science of abnormal mental functions, studies the individual patient's behavior. Much stress has been put on certain symptoms which were assumed to be of fundamental importance and theories frequently developed from their occurrence. With environmental changes, including therapeutic and cultural influences, some of these symptoms have become less frequent, others varied their character, while a third group has become more obvious. It is of scientific interest to study these changes and important for treatment to determine how the frequency of psychopathological symptoms can be decreased.

"Hysterical reactions present a well-known example. In medieval times and until the eighteenth century, these symptoms frequently related to religious aspects and to witchcraft. In the nineteenth century, hysterical convulsions seemed of utmost importance to the physicians. All these symptoms are now rarely seen and phobias, varied physical symptoms which correspond to current illnesses, and sexual difficulties have taken their place. A considerable number of psychosomatic disorders may belong in this group."

Diethelm describes several changes in the characteristic symptomatology of the schizophrenias. Catatonic posturing, including catalepsy, prolonged stupor and other evidences of autistic withdrawal; smearing, echolalia, echopraxia, neologisms, and manneristic activity; and symbolic destructiveness are all rare in modern psychiatric hospitals. The once common involutional melancholia of a decade ago, with "the classic symptoms such as agitation, distorted hypochondriacal delusions, or delusions of excessive sinning are infrequent . . ." He continues:

". . . The acting out of a neurotic and psychopathic nature and the uncontrolled behavior which led to loss of human dignity is less marked. The factors affecting this change may be related . . . above all to cultural attitudes. . . .

"In psychoneurotic illnesses, the obsessions, compulsions, and hysterical symptoms have decreased in frequency while anxiety symptoms, phobias, and psychosomatic symptoms are prevalent. Depressions of psychoneurotic origin seem to be more common than at the beginning of this century. In manic-depressive illnesses psychologic and definite psychoneurotic factors are increasingly recognizable and have affected the treatment."

He concludes that contemporary cultural investigations are required for obtaining a clarification of the "meaning of the changes in psychopathology."

While W. S. Robinson, in his paper on *Ecological Correlations and the Behavior of Individuals*, has argued that a set of ecological correlations tends to overestimate the relation among variables since these same variables can also be more carefully assessed in direct relationship to the individuals concerned, the same claim can scarcely be aimed at the meaningful cultural background of an individual as internalized and interpreted in life experience. In this sense, A. R. Martin, in earlier descriptions of Yorkville cultural communities, described the "emotional climate of the home" for each cultural group not as a fixed quantity of precise mathematical definition, and found everywhere, but as a central tendency or generalized matrix of family relationships, activities and dominant values systems, no two instances of which were presumptively identical. In anthropology even earlier, Edward Sapir in his work, *The Unconscious Patterning of Behavior in Society*,[84] though insistent upon the uniqueness of a given life experience, nevertheless noted the same generically operative tendencies so far as the realm of essentially cultural behavior was concerned. In the expansion of his work to the interrelationships of culture and psychiatry, Sapir still said of the system of *necessary* connections, "A personality is carved out by the subtle interactions of those systems of ideas characteristic of a culture as a whole, as well as those systems of ideas which get established for the individual through more special types of participation with the physical and psychological needs of the individual organism." It was these last that Sapir called the "individual sub-cultures." The implication of a second *necessary* connection between culture and mental illness was stated as in inevitable relation between personal meanings and cultural symbolisms:

> "The personal meaning of the symbolisms of an individual's sub-culture are constantly being reaffirmed by society, or at least he likes to think they are. When they obviously cease to be, he loses his orientation. A system of sorts remains and causes his alienation from an impossible world."

The necessity for psychiatry systematically to gather data on both normative social and cultural backgrounds in contemporary cultures, and to consider these last in terms of the systems of meanings which always configure in the foreground or background of individualized cases, is a function of known and inevitable relationships between culture, personality and mental illness. Humans are unconscious of the grammar of the languages they speak, of the symmetry or formal regularity of kinship systems, though it is there, of regularities in etiquette and custom, though they exist, or of central tendencies in behavioral processes referable as Florence Kluckhohn has termed them, to cultural orientations.[85]

Just as some etiological studies summarize personal and cultural data in their inevitable relationship, so any departure from this principle tends to be etiologically meaningless. The ecological studies which strip down the term, environment, in the context of social psychiatry, to single noncultural factors like nearness to business districts, and the like, ordinarily attempt to argue *post hoc, ergo propter hoc*, and to claim strong etiological significance for these detached items of larger complex variables. We have already alluded to H. Warren Dunham's interesting work on the social personality of catatonics in slum areas. This paper, in 1944, was important in describing the plight of sensitive, self-conscious, schizophrenic individuals in poorer districts, as well as in flagging our attention to the "quiet ones" of such districts.[86] The claim, however, was that the slum area intensified such anxieties in such individuals, and in this sense had special impact on those who became ill. It is questionable, on second glance, whether catatonics are merely so produced; ordinarily, their illness is of a sort where impingement of practically any setting other than the protected hospital environment is often greatly disturbing. There is no study of the relative incidence of childhood schizophrenias from this and other sections of a city and no studies of particular, early developmental problems associated with such settings. While it is possible that the person with timidity and sensitivity responds poorly in this most unprotected of environments, it seems equally likely that parental overprotection and solicitude, plus worry and rejection over mishaps, may contribute more to the original response of self-conscious timidity than the grosser characteristics of the slum environment. From the clinical point of view, the factors having direct and character-forming influence in early development are more basically etiological, the others merely exacerbating in the light of already established and deeply founded features of personality. The question of where deviancy or psychoses begin is clearly one in which data on the earliest development of psychotic patterns, a problem of incidence, are required.

At this point, it would seem that withdrawal, isolation, deviancy or psychotic patterns, in order to worsen, would first be exacerbated in emotional home climates and in family settings primarily, and only further intensified if at all in the neighborhood and district. Obviously, the cultural viewpoint, as exemplified by meanings and values, attitudes and goals resident in socio-economic status and sociocultural, or ethnic, groupings, must be tested before single factor analyses may be taken seriously. This is not to say that the experience of social isolation, or narcissistic hostility, or anxious and dependent emotions do not fit into the development of schizophrenia. How they do, or how they are engendered in family, in socioeconomic and in cultural matrices is the real question.

As John A. Clausen and Melvin L. Kohn have recently pointed out:[87]

> "It is now generally recognized that ecological processes tend to sort out not only sub-communities but also sub-cultures . . ."

Selecting ethnic group membership and social class as most relevant in determining the indices for a cultural frame of reference, they continue:

> "Studies of the personality development of children from the lowest levels of the status system of American society have indicated several intense value conflicts to which they are typically subjected, especially from the time they enter the middle-class-oriented school. The instability of the

expectations developed by such children (and the deprecatory self-conceptions built up through internalizing the judgments of others) likewise may be expected to lead to the development of personalities which are highly vulnerable to stress."

They add that, "Though the difficulties peculiar to lower-class status are most striking, it should not be forgotten that the middle and upper classes produce their own varieties of stress." This view of social class as a species of subculture in the American scene has considerable importance provided ethnic variables are considered along with social status differentials. As they say: ". . . Ecological studies can serve as a stepping stone, but . . . too often they have left the investigator stranded in the middle of the stream." That social stratification in part governs "what happens therapeutically to a person who becomes a psychiatric patient" was recently demonstrated in a study by Leslie Schaffer and Jerome K. Myers.[88]

Talcott Parsons has not only discussed medicine as a part of the social system, but like Leo Simmons and Harold G. Wolff has investigated the social roles of professions concerned with illness as well as the attitudes towards illness which appear in social structures. Since mental illness is as much, if not more, a type of participation in, and reaction to, social processes, as it is "an entity" residing in a person, such studies as these which describe and analyze the therapeutic milieu in terms of realities of social structures throw light upon the total environment into which the individual is born and in which he grows and lives. Franz Alexander and Thomas Szasz, in elaborating on psychosomatic medicine, have included both the biological concepts of medicine, and psychosocial concepts in explaining such illnesses.[89] Even earlier, Alexander added to the usual factors like infant care and childhood experience, the "emotional climate of family," the later "emotional ex-

periences in intimate personal and occupational relations,"
specific personality traits, and relations with parents and
siblings.[90]   The work of Jurgen Ruesch, done in collaboration with the anthropologist, Martin B. Loeb, at Langley-
Porter Clinic, noted statistical series supporting the theory
that delayed recovery and psychosomatic diseases together affected more middle class people and those up-
wardly mobile, as contrasted with conduct disorders
"affecting primarily" lower class members or those down-
wardly mobile.[91]   Caudill, Redlich and associates have
similarly studied social structural and interaction processes
on a psychiatric ward.[92]

The point that behavior is patterned, and has cultural or
structural contexts, is not novel in anthropology.   That
the latter concepts of social causality are increasingly used
in psychiatry seems also evident.   The tendency of psychiatrists, in clinical research or theory, to discount such
essentially circular explanations of behavior as "habit," or
such fateful ones as climate, race or geography, is partly
due no doubt to the constant and healthy contact with
changing and dynamic human problems and the steady
flow of successes in therapy which argue against too much
fixity and rigid determinism in human affairs.   Possibly
because of these skills and successes, less attention has been
paid to the non-biological factors which limit systems of
behavior and selectively structure it in one direction or
another.   Devereux, in noting that these delimiting factors must be of special interest to psychiatry, while not
wholly discounting habit in the relation of biological needs
and experience, adds a third axis of behavior, the cultural,
as one "which organizes behavior" through "the subjective experience of culture."[93]   It must be remembered,
however, that both the objective reality of culture and its
subjective impact on the individual in actuality organize
experience and even human needs as they are commonly

met, so that no reduction of culture to biological need satisfaction, as was essentially the theory of Malinowski or to raw experience as was the view of Dewey, really suffices. As Devereux states the case for psychoanalytic anthropology, "Culture is primarily a system of defenses and is, therefore, related chiefly to the ego-functions." It is, provided economics is viewed as being more than just a "nutritional institution," law as more than just a "safety institution," or marriage as more than just a "sexual institution," though clearly all have biological (and *id*) connections. The necessity of recognizing cultural factors as setting more general and pervasive limitations on human behavior than biological needs which, in humans, never act alone, or experience which is never without context, is of crucial importance in the understanding of both normative or aberrant behavior patterns. As Devereux wisely notes, "Symptoms are a result of the reorganization of behavior while the individual is in a state of conflict," but they themselves serve further to organize the "totality of behavior." Such frantic and misguided reorganizations of behavior, no matter how inappropriate and distorted they are as attempts to achieve emotional balance, are developed in the same settings which produce states of recognized conflict, normative behavior patterns, and organizations of a healthy, asymptomatic sort. To separate out the factors, cultural, experiential and biological which operate in unison may be proper for purposes of analysis, provided they are weighted accurately as to importance, are tested in actual interconnection, and are not presumed to be resolvable into airtight compartments, or reducible to the most idiosyncratic and least generally delimiting of their number.

While force-energy concepts certainly operate in all biological (and human) phenomena, they are not delimiting factors which alone direct behavior in either a constricting or releasing form. On the other hand, cultural experience may operate to produce qualitative and quantitative behavioral differences cross-culturally, or within a given cultural system may set the preconditions for the accumulation or release of tensions, the creation of balances and imbalances, the depth of conflicts, and the production of reorganizations or maturity and growth in conduct. That the analysis must be made on both cultural and personal levels in the individual case is true; but in the assessments of types of disorder and cultural background, in epidemiology, the range of such analysis beyond the individual case is equally necessary. The relative durability and rigidity of symptoms in an individual who has developed psychopathology make the task easier, no doubt, for behavioral and cultural analysis in single cases; and by extension, studies of psychopathology in cultural groups are not any more or less formidable, perhaps, than would be complete and rounded studies to a similar depth of normative, healthy behavior.

VARIATIONS IN CULTURE AND PSYCHOPATHOLOGY

Striking evidence of differences in the psychopathology of cultural groups has been described by psychiatrists working with African materials. These differences amount to variations in the form of major functional psychoses (the schizophrenias and affective disorders) or in the symptomatology of these diseases and their relative incidence as compared with American and European data. Commenting on the inadequacy of Western standards in application to African psychiatry, D. Mackay wrote in 1948:" . . . We in Africa have not got a Normal for our basis, because we have never taken the trouble to study African normality . . . We have so far judged our cases on their departure from a European Normal, if we have judged

them at all.   Or else we have judged them on their departure from a Normal which we do not know . . ."[94]   J. C.
Carothers, in the fullest survey of African mental health
conditions, adds that while some African patients exhibit
patterns of reaction "similar to those included in neurotic
categories in Europe, the diagnostic criteria applicable in
Europe cannot be stretched to include many other patients" suffering from specifically African cultural forms
of psychoneuroses.[95]   Laubscher's account of extremely
low suicide rates in rural Africa (one per 100,000 per annum,
compared with figures for the United Kingdom of 10 per
100,000 in 1950 and over 11 per 100,000 in the United
States in 1948) rounds out the variation for the cultures of
that continent.[96]

In the form and frequency of psychoses, in the overlap
and divergence in certain psychoneuroses from European
types, and in the incidence of suicide in Africa when compared with modern urbanized nations, the data from this
continent vary from Europe and America.   In addition
to Laubscher's major study of South Africa, there are
Carothers' earlier studies in East Africa (Kenya) of 1948
and 1951,[97] and his more current ethnopsychiatric survey
of African materials.   Tooth, in West Africa, has ably
summarized the Gold Coast data.[98]   A closer scrutiny
of these four studies by psychiatrists is instructive of detailed
regional differences in incidence and symptomatology.
Besides these four, Brock and Autret have described one
variant mental illness found in Africa and known generally
as *Kwashiorkor*.[99]

Actually, *Kwashiorkor* is basically a disease of malnutrition.   It was so described by H. C. Trowell and J. N. P.
Davies in the *British Medical Journal* of 1952.   However,
M. Clark, in the *East African Medical Journal* of the year
before, while noting that *Kwashiorkor* appeared most often
between the ages of two and four, emphasizes the peevish

apathy and catatonic-like inertia and dullness of these children which separate them off from other cases of undernourishment and point to crucial changes in the emotional life. As J. N. P. Davies put it, in the *Annual Review of Medicine* (1952) such a child is "too often a whining, apathetic invalid," permanently handicapped in his development. Trowell and Davies draw attention to the point that Kwashiorkor is described for several cultures of Africa, Asia and America; Davies (1952) describes the relation of "Mehlnährschaden" in Budapest to *Kwashiorkor* in Africa.

Tooth notes that schizophrenia among adult Africans of the Gold Coast does occur in the familiar European patterns of simple, mixed, hebephrenic, catatonic and paranoid and is the chief chronic form of insanity. However, Tooth adds:

". . . But whereas in Europeans, the distinction between an affective state with schizophrenic features, and a depressive phase in a primarily schizophrenic psychosis, is a common stumbling block in differential diagnosis, in Africans schizophrenia is more liable to be confused with one of the organic psychoses. Among the bush peoples, a typically schizophrenic picture is most likely to be due to organic illness, while schizophrenia itself appears as an amorphous, endogenous psychosis. But the schizophrenic psychoses occurring in the urban, literate section of the population show more nearly the same forms as are found in Europeans."

Moreover, Carothers, quoting H. L. Gordon (1936) and M. Minde of the Sterkfontein Mental Hospital in Johannesburg (1953) finds that paranoia, paraphrenia and even paranoid schizophrenia are relatively rare in Africans.[100] On the other hand, he states as common "a type of twilight or confusional state," sometimes a matter of hours or of weeks but always tending to spontaneous recovery within a limited time; these states appear against backgrounds of physical disease, neurosis or psychosis precipitated by a variety of mental and physical traumata. Anxiety of short duration marks the onset of the more acute cases. "It is always related by the patient to bewitchment and he is fully cognizant of the latter's origin and object. Premonitory symptoms of a Ganser syndrome type, with childish and unaccountable behavior, precede the onset of the major episode, as shown by several writers." Carothers' account of these episodes feature a confusional dominance of action by emotion, an uncontrolled state of fear (panic reaction) or of hostility, a final peak of self-directed violence ultimately visited upon others, and reality distortion with or without hallucination. Recovery follows though a Ganser syndrome or various hysterical symptoms may be left. The entire episode may end with amnesia, once and for all, with apparent normalcy restored and no repetition "unless the cause of the trouble continues in an active form or some new one arises."[101]

Before proceeding with typology in African cultures, it is helpful to consider incidence. Laubscher's 1937 report described a hospitalized population in Queensland of over 550 patients, with some 1700 admissions over a 15 year period. Unfortunately, the descriptions are generalized and not statistically applied to the total 1700. Carothers, as medical officer in charge of Mathari Mental Hospital in Kenya, had opportunity to present admissions data over a five year period concerning 558 patients. He gives an annual rate of 3.4 per 100,000 comparable with Tooth's figure of 3.3 per 100,000 based on the Accra Asylum of the Gold Coast. For Negro-White comparisons in the United States, Malzberg's classic on first admissions to New York State mental hospitals over a three year period remains the definitive work.[102]

In New York, a total annual admissions rate of 150.6 per 100,000 for Negroes and 73.7 for Whites (standardized for age becoming 224.7 and 97.4 respectively) dwarfs the African figures and compares with Carothers' earlier contrast of low figures in Africa and the high annual rate of 161 per 100,000 for American Negroes in Massachusetts. In this period, before antibiotic specifics for syphilis were discovered, the Negro rate of general paresis was 4.1 times higher than the White; that for alcoholic psychoses 3.4 times higher; for cerebral arteriosclerosis 2.9 times; senile psychoses 1.9 times; schizophrenia 2.0 times; and depressive disorders 1.5 times. When allowances are made for urbanization and migration which affect such rates, the differences in rates diminish. For general paresis and alcoholic psychoses in Negroes, Malzberg's finding was that "social factors were largely, even primarily, responsible"; for schizophrenias and depressive disorders, he claimed to find correlations with low economic status, concluding that "the lower economic status of the Negro must contribute directly to his higher rate of mental disease." Only hospital admissions formed the basis of such claims. In connection with his finding that rural Negro rates in America stand intermediate between those of rural Africans on the one hand, and urbanized Negroes and Whites in America, Carothers quotes Wexberg's study of approximately seven thousand Negro and White patients in New Orleans; the major conclusion is that "no evidence could be found of the relevance of biological-racial determinants for the incidence of neuropsychiatric conditions."[103]

Such authors as Carothers, Laubscher, Tooth, or Shelley and Watson were attached to mental hospitals in which circumstances affecting admission are not comparable to *incidence of illness in a community*. However, both Tooth and Carothers made earnest efforts to collect data on the non-hospitalized through surveys conducted by resident officials.

In addition, Tooth's study of the Gold Coast was based chiefly on rural survey in the manner of the Scandinavian community studies, including personal examination of as many reported cases as were accessible at the time. Approximately two-thirds of all reported cases were so examined. While Carothers cites an incidence rate of 35 per 100,000, Tooth reports 96 per 100,000, 60 per 100,000 being examined in the field or in the institution; this ratio of 60:96 examined is high and the disparity of the two figures is accounted for by insurmountable language barrier, native resistance, migration and the like.

Carothers notes that rapid acculturation in the form of detribalization, immigration to urban centers, and employment away from home results in increasing rates of hospitalization for mental disorders. H. M. Shelley and W. H. Watson, reporting in the *Journal of Mental Science* for 1936, add: "When it is remembered that Europeans do not present a united front in matters concerning the treatment of natives (with) one kind of treatment from missionaries, another from officials and another from those engaged in commerce, it is small wonder that the native sense of values is confused and often completely distorted." In support of the factor of acculturation, as affecting illness, Tooth discovered a higher literacy rate than average among psychotics and a semi-rural survey rate similar to that for New York state hospital admissions alone in the one relatively urbanized district of his area (Western Dagomba with its rate of 156 per 100,000). With exclusions of such urban areas, the ninety-six person rate in West Africa would fall considerably. Carothers, in his ethnopsychiatric survey of all the existing African data, including over one hundred and ninety references, concludes: " . . . There is evidence of a disparity between the total incidence of mental derangement in Africa, on the one hand, and in Western Europe and North America on the other." The rate in Africa, except where acculturated to Western standards, is always lower, and this despite conditions of considerable poverty and physical illness.

According to D. K. Henderson and R. D. Gillespie, in their *Textbook of Psychiatry*, the total incidence of mental disorders as a whole differs but slightly in the two sexes. In Africa, however, the hospitalized patients show a large preponderance of males. No doubt, cultural factors again must be taken together with admissions policies, modes of detection and differential uses of the sexes of existing facilities. Yet admissions policy and the detection factor alone could not account for a rate at Accra in 1950 and in Nigeria of six males to every female, or the difference in South Africa (1950) of more than two to one. If the high male rates were heightened by admissions from men's labor camps or army barracks, Tooth's rural survey of the Gold Coast countryside still found a ratio of 1.7 males to 1 female and Carothers' regional survey was similar. No doubt the acculturation process, even in rural circumstances, affects the sexes differently. Further, a comparison of age of admission in Kenya and in the United States would show 78 per cent of African patients between the ages of 10 and 40, whereas in the United States only 42 per cent are so admitted.

In regard to specific symptomatology in patients from areas of Africa, the picture for schizophrenias is most interesting. We have commented above on the rarity of paranoid forms. Carothers adds that this type occurs more frequently among those who have received a "European" education or an "equivalent type" of sophistication. Over 60 per cent of Laubscher's South African patients were diagnosed as schizophrenic (of 7,782 diagnoses to January, 1951). Laubscher, in separate clinical discussions of over a hundred of these agrees with Aubin[104] that auditory and visual hallucinations are rarely systematized or fixed and have a predominantly changing religious mythological content. Laubscher agrees with Carothers also that the "picture of mental confusion stands out clearly above any other syndrome." He had not found "homosexual masking by means of rationalizations and projections among male native paranoids to reach the same degree of defense complexity as abounds among European paranoids." Further, delusions of being poisoned or being bewitched are the most common. Both Tooth and Carothers (1948) are explicit that persecutory delusions are common, with delusions of grandeur rare. And Carothers (1953) quotes Gallais and Planques: "It is nearly always a question of bewitchment, of ill-wishing, of condemnation to death . . ." Tooth observes that schizophrenia in literate, acculturated Africans was found to take forms more similar to those seen in Europeans. Laubscher concludes that schizophrenia is the common psychosis of the rural African and that it occurs despite cultural safety valves; moreover, culture influences mental content in these psychoses. In African cultures, this mental content is determined by "the cultural pattern to which the native belongs." In 1937, Laubscher felt that the structure of a mental disorder was somehow immune from this influence. In 1953, after surveying the literature on schizophrenias in Africa, Carothers answers:[105]

> "The present writer cannot agree with this; the structure too is altered. The lack of integrative elements seen in rural African schizophrenia is something more than 'content' and may well have connotations for prognosis. Other reaction types show even stronger evidence of this . . ."

Tooth, describing the schizophrenias in the Gold Coast area, writes: "Among the 'bush' peoples the delusional content was almost invariably concerned with the ramifications of the fetish system . . . An offense has been committed either against the nature spirits who then trouble the offender in the form of dwarfs or fairies, or against the ancestral hierarchy who appear and influence the sufferer in person." As with Laubscher's clinical notes on over a hundred patients, Tooth's material reveals that only the most literate and urban Africans tend to develop ideas of influence of the European type, that is, *grandiose* delusions of identification with Christ or God, or influences involving electricity, wireless, telepathy or hypnotism. Of these, Tooth observes, "Schizophrenia in literate Africans was found to take very similar forms to those seen in Europeans." For the rest, his data like Laubscher's, concern persons poisoned or bewitched by real individuals, confusional states, marked blunting of affect, loosely organized, autistic thinking, and bizarre, impulsive acts. Laubscher's observation that 80 percent of the hospitalized practiced overt homosexuality with no masking or systematized defenses, the bulk of these classed as "dull schizophrenics" accepting a passive role, is interesting in view of Freudian formulations that systematized paranoid mechanisms arise chiefly as defenses against homosexuality. Carothers and Tooth both describe as predominant, categories which, by conventional standards would be termed simple or catatonic schizophrenias, modified by different cultural background.

In regard to the affective disorders, Carothers' survey is consistent with H. L. Gordon's paper of the early 1930's: there is a remarkable absence of such diagnoses, except for a few of the elated type. However, Carothers feels that the distinction between depressive disorders and anxiety neuroses, well founded in European psychiatry, has had "far more questionable value" in the African. On the whole, the figures are low, but even more interesting, in the accounts of Aubin, Tooth and Carothers, brief states of elation are usually described. Though excited, restless, noisy and irritable, there is little sustained elation, little tendency to develop grandiose plans, and quite often, in Carothers' account, a tendency to show "schizophrenic features especially bizarrely exaggerated movements and facial expressions." To Tooth's and Carothers' statements of low rates for truly depressive states, Laubscher adds that self-mutilation is extremely rare in this disorder; of the 1700 admissions to Queenstown Mental Hospital, only one case in fifteen years was a depressive involving suicide. Concerning etiology, Tooth writes: "One of the most characteristic elements in the depressions of European psychotics is self-reproach . . . but it is certainly true that self-reproach is rarely met with in the content of African psychotics." The tendency in most African cultures to minimize free-will, guilt, and choice in human affairs, and to shift responsibility more to group than personal levels, or grief from isolated to group ritual surroundings may be among the reasons for this resolute turning away from personal fatalism. On this point, Carothers writes:[106]

"Self reproach and the delusional systems that arise from this are often regarded as secondary manifestations of a fundamental disorder of affect, but it seems that this affect is not sustained without this element and that psychotic depression in the familiar sense can hardly develop in its absence. In fact, organization seems, in mental as in other provinces, to be the determining factor in persistence."

This feeling that the cultural bases in African behavior are different from the European and affect incidence, symptomatology and structure of disorders is borne out in regular variation of psychoneurotic as well as psychotic cases. Aside from the Bemba of Northern Rhodesia whose customs demand a prompt performance of counter-ritual, low rates of obsessive neuroses are uniformly reported. Laubscher notes that a study of various customs shows a factor of atonement towards ancestors enacted in ritual and sacrifice. Anxiety states, likewise, are frequently an outcome of bewitching and poisoning. Phobias related to witchcraft, and physical symptoms in the forms of cardiac or gastric neuroses, or of impotence, refer to putative threats to one's personal and procreative life. Fears of food poisoning and anorexia nervosa, sometimes fatal, suggest what we might call elements of an acute schizophrenic episode. In addition, Dembovitz in his work with West African troops, noted that hysterical symptoms and conversion mechanisms appear so readily that not only neurotic depressions of the reactive type, but even anxiety states and true psychoses are colored by them. The physical symptoms run the gamut of globus hystericus, aphonia, paraplegia and monoplegias, deafness, blindness, tremors, rigidity, and hyperventilation tetany. The predominant mental symptoms include amnesias, fugues, fits and stupors.

Elements of acute schizophrenic episodes, possibly catatonic, are indicated in twenty-one cases of 609 first admissions diagnosed by Carothers as "frenzied anxiety." Such cases, and others described by Laubscher and by Shelley and Watson resemble the classic Malay *amok*. Laubscher has described "acute hysterical attacks, resembling Charcot's grand hysteria . . . but the picture presented is typical of emotional abreaction and follows a dramatic frustration and thwarting of impulses and desires. Of course, this is attributed to some possessing power; this is more the recognized way of reacting to such disturbances than a spontaneous, unconscious discharge of libido in motor acts without conscious plan or design."

Yet Laubscher, Shelley and Watson, and Aubin all describe high homicide and low suicide rates in connection with such impulsive and furious attacks, Laubscher characteristically translating into such Freudian terms as "less introjection of sadism." Aubin's description of paroxysmal manifestations (motor and psychomotor, sensory and psychosensory, ideational and affective) and the episodic fury and terrifying hallucinations which sometimes accompany them, again suggest transitory phases in a schizophrenic process in which the acting out of emotional impulse is freer than in European models, and the disorganization potential is less. After recovery from these states, or in periods between them, seemingly normal conduct is possible.

Dembovitz writes at length of running amok in West African troops, distinguishing the true berserk who fights to the end from the hysterical form, who hurts no one and is readily subdued. Recurrent confusional states and common hallucinatory experiences are spoken of as occurring in anxiety states which do not necessarily imply a psychotic episode. "Normal Africans see and speak to their dead parents." Different from denial is the "disavowal" (*reniement*) of Aubin, "which excludes from consciousness all situations seen as dangers" whether real or magical and including dangers concerning the group such as the breaking of taboos and customs.

This central core of confused, excited, incoherent and emotionally labile ideation and affect is found in most disorders whether they pass under the European labels of hysteria, anxiety states or schizophrenias. "In short," Tooth concludes, "the cultural environment is such that short-circuit reactions . . . released from the inhibitions of intellect are not only tolerated but encouraged." Perhaps this is too strong. Gallais and Planques note that the intellectual and affective factors are closely interwoven. It remains to point out that these are of a different order, understandable only in the light of a different cultural background.

Carothers' summary for recent African psychiatry is

succinct. In elucidation of the difference, he writes:[107]

> "In general it seems that the rather clear distinction that
> exists in Europeans between the 'conscious' and 'uncon-
> scious' elements of mind does not exist in rural Africans.
> The 'censor's' place is taken by the sorcerer, and 'splits' are
> vertical, not horizontal. Emotion easily dominates the
> entire mind; and, when it does, the grip on the world of
> things is loosened, and frank confusion takes the place of
> misinterpretation. All the neuroses seen in European indi-
> viduals are here, as a rule, resolved on social lines; and the
> structure of psychoses is so altered by the lack of conscious
> integration that these are apt to take amorphous or abortive
> forms."

Perhaps this sort of summary is just the beginning of a
statement of differences, not the end-product. There are
certainly far too few discussions of specific psychopathology
within the boundaries of particular cultures and with
reference to specific degrees of Europeanization or detribalization. Nevertheless, the accounts to date from widely
scattered provinces of Africa, including the Cape, East
Africa and the Gold Coast are remarkably contrasting
with Europe and North America and surprisingly similar
one with another. If we list the differences, they are: the
paucity of paranoid forms and masked homosexuality,
unless Europeanized; the confusional or excited catatonic
phases of schizophrenia; the so-called "frenzied anxiety"
with hysterical elements (Carothers and Aubin); the lack
of truly affective disorders of the depressive type, or of
long-lasting and systematized delusions; the fact that
Tooth stresses the lack of certainty in assigning schizophrenic patients to one European category or another,
and his observation that under "home care they did not
exhibit the clinical variations as clearly as those that were
seen in the asylum"; and finally, the variations in delusional content by culture. These differences all point to

a gross but regular variation in psychopathology. On specific points of agreement in the three regions, as with the relative rarity of affective disorders, statements are exactly comparable, Laubscher stating that depressive forms are rare (6.7 per cent for males, 6 for females and only 3.6 for Queensland Hospital patients), Carothers finding a comparable 3.8 per cent in Kenya for 1939-1943 later rising to 6.1 per cent, an incidence figure similar to Laubscher's. Tooth's field survey of necessity yielded higher figures, diagnosed as "mania" or "hypomania," but some probably are schizophrenics in acute episodes (hear voices, are manneristic, show bizarre ideation). At any rate, Tooth writes of Accra: "The absence of depressed patients is most strikingly demonstrated by a visit to an African mental hospital where, under infinitely more depressing conditions, the atmosphere of tense unhappiness usually found in European mental hospitals is replaced by one of unrestrained and misdirected exhuberance of spirits." In contrast to the African patients at Mathari, Carothers notes elsewhere for this area that of two hundred twenty-two admissions of Europeans, a high of 22 per cent were depressed.

Turning from Africa, analyses of mental hospital admissions for New Zealand and Hawaii have been supplied by the anthropologist, Ernest Beaglehole. In each case, the interest has been in comparison of native groups, Maori or Hawaiian, with migrant populations from Asian, European or American cultures. In his first study, in New Zealand, admissions for a 10-year period, 1925 to 1935, were made for Europeans on the one hand, and Maori or part-Maori on the other. Unfortunately, congenital disorders like mental defectives or those having relatively low intellectual endowment were not distinguished from acquired defects, so that incidence of functional psychoses may be blurred; moreover, Maori culture was decidedly modified by the time of this study, the Maori being an indigenous population long subject to acculturation. When the rates were standardized for age, however, they were 8.37 per 10,000 for Europeans and 4.19 for Maori. These rates applied only to hospitalization, *not incidence* in community settings. As such, however, they are of considerable interest inasmuch as there is no good evidence that by the late 1920's and early 1930's there was this large a difference in attitudes towards hospitalization or accessibility to facilities in the two cultural groups.

Concerning symptomatology, the Maori of New Zealand contrast with the data from various African cultures in having a remarkably high rate of "manic-depressive psychoses" not shared by the Europeans. Maori females showed a rate of 52.6 per cent in this category of all first admissions in a 10 year period. One might suspect variance in "schools" of psychiatry to account for these differences in diagnostic category, but fortunately for the contrast, British psychiatry has dominated both the New Zealand and African scenes. The relative incidence of schizophrenias (not differentiated as to type) was roughly similar for Maori and European. Official Fijian figures for 1936 which are included show a hospitalization figure of only 1.6 per 10,000 for Fijians, 4.05 for Europeans; the differerences between New Zealand and Fiji in facilities, modes of detection and community attitudes toward treatment may be reflected in these results. At any rate, for those interested in the problem of the rapidly acculturating alien in an inimical environment, the comparative crude totals for Chinese and East Indians are 530 and 161 per size of population (100 being the proportionate share according to population size.) These figures are not standardized for age and can only tentatively be compared with the corresponding per population figure of 40 for Fijians (1.6 per 10,000) and 96 for Europeans.[108]

Beaglehole's comparative Hawaiian study uses the sample years 1930, 1935 and 1936, employing the same ratio of 100 as being the proportionate share of mental illness according to population size. Here native and part-Hawaiians were distinguished, the former having a ratio of 200 per population, while the latter ranged from about a fourth to a third of this figure. Native Hawaiians had not only twice the expected amount of psychoses, but figures ranged to three times the expected or proportionate amount for Puerto Ricans and five times for the tiny Korean population. A large population in the Islands, like the Japanese, were comparable with the part-Hawaiians (about 75). First admissions figures in this study showed the same comparative rates as prevalence figures. This study centered in acculturation phenomena and both Hawaiians and part-Hawaiians, despite the differences between them in general incidence, showed variations in incidence of particular disorders. Hawaiians had the lowest rates of schizophrenia (30 to 43 per cent); part-Hawaiians an average proportion. Hawaiians had a high proportion of depressives ("manic-phase," in this report); four-fifths were "manic." Part-Hawaiians had the lowest incidence of such affective disorders, with no recorded excess of the "manic" form.

Beaglehole concludes that the incidence of psychoses rises in cultural groups confronted with the necessity of adapting to "Western forms." This is more the case, he holds, for Hawaiians, Puerto Ricans and Koreans. The case is distinctly unclear unless it is meant that the major Japanese migrations were earlier and more sizeable than those affecting Puerto Ricans and Koreans. The Hawaiians, while indigenous, were certainly dwarfed by successive waves of migration to their shores. More interesting, perhaps, is that the acculturation process for part-Hawaiians here decreases the chances for paranoid forms of schizophrenia to arise, and likewise decreases markedly the incidence of affective disorders in the "manic" form. Together with the high rates of hospitalization for the native population, these results contrast surprisingly for the findings from Africa which are diametrically different on each score.

When it is remembered, however, that the "native Hawaiian" represents a minority, not an indigenous majority, and one schooled for decades in American and Euro-Asian cultural practices, the mystery disappears. Far from being a native culture in the beginnings of the acculturation process, it is, as Beaglehole rightly felt, the longest acculturated, problematic minority of the Islands. However, with the Puerto Rican predominantly a Spanish cultural form and the Korean an Asian, "Western patterns of culture" would seem too narrow a term for the several patterns which dominate Hawaii. On the other hand, Puerto Rican, Korean, and more recently Filipino rates of disorder have illustrated more current struggles to adapt, and a faster current pace of acculturation in each case reflected in far greater incidence rates than is the case with the relatively settled populations from Japan, from Okinawa or resulting from part-Hawaiian miscegenation and acculturation.[109]

In North America, Hallowell's study of two groups of Salteaux Indians of the Berens River District was based on field research which disclosed one to be highly acculturated, the other less so. In the acculturated "Lakeside" group, according to intensive Rorschach investigation, 81 per cent of the best adjusted and 75 per cent of the maladjusted had their place of provenience. His conclusion is that under conditions of acculturation, some individuals make "excellent, even superior adjustments; others fail to make as good adjustments as under the old regime . . ." The more restricted range of adjustment, he feels, is consistent with the fewer choices or conflicts of the less acculturated society. While not all persons are prone to feel the destructiveness of such conflicts, their presence in an intrapsychic sense may, according to Hallowell, precipitate disturbance in those susceptible individuals represented in the 75 per cent of maladjustment at Lakeside.[110]

For the same cultural area, both Ruth Landes[111] and J. M. Cooper[112] have reported on the *windigo* psychosis of Ojibwa and Cree Indians of Canada. This disorder combines homicidal behavior with cannibalistic fears and tendencies in a culture where life-long food frustrations and oral sadistic behavior appear to be outstanding features. For the same setting, Hallowell has taken pains to show how language, belief, art and mode of life in a culture are related to perception, "how they become involved in the perceptual experience of individuals, the role they play in the total structuralization of the perceptual field and the consequences of this fact for the actual conduct of the individual." As Hallowell notes:[113]

> ". . . Entities that have *no* tangible or material existence may become perceptual objects in the actual experience of individuals . . . In the foregoing anecdote there are thirteen references to *hearing* the windigo . . . The sounds heard by A "meant" *windigo* to him. But this was possible only because cannibal monsters were among the traditionally reified concepts and imagery of his culture. Furthermore, just as a word or a sentence may induce an affective response or immediately define a situation as dangerous and thus call forth appropriate conduct, such was the case here. Once the situation became perceptually structuralized in this way, subsequent sounds likewise become meaningful in terms of the same pattern. . . . "

For some time, the manner in which *certain types* of autistic auditory and visual hallucinations arise in psychotics of given cultural background has remained a mystery.

This applies to the stylized hallucinations, auditory and visual, in the African data, in European or American patients (Christ, God, radio, telegraphy), in non-psychotic vision quests of Plains Indians, or here, again, in *windigo* (named for an Ojibwa-speaking monster with cannibalistic tendencies). That a culture can affect visual perception, and concepts about spatial relations in the "tangible or material" world, varying perception in the normal and abnormal dimensions of conduct, was shown by Hallowell elsewhere in his discussion of perception and spatial concepts among the Salteaux. There he wrote:[114]

". . . The level of abstraction utilized in dealing with certain spatial attributes is not a simple function of maturation or intellectual capacity on the part of individuals. It is a function of the status of the cultural heritage as well. For the cultural heritage of a people, among other things, limits or promotes the manner in which and the terms in which the individual deals with the spatial attributes of the world about him. If a culture does not provide the terms and concepts, spatial attributes cannot even be talked about with precision. Individuals are left to fend for themselves, as it were, on the level of elementary discriminatory reactions. This limits the possibilities for the mental manipulation of more refined and developed concepts that require symbolic representation in some form. Without such instruments in the cultural heritage certain areas of action are excluded and the solution of many practical problems impossible."

On the other hand, as comparative studies of art from modern and nonliterature societies will indicate, a cultural pattern will reify not only types of concepts, but forms of imagery even as to intensity, realism, emotional impact, distortion, rhythm, balance. What it *promotes* in types of emotional expression is of equal importance to what it limits, omits, or suppresses. The same observations apply to the auditory and visual ranges of perception. Thus Joseph and Murray write of Rorschachs of any isolated rural population in a manner which reminds us of the contrast between rural natives and Europeanized subjects in Africa. Discussing the psychological test materials of Chamorros and Carolinians of Saipan, the authors state:[115]

> ". . . A high degree of associative concreteness is to be expected in any people who have not at their disposal the general and abstract associations which are provided by a 'higher education'. We may, for instance, anticipate much concreteness in the Rorschachs of any isolated rural population . . . "

The lack of delusional systematizations in a wide variety of mental disorders of nonliterate peoples: the "running wild" of Fuegian tribes (Cooper, *op. cit.*), the Greenland Eskimo *piblokto* (women running about naked, Cooper, *op.cit.*), the "Arctic hysteria" of Lapps, Eskimos, and northeast Siberian tribes (Cooper and Yap, *op.cit*), and the similar forms of psychosis, Latah of Malays and Imu of the Ainu tribes of Hokkaido (Yap, *op.cit.*, and Aberle),[116] all point to atypical forms of schizophrenias varying from the Western standard. Like the "frenzied anxieties" with hysterical elements of Carothers and Aubin, they remind us of schizo-affective disorders as discussed by Adolf Meyer, but more loosely organized, more episodic, and more bound to action modes of emotional expression than to fantasy. In "Arctic hysteria," Latah, running amok, and Imu, both startle and surprise reactions are common, echolalia and echopraxia predominate, and trances, convulsions, coprolalia, and catathymic outbursts occur. The running amok forms are marked by sudden, furious aggression and hostility visited upon oneself either in the initial or final phases. Erwin H. Ackerknecht early noted similarities in Malay Latah and Siberian "Arctic hysteria" (as reported by Czaplička and others) in which the loss of will and automatic obedience often took forms of echolalia and echopraxia; these symptoms corresponded closely with a type of catatonia once seen commonly in the West but now comparatively rare.[117] Amok, in the Asian, African, and possibly the Fuegian forms refers to violent homicidal aggression with ideas of persecution and possession. While hostility towards a given individual is often in evidence, it radiates indiscriminately and with little delusional systematization towards practically any victims who come to hand. African forms of amok are often self-mutilating initially, the Asian self-destructive ultimately. To the states of homicidal confusion and excitement, *windigo* among the Ojibwa and Cree may be added. Carothers' "frenzied anxiety" certainly belongs to the same list; and H. G. Van Loon's observation, as early as 1928, that dementia praecox "announces itself amongst Malays very often by aggressive confusion" places the classic form of running amok in Malaysia in the same category as that found in North America, South America and Africa.[118]

This category is undoubtedly a variant of Western forms of the schizophrenias, best classified provisionally as schizo-affective disorder. Seligman's "brief maniacal attacks," for the unacculturated natives of New Guinea; similar reports in the incidence figures ("hypomania," and "brief manic phases" of affective disorders) of Africa likewise point in the same direction. The author's experience with epidemiological data in Hawaii in 1949 paralleled Beaglehole's: a stable, large, and long-acculturated population like the Japanese showed few surprises from a Western point of view and generally speaking low incidence, whereas the people most in the throes of initial acculturation, the Filipinos at the bottom of the social scale, showed a high proportion of affective disorders ("manic depressive psychosis") and catatonic confusional states among the Hawaiian hospitalized. In Hell's Half Acre of Honolulu, where immigrant Filipinos undergoing urbanization chiefly dwelled, several classic cases of running amok, and ending in death of onlookers and the aggressor alike, occurred in a brief period of time.

These data, from Asia, Oceania, Africa and the Americas uniformly mark a high incidence of states of confused excitement, with disorganizing amounts of anxiety, fear and hostility present, and frequently associated with either indiscriminate homicidal behavior or self-mutilation, or both, in a setting of catathymic outbursts of activity. The contrast to the West of these nonliterate peoples, Eskimos, Ojibwa, Cree, Fuegians, and various cultures of Asia, Africa, northern Europe, and the Pacific, with their relatively low incidence of depressed and suicidal states suggests that in addition to their marked associative concreteness and high activity and motility orientations, these psychotics more typically direct hostility outward and express it with greater freedom and directness than in European models. That they express it outside of tightly organized family or kinship scenes is also interesting. In European patients, not only will the confusions in sexual identification (homosexual or asexual) be masked by systematized rationalizations, but basic hostility and anxiety will themselves be disguised and internalized with less expressive outlet. In this light, it is entirely conceivable, as Carothers, Seligman and others have documented, that "brief, maniacal attacks," often self-terminating in natural course, are a result of lack of systematized fantasy or delusions acting as ego-defenses and in place of them action and motility functioning. In the West, there are superimposed layers of fantasy.

In a parallel sense, in Western cultures, those emphasizing emotional expression and outlet or placing a high valuation on heterosexual potency, like the South Italian, may be nearer these models of fantasy constriction than those restricting emotional expression by and large, and containing double standards for sexual conduct. In a paper on "Mental Illness in Primitive Societies" by Paul K. Benedict and Irving Jacks, the manuscript emphasizes "the role played by the Judeo-Christian preoccupation with guilt and its consequent channeling of hostility towards rather than away from the self." This is true of the distinction noted earlier by Ruth Benedict in the difference between cultures which emphasize guilt and thus center individual choice and responsibility versus those which control behavior by defining conduct in its context of custom and applying the sanctions of shame to any transgressor. But this distinction of Ruth Benedict in *Chrysanthemum and the Sword*, between what she termed "guilt cultures" and "shame cultures," is only one side of the coin. In psychodynamic terms, we must still know the amount and complication of defenses used against stress, whether rationalizations and delusions are present to constitute a secondary defense system or whether motility and fantasy act together in a more direct sense. In the same way, the psychiatrist must know when, culturally speaking, to expect more associative concreteness to operate in patients, where hostility is turned to self-destructiveness or against others, where the affective life is dulled or made labile, and the roles played by motility and fantasy.

The anthropologist, too, could benefit by knowledge of these distinctions since schizo-affective states of confused excitement have too often in their literature (like Tooth's "mania" and "hypomania") been misdiagnosed as hysterias or as manic states. Joseph and Murray, in their work on Saipanese, stop to note that six Alorese cases in Dubois' *The People of Alor* are diagnosed in error as "manic states" or manic-depressive psychosis. The same authors, in their work on Saipan, are impressed by a higher rate of psychosis among the more acculturated Chamorros in contrast to the native Carolinians. It would be interesting to know whether this is because of deeper seated and long-lasting disorders among the Chamorros in consequence of their greater Europeanization and acculturation.

The work of C. G. Seligman in New Guinea, C. Lopez in Brazil, J. Dhunjibhoy in India, A. I. Hallowell among the Salteaux, and the African specialists, all suggesting higher rates of incidence and greater conformance to Western models in consequence of acculturation no doubt influenced Beaglehole's theories of the late Thirties concerning cultural breakdown and mental disorganization. Actually, five years earlier, George Devereux in 1934, impressed by these world areas materials which were fast accumulating, and perhaps mistakenly emphasizing the rarity of any forms of schizophrenia among them, proposed a "sociological theory" of schizophrenia as resulting when the culture became "complex enough" so that the individual became disoriented as to his social role.[119] Apart from the lower incidence rates of long-lasting disorders, which now seems probable for nonliterate cultures of the world, the present theory of schizo-affective disorders of shorter duration is more consistent with current anthropological knowledge that all cultures are almost equally and infinitely "complex."

The Spencerian notion of Western Europe's greater "complexity," individuality, and personality-heterogeneity; the primitive as custom-ridden, conforming, and evidencing a dead level of uniformity in personal characteristics, is a Western stereotype long since abandoned in anthropological circles. In place of either notions of a Rousseauan lack of worry, or of widespread personality disorganization among nonliterate peoples, or the Spencerian idea of magic-ridden and illogical irrationality among them, it is necessary to note the distinction in cultural types where in one associative concreteness is present, in another lacking. In one scene, more direct expression of emotions is promoted, in another prohibited; in one culture, action and motility in social, economic and artistic life is required; in another ratiocination, fantasy, guardedness and rationalizations abound. As John Dewey stated the matter in *Philosophy and Civilization*, the distance between nonliterate cultures (the so-called "savage mind") and our own Westernized societies is the difference between basically contrasting conditions of existence, modes of life, values and percepts. As he discussed the question methodologically:[120]

" .. The tendency to forget the office of distinctions and classifications, and to take them as marking things in themselves is the current fallacy of scientific specialism . . . This attitude which once flourished in physical science now governs theorizing about human nature. Man has been resolved into a definite collection of primary instincts which may be numbered, catalogued and exhaustively described one by one . . . But in fact there are as many specific reactions to differing stimulating conditions as there is time for, and our lists are only classifications for a purpose."

The data on varying normative cultural behavior, and on differential psychopathology in these other cultural scenes demonstrate that the largest unresolvable "differing stimulating conditions" affecting human conduct are cultural in essence. The reach of the cultural factor in any scene, acculturated or not, is undoubtedly great and can affect behavior on normal, neurotic or psychotic levels of expression precisely because of the duration of culture. Its effective stock in trade is massive in proportion to an individual life course and to one's personalized experience and accomplishments. When dealing with the problems of human organic and social life, we must free ourselves from what Whitehead aptly termed the fallacy of "simple location." The human being is never located in a single instant, once cultural forces have taken hold as inevitably they do. In his social and even organic development, the three modes of time, past, present and future, are to be reckoned with as they naturally converge in human thought. Ernst Cassirer, in *An Essay on Man* quotes Leibniz to the same effect: "The present is suffused with the past, and pregnant with the future." Especially where psychodynamic questions are involved in human conduct, the supreme ability of men to bring to bear upon conscious and unconscious motivations the past, present and future, as if these were immediately available, places their mental and emotional functioning in a common setting amenable to the cultural influence of others. In this sense of constant interaction and uninterrupted communication with others on mental and emotional planes, all cultures are equally and infinitely complex. It is this which commends the entire world of culture to our notice for comparative study with attention to specific differences, the specific ideational and emotional conditions of cultural existence.

In *The Future of an Illusion*, Sigmund Freud argues that it would be an advantage to leave absolute values and ideals out of consideration and admit "honestly the purely human origin of all cultural laws and institutions." It would also be helpful to abandon the idea that these cultural values are themselves immutable or rigid in any cultural history. Freud's notion that cultural rules and institutions should serve people, not rule them, or that growth required overcoming fixed conceptions of either rules or institutions is brave advice indeed. "Man cannot remain a child forever; he must venture at last into . . . 'education to reality'," wrote Freud.

However, whether we are dealing with individual superego formation, or with the growth and change, under acculturation, in whole cultures, the simple fact is the immediacy of cultural laws and institutions, and their overwhelming importance as a way of life to whole groups of people. There can be no other interpretation to the facts presented that native peoples tend to be hospitalized less frequently than Europeans from the same areas, that the rates rise with cultural dislocations, and that the forms of disorder vary with cultural background. All peoples are cultured, so to speak, and the point is not abandonment of these modes of life which are, essentially, the ways they live. Instead, for psychiatry, there is here afforded a matchless laboratory in which to study the effects of differing organizations and patternings of the life course. This does not mean that valuation, in the sense of scientific and humanistic judgments, is forbidden. Since social psychiatry is concerned not only with the raw data and findings of prevalence and incidence studies, but probes the significance of socio-cultural factors in the etiology and dynamics of mental disorder, it belongs logically to public health and preventive medicine with the need for collaboration with psychology, the life sciences, and social science. It cannot be abandoned to purely personal standards of emancipation, nor is there any indication that it will be.

Psychiatry has scarcely begun to investigate the levels of fantasy and motility usage in different cultures, although Flora L. Bailey[121] and Margot Astrov[122] have reported on the importance of motility, activity and mobility as dominant themes in Navajo literature, economic way of life, linguistic structure, habits and customs. Even earlier, Jane Belo[123] reported on characteristic motor habits of the Balinese, and George Devereux,[124] in 1951, provided a third contrast from the Mohave. For fantasy, there are scattered references, Victor Barnouw's study of the fantasy world of a Chippewa woman,[125] Hallowell's of a dissocial

Indian girl,[126] and Margaret Lantis' and Katherine Spencer's recent accounts of Eskimo and Navajo personality, respectively, as revealed in folklore and myth. J. S. Lincoln,[127] D. M. Spencer,[128] and Dorothy Eggan,[129] among others, have shown that the manifest content, form and interpretation of dreams are largely culturally patterned. Both W. J. Wallace and Devereux have reported on Mohave dreams in much the same sense. Finally, David Efron published a comprehensive study in 1941 on changes in gesture and motility patterns of second-generation American Jewish and Italo-American populations showing a gradual inhibition of motility of the first-generation type, including gestural languages, under conditions of acculturation.[130] The point was not only that specific cultural groups had distinct types of gestural communication carrying qualities of emotional expression, but that these were modified under conditions of cultural change.

Besides acculturation phenomena, wherein new and variant forms of a culture make their initial historical appearance, there is the matter of already existing regional variants of a basic cultural form. For the Italian, and even the acculturated Italo-Americans, Robert Lowie in his *Social Organizations* has applied the term, *campanilismo*, for the narrowly defined solidarity of a rural region and village which may sometimes be extended to town and provincial limits but rarely farther.[131] The existence of these regional differences which are crystallized in economy, custom and traditional history can be traced out, though only roughly at present, in mental health data as well. While Italy's overall commitment laws of 1904 and subsequently, aimed at protection of the general population, and not at patients' needs, Italian admissions rates even in the peak years of the early 1940's ran about 50 per cent lower than the United States. Yet from a regional standpoint, Rome and the area north of it had an annual rate of 168 per 100,000 hospitalized, while the area south of Rome plus Sicily and Sardinia had 95 per 100,000 by the middle of the decade. Paul Lemkau and Carlo de Sanctis who have presented these data show care in distinguishing between North Italy, South Italy, and the islands as to cultural variants affecting the annual hospital admissions rates for mental disorders.

Even the over-all figures for Italy in the Forties which Lemkau and de Sanctis present (a generalized rate of 59 to 62 per 100,000 population) while it is only a third of United States rates, or a fourth of Swiss rates for comparable periods, must be considered along with such Italian customs and attitudes as the care of older, ill persons in the family household, the blot on family reputation which may lower a daughter's or son's chances for suitable marriage, and the tendency to equate illness of any variety with both sexual and personality weakness.[132] In the *American Journal of Psychiatry* for the year preceding the Lemkau-De Sanctis article, Eric Berne pointed out in his survey of Oriental mental hospitals that in Ceylon, fully two-thirds of the patients hospitalized are males![133] Berne's further point that Malays do not seem to succumb to schizophrenias so much as to "toxic confusional psychoses," or the suggestion there and elsewhere that frankly hysterical symptoms strongly color the illnesses of India and respond to treatments that incorporate yoga with modern psychiatric practice are reminiscent of the findings of Van Loon in Malaysia, Carothers *et al* in Africa on toxic and confusional states, and Seligman in New Guinea.

The point is that such observations need to be made in more restricted cultural arenas, where both socio-cultural backgrounds and policies affecting hospitalization are well known. Until this is done, regional cultural variants, and shifts in illness typology occurring with cultural change, will not begin to be studied. The search has led toward scientific differentiations of types not commonly emphasized in psychiatry as representing its chief traditional distinctions in nosology or diagnosis. Before proceeding, it will be helpful to attack certain questions in typology directly from the point of view of the kind of social psychiatric theory involved.

"It is a well-founded historical generalization," wrote Whitehead, "that the last thing to be discovered in any science is what the science is really about."[134] In psychiatry, in the Kraepelinian period of symptom-cluster description, and bounded for the main part by Western and Northern European models of such diseases, the disease process itself, far from being thought psychosocial in essence, was regarded as being founded in biologic and individual psychological event-sequences. While Adolf Meyer substituted a more functional and environmentalist view of personality as man in action, and Freud and his followers took interest in the family matrix of such activity, wholehearted descriptions and analyses of reaction patterns and formations, according to total contours of the setting and influences which produced them, belong to a later date. In the brilliant, original work of Freud, for example, the origin of illness in indelible, if often unconscious, memory-traces and in conflicts of *id* and *superego* as individually-centered apparatus pointed back to the start Freud himself had as neuro-anatomist, as an individualist in a setting of then-successful mechanically materialistic philosophies. The establishment of the significance of dreams, the unconscious, censorship, resistance or infantile sexuality are at best individually-centered concepts.

However much these concepts have reference to family structure in the total Oedipus theory, that family structure is a mechanically-operating invariant, at points similar and at many more distinct from the actual realities and constantly growing data on family structures across the world's surface. Even so, while conflicts of *id* and *superego* go far, as in original Freudian theory, in the explanation of hysterical and obsessive compulsive disorders, the generalization and the restrictive shorthand this theory imposes hardly contain the cross-cultural data. Indeed, it hardly begins to describe the blindness or leg paralysis of two Ute Indian patients, responsive in a matter of days to dream analysis and shamanistic suggestion versus the long-lived and heavily invested hysterical symptoms of an East Indian mystic.[135] They are not the same illness, most often, in the light of genesis, etiology, differences in the setting for growth, and even in reference to the biological and sexual components of their individual features. Even the appropriately called *mechanisms* of defense, for the hysterias, of condensation, displacement, symbolization and secondary elaboration; or for the obsessive compulsive neuroses, of the use of opposites, denial, undoing and repetition, these are circular explanations of symptom entities, or, as Meyer pointed out, not descriptions of *total* personality or reaction patterns.

Identification as a method of learning, again internally descriptive of individual motivations, does not really tell us how those motivations, and not others, first arose. Projection as a method of handling anxiety, stress or frustration is again descriptive shorthand, invaluable to be sure, but known even before Bleuler, and still not adequately defined in terms of the total setting in which it will arise, the ways in which it operates, and the means by which it will cease. While schizophrenias, in Freudian terms, are weaknesses of ego-structure, we are not told, specifically, of what types and how these, too, may arise. Whereas oral and anal, or narcissistic infantilisms are suggestive in some instances, schizophrenias occur in some quarters of the globe in settings of unabated heterosexuality. Throughout the whole Freudian system, culture, human values, and the quality of human relationships in an individual or in a group are epiphenomenal and consequently the descriptive shorthand turns out, all too often, to be not broadly analytical.

In Carl Jung, the test of good intentions fares better for there is definite interest here in the cultural, religious and aesthetic backgrounds of human beings, as well as in the cultural meanings of symbols. Impressed by the presence of opposites, as these occur in fantasies, and especially in the conflictual products of schizophrenic patients, Jung saw in these the archetypes, or images of a "collective nature" sealed in the unconscious of the race. Obviously, the Durkheimian notion of cultural conditioning, of "collective representations," was being used, but now in relation to a new theory of the unconscious, and one having traditional roots. With little anthropology available, free associations were used to discover how individuals failed in reaching life goals. While on the brink of discovering something concerning the differing quality of human relations in different cultural traditions, the delimited area in which Jung worked kept him, despite provocative discoveries from the Freudian quarter and the pervasive influence of Wundt, from breaking with older typologies.

The direct attack on rigidity in typology was reserved for Adolf Meyer, and has been continued by his lineal descendants. Influenced at first by a broader grasp of neuroanatomy and neuropathology, diagnostic terms changed in the direction of reaction types being stressed, with prognoses altered by a somewhat Freudian-genetic and dynamic approach. In therapy, the use of distributive analysis broke the rigidity of the Descriptive School, with the study of the individual and his specific reactions, including his social relationships, taking the place of fixed classifications, or in contradistinction to Freud, in place of the reduction to infancy. With Meyer as with Jung, increasing emphasis on age levels in the life cycle, each age playing its part, and on the cultural and social organization of the family, left but a short step to be taken in defining this part of a science of human relations which could include values and ethics.

Only by a fallacy of simple location do we erroneously regard mental illness as being, on the one hand, biologically ordained, or on the other, individually centered as individual failures. All such disorders, except the narrowing number of those which are overwhelmingly organic in origin, are failures in human relations to be sure, but again, failures which are as attributable to the individual characteristics of the society and culture as they are to the social characteristics of the individual.

Both Karen Horney and Erich Fromm, in separate ways, proposed orientations to psychoanalytic theory which reversed Freud's contention that sexual development determined character, and instead contended that character guides all behavior, including the sexual. Horney, in her discussions of reaction formations in female patients, or in tracing widespread evidences of neuroticism in contemporary American culture, indicates points at which the perpetuation of faulty neurotic solutions to the problems of the feminine role, or the competitive role, occur because of invariant conditions in cultural environment. Fromm, in an even more generalizing vein, has defined and recently redefined social character. In the latest statement, he writes:[136]

". . . By 'social character' I refer to the core of the character common to most members of a culture, in contradistinction to the *individual character* in which people belonging to the same culture differ from each other. A society is not something *outside* of the individuals which it is composed of, but it *is* the totality of these many individuals. The emotional forces which are operating in most of its members become powerful forces in the social process, stabilizing, changing, or disrupting it... One has relied much too exclusively on gathering data on what people *think* (or believe that they are supposed to think) instead of studying the emotional forces behind their thinking.   While opinion polls are significant for certain purposes, we need to know more; they are not the tool for understanding the forces operating underneath the surface of opinion.   Only if we know these forces are we able to predict how the members of a society will react . . . From the standpoint of social dynamics every opinion is worth only as much as the emotional matrix in which it is rooted."

Theories of social character do not supplant those of psychogenesis; they are supplementary to them.   Paul Lemkau, Benjamin Pasamanik, and Marcia Cooper, approaching the same question from the standpoint of psychogenetic theory, have reached essentially the same conclusion.[137]   Pointing out that psychiatric acceptance of the psychogenic hypothesis implies a "bridge" of causation between prior experience and later illness, the authors add:

". . . This does not, of course mean that we must also accept any particular theory of dynamic mechanism, or even any of the suspiciously direct concepts of personality type such as the oral and anal types . . . It is not necessary to concern ourselves with dynamics according to Freud, Jung, Adler, Meyer, or any other system.   All that is needed is to accept as valid the simple statement that life experience not directly affecting the structure of the organism can influence later behavior, and, in extreme cases, lead to symptoms identifiable as psychiatric illness of one sort or another."

Lemkau *et al* note that unless this temporal concept is true, there is no basis for the prevention of basically non-organic mental illness and no hope that mental health can be promoted.   If on the other hand, the psychogenetic hypothesis is true, then there logically follow responsibilities for preventive efforts that psychiatry cannot escape, among these the prevention of damaging circumstances or the change in their impact upon personality. The consideration of the Freudian position, in turn, yields the same familiar critique:

> ". . . Freud stimulated interest in the effect of cultural concepts on the individual, but he made few if any suggestions beyond rather vague ones about sex education . . . Indeed, in his *Civilization and Its Discontents*, a product of his matured thinking, he states that civilization can grow only by increasing repressions and consequent neurosis. Freud's major hypothesis is that basically, the human being is ruled by instinct and by innately determined developmental patterns."

Freud said little about prevention of "the disasters he demonstrates so clearly," or, in Fromm's words, he consistently interpreted the dynamic nature of character traits as an expression of their inevitable and often self-destructive libidinous source. The interest of Fromm in a psychiatrically elaborated, and interdisciplinary, science of human relations is paralleled by Lemkau, Pasamanik, and Cooper:

> ". . . Most psychiatrists nowadays either boast of a knowledge of anthropology or apologize that they do not have it. What is such knowledge for? Surely it is not just to contribute to pathology, a dissecting of the threads of an illness to see how it came about. It must also have some value in a more constructive sense, to help explain the process of the construction of the personality as well as to furnish a diagram of its present status. It must be to give hints from comparing different developments in different cultures, so that something may be done to improve personalities in our own land."

In this sense, and in the *American Journal of Psychiatry*, these authors speak of the "eventual prophylactic intent of anthropological studies." Indications that the eventuality is more immediate than appears at first glance are the astounding number of sub-cultures and cultural enclaves in the United States, the endless stream of ethnic minorities, the presence of acculturation, culture conflict and social change phenomena, and the interdisciplinary interest in the populations of our present day mental hospitals.

POSITIVE EMPHASES OF THE BIOSOCIAL POSITION

The question of whether the psychosocial position is founded upon, or even proceeds from the basis of any particular set of psychiatric theories, whether Freudian, Jungian, Rankian, Meyerian, or any other,—is an idle query. Today, such a view is open to objection because it is divisive and limiting. While a biosocial or psychosocial position is more selective than a mere amiable eclecticism, it is not conceived of, or intended as, an exclusive approach. A scientific method such as this attempts, by its very nature, to combine certain kinds of data and to synthesize relevant information.

Consequently, the biosocial position selects from among behavioral studies of man those which are well-founded in psychiatric knowledge, and, at the same time, are interdisciplinary in range. Immediately this rules out those psychological theories which run hopelessly aground on socio-cultural facts, or which limits their logical combinations and interpretations in theory. With equal force it eliminates socio-cultural theories which cannot make psychiatric or psychological sense. As a result, the reach of the psychosocial position, or its applicability, is not intended to promote any tendency to form "schools" in the form of special, delimiting viewpoints in psychiatry. There is even less intention to impose single methodologies, or insist upon predominantly specialized practices of treatment.

In this sense, the position merely serves notice that a body of fact, method, and theory does already exist which is interdisciplinary in character. As method, it may be used among others, or in judicious combination with others. In brief, the force of this theory and method is to view total personality in its total context, the latter con-noting psychiatrically relevant aspects of socio-cultural background. Indeed, this last concept is as important and novel today as were conceptions of the importance of the total contours of personality in the time, and the position, of Adolf Meyer.

Any such clearly defined position should announce its own particular methodologic cautions. In the first place, the psychosocial position warns that without this correction in perspectives on mental health, a certain myopia, noted by J. L. Halliday for other fields of medicine, can take hold and set limits to both the techniques of treatment and of prevention. On the other hand, a psychosocial synthesis in psychiatry, while opposed to overly-imaginative or oversimplified organicist emphases, does not simply ride a tide of psychological emphases in the mid-century psychiatry of the United States. Instead, it argues for scientific explorations on every conceivable front, neurological, experimental, physiological and biochemical.

A philosophy of science acknowledges historical and current progress and welcomes continued and balanced maturation in useful fields of inquiry. As is known, no field in medicine can proceed without organicist viewpoints and various kinds of experimentation. More positively, however, it is now known that certain methods of treatment, such as the psychoanalytic, the institutional push-therapies, biophysical and biochemical treatments, or supportive therapy are at one time, or for one patient, entirely appropriate, and at another time in a given course of treatment utterly inapplicable to him. For another patient, with a different illness, or the same general illness with different prognosis, the same course of treatment may be utterly inappropriate to his needs. For one, free association may be most destructive; for another, supportive therapy or push therapy may be wide of the mark. In the light of an enormous array of personality and illness variation, existing on the individual level, the psychosocial methods and insights apply throughout the range of mental disease phenomena, therefore, chiefly in the *planning* of a course of treatment. In addition, preventive psychiatry has much to utilize here in the improvement of marginal personality functioning, or in the possibility of the prevention of psychological disaster, as Lemkau and his associates envisage it. Rennie's work on prognosis in the psychoneuroses is, in this sense, a contribution in the realm of preventive medicine, as much as it is a comment on the possibilities of malign and beneficial results of certain kinds of treatment. The problems of treatment in psychiatry gain in perspective, according to Lemkau, when we begin to relate the hidden needs and status of a case, ordinarily adjudged in the light of psychodynamics, pathology, or personality functioning alone, with those external conditions, past and present, which have influenced individual personality.

At any rate, current methods and theories, founded in single disciplines, are often inadequate to the needs of institutional therapy which must cope with a variety of personalities, and disorders stemming from a variety of cultural contexts. Such methods are even more inadequate, when used singly, to the still larger task of providing data and practical techniques in the more challenging dimensions of preventive psychiatry.

A single example is apposite. In our discussions of certain African variations in incidence and psychopathology, we noted the Freudian theory of homosexual masking and paranoid projection and its possible wider application or greater relevance in Western European and American data from contemporary cultures. For the most part, African or even Brazilian or Bahian peoples lacked these symptoms. While such generic groupings as schizophrenias were still common in both settings, paranoid reaction forms were found frequently, in systematized types, only in the Euro-American data. Any reader of the two Kinsey reports, no matter how critical of their sampling and other statistical and conceptual shortcomings, (e.g., the use of orgasm as a unit measure of sexual behavior), will hardly fail to note the amount of homosexual behavior, temporary or sustained, which these reports record for American males and females. Apparently, this is not always latent, much less masked in interview, when it can become a coded and quantified part of a questionnaire method used by Kinsey and associates. If one is aware of the extent of these phenomena, overtly discussed by a large part of this non-randomized and geographically scattered population, subject to interview, he may only guess, in the absence of psychological and personality tests, how much latent or covert, masked homosexuality would exist in a stricter sample or cross-section of American population when studied more intensively.

Consider then, the latent and often covert homosexuality noted in many American psychiatric patients. This is frequently, without correcting for sub-cultural differentials, noticed as associated generally with a wide range of neurotic and psychotic disorders, and has been remarked especially for the schizophrenias showing paranoid reactions. But scientific curiosity, or demonstration and investigation cannot end here. For some time, such anthropologists as Clellan Ford and G. P. Murdock of Yale, working in the field of sexual behavior across cultural boundaries have pointed out that maturation and differentiation of the sexual drive is a matter, very largely, of social and cultural norms and standards. In other related contexts, cultural anthropologists have substantiated a corollary of this first principle and one which goes far beyond a mere Freudian pan-human approach. They have found, in a number of cultures, that children of given sex are virtually reared to identify with parent or with relatives of the same sex, but under such *varying* conditions in child-rearing and cultural practices as quite often produce within a group of children by-products of ambivalence or hate or fear. In some cultures, quite the opposite, the security of love and respect, and positive personal and sexual identifications become a strong central tendency in the psychology of the group. Frequently too, where the psychological valences are negative and destructive of positive identification, the cultural settings as they affect the socially sanctioned, adult sexual models (father; mother; or the mother's brother in a given clan system) are such that these adults are involved in settings, socially speaking, which produce discontinuities or negative emotions in the affective responses of the child.

Such a discontinuity in male identification, for example, was pointed out by Bronislaw Malinowski in one of his many Trobriand Island studies, *Sex and Repression in Savage Society.* Here initial acceptance by a father and positive male-child relationship to him were complicated, in the pubescent period, by the imposition of a mother's brother's authority with its strong overtones of sudden male authoritarian control and rejection. The entire Trobriand myth of the existence of a *Vada* cult, a projection of notions of organized female sorcery, is interesting in the light of this jarring of positive male identifications. So, too, are the "love magic" mechanisms which accompany male trading in inter-island *kula* trade-expeditions, and reported in *Argonauts of the Western Pacific* for males of this same cultural group. In the Trobriands, the same problem is traceable in the cultural notions of a somewhat feminized ideal male type; in the actual sexual practices; in the culturally elaborated denials of physiological paternity; and even in the religious system whereby *baloma* or spirits of the dead impregnate females in their reincarnations by entrance through the woman's head!

Returning to the African materials from certain regions of that continent, the suggestion is tempting that sexual non-identifications and misidentifications are there, by contrast, all the more absent, leaving such problems to Trobrianders or to Americans, chiefly because of differences in kinship structure and social organization which *vary* more in the areas of Africa considered from the model of the classical Oedipus complex. If Malinowski was hoping to speak for nonliterate cultures (in the sense of the title of his book), he chose a poor example, and one which understated his case for differences. He had reason, however, when he protested against pan-human Freudian appraisals. In BaThonga culture, where males also are chiefs and dominate the political and economic sphere, a case of masculine protest against women even more exaggerated than the *Vada* cult is found in their *Beloi* cult. Here too there are serious discontinuities in male identification. Other nonliterate cultures will show, variously, masking, or less overt homosexuality, or even a striking and healthy ignorance and disinterest in homosexual practices.

Our point is simply that research models in the life cycle exist for study in various cultures. All cultures do indeed balance off their statements of the situations bearing on sexual identifications, male or female, with parallel and, at the same time, different models of relationship with parent, siblings or relatives of *opposite* sex. Obviously, the actual balance of relationships to *same* and *opposite* sex operate together. This seeming preoccupation of anthropology with these family and kinship models of relationship, each in every culture with its inevitable guide to duties, obligations and feeling tones, has provided more grist for mills of doctrine on kinship and social organization than for carefully guided studies of the psychological consequences of such systems in which psychiatry and anthropology both participate.

Even though the Freudian system of generally invariant family relationships and dynamics needs to be reviewed and corrected, it appears that Freudian theory has nonetheless opened the door on a most important area of research. The relationship to parent of like sex is important for the individual, especially where conditions promoting identifications, misidentifications, or nonidentifications are culturally structured in easily recognizable form. G. W. Henry's study, *Sex Variants, a Study of Homosexual Patterns*, portrays case after case of such nonidentifications and misidentifications.[138] Even here, in a sample for which cultural background is not discussed or revealed, there are gross differences, for example, between the male *repelled from*, or hostile towards, the masculine role, and one whose emotional interests have been directed exclusively to members of his own sex. One is reminded of Horney's terminology, in another context, of "moving toward," "moving away from," or movement "against" other people, with its connotations, respectively, of warmth, withdrawal, and hostility. Here the misidentification pattern (the one whose interests are directed, in psychosexual behavior, away from those of members of his own sex) may engage in sporadic or active homosexual patterns or have such latent interests. In the two volumes of Henry's study; the first on male, and the second on female vari-

ants, the family constellations contributing to such groupings as he uses (bisexual, homosexual active and passive
and narcissism) are unmistakable in deciding the balance,
or difference, between those repelled from assuming a
mature bio-social role, and who therefore positively identify with the psychosexual role of the opposite sex (mis-
identify, in our terminology) and those who are nonidentified. There are also those who are confused as to
psychosexual role in the sense of being nonidentified, in
our terminology. In addition there are some whose
identifications and psychosexual affects are merely blurred
by lack of any truly satisfying relationships with the opposite sex in their prior history (partial identification). No
doubt the latter do not suffer the same degree of confusion
or distortion as to their basic identity.

In a recent British study of marriage and the family, a
research of considerable methodological sophistication,
J. H. Robb has presented the same guiding theory, namely,
the need to see *how* the family functions as a group, the
psychological relations which exist among its members,
and the resulting personality balances of its component
individuals.[139] Whether one accepts, in whole or in part,
a Freudian theory of identifications and misidentifications
(or the relation of these misidentifications to hostile paranoid projections), it is already abundantly clear that there
is no single model of family organization, cross-culturally,
which alone and inevitably operates for the entire human
species to bring one type of normalcy or one of sexual
aberration to the fore.

Since there is no intention here to confuse clinical cases
with normative cultures, let us say simply that a concept
of normality always varies with a cultural setting and the
conditions under which it functions. It is this setting which
determines the normative aspects of social and sexual roles.
The range of such variation has, as outer limits which pre-

vent an absolute relativity from operating, certain minimal needs of human beings. These are needs of both a biological and psychosocial nature. In every culture, even the most barren, there are means for obtaining a modicum of recreation, relaxation, and the harnessing of human expressive tendencies whether in art, music, drama, the social uses of leisure, games and sports, mythology, literature and the like. All societies regulate sexual, economic, religious, and social relationships. All contain family systems and classifications of kin as inner limits, while at the same time denoting wider systems of association, which, though having less affective force, particularly in formative years, are by no means always negligible in effects upon the family and the individual. Because of these variations, which are essentially differences in culture, there is no single family model, cross-culturally, bringing one type of normalcy, alone, or one of aberration to the fore. Within a culture, while family types are not absolutely identical, and while individuals differ in sexual, economic, religious and social behavior, there are nevertheless central tendencies in each of these phenomena which make them interdependent, roughly harmonious, and finally a system or type.

On the other hand, a cultural system, by its own inadequacies and "problems" (such as economic uncertainty, war, or kinds of inhumanity or hostility built in it) contains its own historically ordained ineptitudes or incomplete solutions. These problems may allow for the appearance of a range of acceptable social character in most persons, but produce notable aberrations in others. Of importance for social psychiatry is to plot the course, in the phrasing of Lemkau and his associates, for "comparing different developments in different cultures, so that something may be done to improve personalities in our own land." Different cultures contrast in the manner of promoting identifications with adult roles, and their statistical degree of success or failure points to specific variations in the structure and functioning of family and social group organization. We add that these particular social structures depend, for their success or failure, not merely upon universal intrapsychic mechanisms and functions, but upon the culture within which the specific family or group operates. Obviously, where one finds such symptom clusters as homosexual trends, aggressive wishes and projected hostility, the combination is intensely threatening to the patient. He, least of all, is in a position to assess the cultural factors without assistance. Yet even how he handles such trends varies from group to group, as Tooth's and Laubscher's data from Africa indicate. The latter component, which is in reality the basic psychodynamics of a case, depends equally upon the culture, one's experience in it, and the course of illness. This is what is meant by a careful assessment of the cultural factor in each case, and its contribution in restoring a greater sense of self-esteem, of kinship and belonging with others.

In discussing nonidentification and depersonalization trends, or indeed the feelings of unreality which accompany serious "loss of reality contact," it already appears that conditions of ambivalent love or hate in parental, or parent-surrogate roles, may be related to nonidentifications or misidentifications in the intrapsychic relationships as they are experienced between a child and parents (or parents, siblings, peers). But family systems, or their equivalents, do not end here. Family types not only contain within them the possibilities of this degree of systematization, but they contain as well a microcosm of all the prevailing relationships, which parallel or accompany these. Here it appears to students of mental hygiene that maternal relationships often are more important, and overshadow the case, apparently regardless of the sex of child and the total history of his adult role identifications. But the total balance of relationships with family members have a way of becoming mirrored in other extra-familial relationships. The phrasings, or content of theories about "schizophrenic patients of schizophrenogenic mothers" seems to eliminate the actual balances of relationships with both parents as experienced by a child of given sex and the extensions of relations to others. Bowlby's excellent work on the importance of maternal love in child care has overtones of such one-sided emphasis.

A cross-cultural investigation into family types associaated with serious psychopathology must be undertaken to determine, in schizophrenias, where both parents (or their surrogates) are so frequently hated, whether more intensified hostility toward parent of opposite sex is statistically favored. Possibly this is the case in more fundamentally disorganized schizophrenics since greater hatred of the parent of opposite sex is most destructive of latency-period, adolescence-period, and maturity-period opportunities for developing freely spontaneous libidinal or sublimated love relationships. Yet there are other relationships, to work, to recreational groups, and the like. If the theory of degrees of identification were demonstrable, the Freudian theory of the Oedipal conflict as being based inevitably on infantile sexuality and opposite sex attractions would be modified. With parent of same sex the least resented, in serious disorganization, the simple reading of the Oedipal theory would be open to serious question. Actually, psychoneurotics seem to fit this model of greater hostility towards parent of like sex, and to retain not only a degree of identification, but reality contact as well. In the schizophrenias, quite the contrary, the reality contacting agencies of perception, ideation, and emotional evaluation are all strikingly invaded, as a sense of identity becomes blurred or impaired, and as, frequently, body image, sexual identity, and adult social role performance, or even self-esteem, breaks under a battering of hostility sometimes directed outward, but always internalized as well and depressing in its internalized effects.

This formulation is reminiscent not only of the nuclear forms of the schizophrenias, even the short-lived forms of some nonliterate societies; with confusional blocking, acute acting-out of hostilities (external and internal), affective lability and its disorganized lack of control, repetitiveness in acts and speech, and bizarre, uncontrolled compensations against depression; but here also, according to some African materials, frank misidentifications occur as to sexual and adult roles. In modern cultures, by contrast, the schizophrenias seem to fall into this pattern on occasion, but today much more frequently, and particularly in American and Western European hospitals, the illness typology shifts in more pronounced fashion into patterns of sexual non-identification, or denials of misidentification, masked homosexuality, paranoid projection, and more systematized ideational disorders with the sexual confusions so rare in African hospitals so very pronounced in our own. In the light of the greater distance from reality evident in the latter cases, and their longer duration, or lack of spontaneous recoveries (as occur in African "confusional states"), it is hypothesized that greater hatred of parent of like sex often represents cases which show less systematized or florid pathology, even where acutely disordered. Greater spontaneity in recovering reality contact or fewer less intensively used defenses mark this simpler pathology. The more deeply channeled and jarring hostility towards members of the opposite sex may represent a greater measure of degree of misanthropy. What strikes us so frequently in cases productive of the higher degree of schizophrenic isolation, autism, and fantasy is the presence of a more disastrous illness, with paranoid overflow or projection, and its encapsulizing into a private world of one's own making.

Apparently, what W. A. White called "flight into reality" could better be renamed spontaneous recovery or reintegration in the nuclear schizophrenias where actual identity is less sweepingly challenged. On the other hand, the world becomes torturing, distasteful, and a really unreliable framework for existence in the degree to which a realistic self-identification in relation to others of like and opposite sex becomes unbearable. In this light, it is clear why "free association," probing, and the seeking of frank confessions are least applicable to those whose need for defenses is most frantic. The fallacies of hypostatization in Freudian theory may include not only that of an invariant form of family structure, or a single method for analysis of emotional disorder, but also a failure to recognize fully how easily one type of human relationship may color another. Beginnings were brilliantly made with the doctrines of transference and counter-transference. Yet neuroses and psychoses are indeed different in that perception, cognition and the affective life are invaded in the greater emotional disturbance of the latter. So, too, are human relationships more thoroughly disturbed. Even within a category as broad and general as the schizophrenias, cross-cultural perspective suggests a variance in typology based on degree of disturbance, a range in prognosis together with a variety of backgrounds, and qualitatively different forms of psychodynamics referable, it would seem, to different socio-cultural backgrounds.

There are, then, in addition to the usual intricacies of the physician-patient relationship, in some quarters too often delimited to discussions of transference and counter-transference, the further matter of what Sullivan called the "cultural handicaps to the work of the psychiatrist." These are partly resident in the particular quality of the personality and psychopathology of the patient, which a person of distinct background finds hard to assess; but they are also typical stock in trade, at other points, of the working relationships affecting the operations of the physician himself. While attempting to generalize only a few of these, Sullivan includes such cultural notions as the belief people are taught, in our society, "that they *ought not* need help." In the frankly more religious atmosphere of non-literate cultures, and often because many of these cultures stress cooperativeness in actual social relations, these constant necessities of propping up self-esteem are sometimes absent. Benedict has contrasted two types of modern culture,—the guilt reactions of Western Europe, implicit in individualism and the Protestant ethic (a Horneyan notion as well), and the shame and social-expiation culture such as is posited for the Japanese in *The Chrysanthemum and the Sword*. In our understanding of Japanese culture, the latter "sense of shame" comes within the guilt-framework. But even more important, there are cultures which produce less of the added effects of shame or guilt, or indeed a sense of foolish inadequacy, or defiant resentments. It is fruitless to ask of ourselves *how much* these overtones are basic personality responses and how much they are culturally induced. Anthropological studies, having a wide geographic range and intensive documentation, already indicate they are both at the same time. The answer cannot be given in more precise quantitative or qualitative terms until anthropology and psychiatry truly collaborate.

Destructive emotions are found in inextricable combination in both the traditional cultural or group scene and in the context of personal lives. From the point of view of mental health cross-culturally, these must be dealt with in the individual therapeutic situation, as well as in the field of preventive psychiatry. The further idea Sullivan notes for our cultural stock in trade, namely that people must know themselves "and be able to see through others" in respect to motivation is as reprehensible in the form of probing on the part of the inexperienced as it is in the form of neatly rationalized systems of guarded suspiciousness in urban patients of Western provenience. In turn, says Sullivan, the black and white, or airtight cultural value-concepts, like "good" versus "bad," "right" or "wrong," "the logical, right way," or fixed Horatio Alger notions of how people overcome limitations, mistakes, and misfortunes, impose burdens on the patient and often the unsuspecting physician which were not there originally. It is a fine line between an adjectival description of a patient's personality liabilities or lacks, (objectively defined failures in human relations) on the one hand, and a sense of hopelessness or defeat about his prognosis or management. Unfortunately, because of our own perfectionistic emphases in cultural value system, that fine line is sometimes not there.[140]

Even in the initial acceptance of, and attitudes towards psychiatry and its various schools and positions, there are cultural differences in patients' set and response. B. H. Roberts and J. K. Myers, writing on religion and nationality in relation to mental illness as determined in the New Haven Study, point out several different rates of disorder in ethnic groups which agree largely with R. W. Hyde's findings, in Boston, in the Forties. The data for New Haven, in 1950, suggested that psychoneurotic disorders were more frequent among Jewish people, whereas the rate of affective disorders in this group had fallen to the average of the total population of those in treatment, public or private. Alcoholism was most prevalent among the Irish. Illnesses of senescence, and affective disorders were higher in the foreign-born; while psychoneuroses, under treatment, were higher in the native-born group.

The schizophrenias, or psychoses with mental deficiency were not related to these social variables. However, since the study was limited to those in treatment at a particular time in 1950, and does not include a community survey of families and individuals, such findings are to be scrutinized from a standpoint different from the data of Hyde and associates. The authors note, and this may well affect the above data, that Jewish cultural values are more accepting of and consistent with the tenets of psychoanalytic thought than are, say, those of Irish.

This fact must be reflected in higher rates of psychoneuroses among the Jewish people *if only those in treatment comprise the universe studied.* Yet this finding, while of no epidemiological importance, is nevertheless significant in another light. Where no conflict exists between doctrine or belief on the one hand, and the style of therapy utilized, then the rate of those so treated will rise with no reflection on incidence rates. Therapies prevailing in reference to mental illness have rarely been studied from the point of view of their appropriateness in a given cultural value system. Both the Hyde study and the Roberts-Myers' publication find that Italians have high rates of affective disorders and illnesses of senescence with Irish "devoid of any psychoneurotic disorders." However, Roberts and Myers stop to note in addition the artifacts of the cultural situation in which Irish may very little use the techniques of psychoanalysis. Italians, quite often to effect marriages or maintain family reputation, will conceal such blots on the escutcheon as illness, physical or mental, in a family, or may forego treatment, again for cultural reasons, in such early periods of life. Even the aged among the Italians may more frequently rely upon home care as respected and honored members of the family. Consequently, among Italians, the ultimates of a disease process of old age may take their toll.[141]

Knowledge of a cultural value system is important both in designing epidemiological or etiological research on mental disorders.   It is one thing to note, in evaluating research *results*, that a group of given cultural background are over-represented, or else not represented adequately in the kind of data that has been gathered; it is another step, however, to design the means for locating the incidence or prevalence of psychoneuroses in an Irish population which is, by and large, not under treatment.   Similarly, one must cross-check the apparent over-representation of Jewish population in private treatment against their possibly lesser representation in psychiatric institutions. Even so, these cultural and religious categories can be re-examined in the light of other variables, such as socio-economic range, generation level and acculturation phenomena, or adaptation of the group in a particular milieu. Even the facilities and types of treatment available have local or geographic reference, so that for our American regions, the Jewish data on psychoneurotic illnesses under private treatment might be expected to vary again in the Deep South or American Northwest.   By and large, Irish may also show a greater use of facilities in the New York and New Haven area, where facilities are plentiful and frequently under Catholic guidance.   The same variance would exist in the other south and west regions.   Until these qualifications are noted for resulting data, and circumvented, where possible, in research design, confusions of cultural variations with those that are clinical will abound.   The regional or community sample is the best antidote to this difficulty.

Confusions of clinic and culture exist in other areas as well.   On quite a different level of interpretation, there are those who assume without much psychiatric data that since nonliterate cultures are not instinctual paradises, or are not otherwise perfect in minimizing problems of adjustment, that they therefore constitute a limitless happy hunting ground for the discovery of illness typology. Such expectations are shattered often by the variance from conditions in modern cultures. A schizophrenic with paranoid reaction-formation from the cultures of the Northwest Coast of North America (Kwakiutl, Tlingit, Tsimshian, etc.) was actually not common, according to available evidence, in days before large-scale culture contact. Since then, more such cases have occurred, but apparently in no huge numbers and with no greater rate of incidence than marks the occasional case in the acculturated parts of African and other regions. The author worked with a complete sample of such cases in a federal institution, the Morningside Hospital and Clinic, and found no direct one-to-one correspondence of clinical cases with aboriginal cultures which had been termed "megalomaniac" by Ruth Benedict. Until such far-fetched confusions or identities of "culture" and "clinic" are eliminated, the psychiatric profession will continue to doubt anthropological discussions of cultural ways of life as modeled on clinical prototypes. No real or permanently useful discussions of cultural backgrounds and their influences on mental disorder are available under such impressionistic methods which do not discriminate statistically between the people in society who are reasonably well in any functional rating scheme, and those who function inadequately because of mental ills. Terms like schizoid, paranoid, megalomaniac, or oral, anal, and genital do not begin to describe the healthy functioning in any culture, let alone its probable failures. This, too, is a positive emphasis of the psychosocial position. Again, in clinical prototypes of cultural systems, we are dealing with descriptive shorthand, but in this case a shorthand unfortunately used in application to massive and traditional ways of life built up over time by countless generations of a people.

I I

*The Psychology of Cultures
and Peoples*

3

The Psychology of Culture

IN AN EARLIER publication, the author stated:[142]

". . . From the standpoint of anthropology, *what* is repressed, *who* are or who become cathected targets of projection or introjection, or *what role models* are available for sublimation, —all of these conditions are matters which vary with the culture. In the same way, cultural analysis explores *how* it is that dependent, controlling, rejecting, hostile or brutalizing human relationships can develop in a society, family, or organization. The same analysis may reveal how typical processes of positive or negative identification are begun within cultural settings by studying respondents, informants or even patients as to their background. The failures or successes of super-ego or ego functioning occur in precisely this context. Once such factors are adequately and sympathetically understood, then adequate keys to etiology, therapy and possibly prevention are furnished."

It is doubtful, therefore, that the study of individualized mechanisms of defense, in separate and isolated cases, is enough to throw light on such matters as "typical processes" of identification in a culture, common characteristics of projection or introjection, or on successful super-ego functioning. In addition to specific cultural factors in pathology discussed above for certain peoples and historical periods, there is the whole question of the values and attitudes affecting behavior variations in healthy functioning. We have, as D. Mackay pointed out for East Africa, little conception of normalcy as it varies with culture or of the relativity of the normal. While anthropological literature, in the main, has not attacked the problem from the point of view of psychiatry and its interests, it contains highly contrasting pictures of family and kin organization, differing patterns of child-rearing, parental roles, and the handling of inter-generation conflict, as well as surprisingly variable kinds of expressivity and constriction of emotions on the level of action or the level of fantasy. Even the attitudes about physical and mental illness vary from culture to culture and thus affect both the discovery and the handling of illness.

In his abundant references to the psychopathology of everyday life, Freud showed clearly that defenses are used among the normally functioning, he himself offering a good part of the personal introspective material. On the other hand, institutions for the mentally ill are full of persons firmly convinced of their normalcy in all details and showing, particularly in the schizophrenias, a monotonous sameness in denials of emotional problems. So delicate are these emotional balances, and so extensive the protective and defensive mechanisms that at times an anxious distortion of reality to fit need-satisfying delusions becomes the actual "reality" for the patient. What Freud would call the "reinvesting of energy, the re-cathexis" does not always imply a reintegration of personality in which reality-testing starts up again on more productive and creative levels. Defensive and protective processes are often self-defeating. They not only exist in the normally functioning in vestigial form, but have various *degrees of organization and utilization* in the mentally ill. One has only to think of particular kinds of productivity in some geniuses; the chaotic sexuality of Leonardo da Vinci, the hypersensitivity and masochism of Van Gogh and de Maupassant, and the wrecked lives of Utrillo, Toulouse-Lautrec, Paganini, or Arthur Schnitzler; we realize the difficulty of assigning a functional rating to total personality. In the famous seventh Chapter of his major work on dream analysis, Freud characteristically showed this difficulty as it applied to all men. At the same time, he also evidenced a greater interest in the comparison of neurotic and psychotic functioning as to *similarities in the kinds of defenses utilized,* than attention to the *differences in their organization and utilization.*

No doubt, as Rennie points out, "normal individuals" use defensive mechanisms in rudimentary form to cope with inner conflicts and exceptional life strains. At the same time, he suggests, careful diagnoses based on clinical, psychodynamic evidence and observation are all the more important in venturing prognoses or selecting therapeutic means. The *organization* of such mechanisms and their *degree of mobilization* in the spare adjustive machinery of all men constitute the outstanding differential factor with which therapy actually must deal. Consequently, this is one approach to *differences* in psychopathology, and one important for therapy. While the temptation is great to read off into the everyday life of "normal people" in a culture the same kinds and intensities of defense utilization as exist in clinical cases, these last occur only in pathological form among the ill of that culture. In exactly the same manner, the problem for social psychiatry is to trace how a kind of rudimentary defense mechanism characteristically originates in the setting of "normative" cultural behavior, and how typically, in given conflicts and strained circumstances, it becomes further adumbrated and intensified. Thus preventive psychiatry cannot omit the so-called normally-functioning of a society, and is best prepared by a cultural knowledge of their conflictual needs, environmental stresses, and perpetuated family and community problems.

Rough similarities in the kinds of protective or defensive mechanisms humans use do not necessarily imply identities in total personality organization or functioning for every individual of a given culture. Let us look again at the engaging simplicity which motivates Freud's major work on dream analysis.[143]   By and large it assumes that the kinds of defenses at the disposal of "normal," neurotic and psychotic always originate in the same arenas of personal conflict, with the same action or purpose, the same effect, and presumably the selfsame conditions of environmental stress.   As for dream symbolizations, some of which undergo little distortion, (others to quote Sullivan, showing parataxic or prototaxic disguises and points of reference), these are not systematically studied as to any possible social and cultural points of origin, different characteristic settings for different life periods, or in terms of *particular* kinds of displacement, condensation or repression.   One is reminded of Sullivan's psychotic Italian patient whose father-authority symbol which "dominated" him was at one time "Columbus, admired and adventurous," later becoming The Big Man, and finally "any man." In this work, *The Interpretation of Dreams*, there is really little attention paid to neurophysiological problems like the physiology of sleep, sleep disturbances, or to social phenomena like the range of cultural fantasy materials. The variation by cultural background of distortion in different kinds of illness was not Freud's central interest. Yet it is a legitimate concern of psychotherapy.   There have been no decisive or definitive studies on a cultural level of these remarkable languages of symbolization and imagination in the mentally ill.   While psychoanalysis, then and now, typically subordinates questions of differential diagnosis and variable typology on a cultural basis to its more central interest in *pan-human mechanisms of psychological development*, it does so with insistence upon a particular kind of exploratory and interpretive technique in patients.   This single elaborated methodology is geared

primarily to certain kinds of neurotic illnesses found in
Europe and America, and is sometimes peculiarly inappropriate to other illnesses in other cultures, and even to
some life periods. Today one adds a concern for these
assets or liabilities of a case.

To cite certain obvious examples, among the Ute
Indians of Colorado, where dream analysis is the major
shamanistic technique, this Freudian method of exploration is reality bounded and socially sanctioned within
stated limits.[144] Sexual behavior also may be discussed
freely and frankly. However, methods aimed at reducing
periods of hospitalization in more serious illnesses of this
or any culture, a problem in Freud's time as in ours, are
not promoted by encouraging free associations in a rapidly
disorganizing personality. Where essentially private languages are used by schizophrenics, should one devote
endless time to following the neologistic language of a
desperate delusion? If lack of control over impulsivity,
whether it takes the form of an Irish patient's predilection
for projecting fantasy, or an Italian's for more direct motility and acting out of emotions, are these not *harmful*
modes of catharsis and *false* tactics of abreaction in serious
illness to be guarded against? Only a fuller study of the
assets or liabilities of the case, and therapeutic methods
aimed differently from these impulses will produce personality reintegrations. Knowing how patients may typically react implies knowledge of their cultural backgrounds.

It is futile to select a single method as *the* therapeutic
means. The etiological variations within such grand
clusters of illness typology as "the schizophrenias" require
further discrimination as to cultural background and the
disorders of emotional communication must be investigated in terms of *the kind of symbolic and emotional language
most often used* in each cultural setting. Certainly there are
cultural ranges, if not fixations, which are systems of

thought and action. The specific, individual case, always the start of significant research, may be grouped with others as to etiology and background factors. It is felt that such groupings and classifications are possibly more meaningful than the generous and all-embracing diagnostic labels.

While vast insights were developed in the Freudian movement, and in other psychiatric theories, the drive in the former movement towards a unitary theory of pan-human psychic development was premature. The universal theory did not adequately account for variations in human behavior across cultural lines, or between different disease processes, or even within a range of symbolic mechanisms of interpersonal communication. It had little to say about positive aspects of culture in interpersonal relations for creative and productive purposes. In this light it is curious that many anthropologists attracted to psychiatry (and several psychiatrists attracted to anthropological data) have settled upon theories of infantile disciplines to explain whole cultures in a highly simplistic fashion. If one goes beyond cultural and disease differentiation to an actual study of symbolic mechanisms resident in different types of families by matched samples of well and ill, the psychological impressionism disappears. As a matter of fact, in most existing studies, psychotic, psychoneurotic and "normal" are rarely distinguished, let alone sampled, matched for control of variables, or studied by family type at all.

In spite of this, one can speak of the existence of various useful therapeutic methods, and indeed, of the "peaceful coexistence in our times" of techniques which are in one case physiological, in another neurological, in another environmental or psychological. No one of these, as technique, type of analysis, or approach to human behavioral problems, is alone sufficient to cope with what

Malraux once called the human predicament in general. The fact is that man *is* an animal of great biological and psychic complexity. Exclusive reliance upon a single tool of analysis, whether biological or psychological, can be greatly misleading. On one level, that of the general psychic unity of mankind (popular in German anthropology in the time of Adolf Bastian), a rigid "Freudian" can overlook the crucial difference between an individual whose *past* defense structure can be maintained even where it now looks fragile, a second person capable of reeducation and a third who has already moved, or may move, full-arc from rigid and obsessive maintenance of constricted, hostile and compulsively-stereotyped relations with others, on to withdrawal, depersonalization feelings, further loss of reality contact and self-esteem to full projection of inner conflicts and delusional ideation. The former may be a way point, potentially, to the latter more disorganizing and paralyzing sort of illness, but the integrations are of three types, their styles of functioning quite different, and the three patients have needs, personality structures, defense organizations, and general adequacy for one kind of treatment or another that will vary.

In Kardiner's works, *The Psychological Frontiers of Society* and *The Individual and His Culture*, we learn that cultures also produce or promote forms of emotional expressivity, folklore, arts and religions, even where these have the character of group *projections*. Whether these are cultural safety valves, in the Freudian sense of displacements, compensations, or distortions, or whether they represent within the boundaries of modified Freudian theory, productive and creative urges, is, of course, a crucial question. Certainly the arts often exist far beyond the bounds of distortion, and may indeed transmit humor, insight, education, relaxation, or the creative mobilization of energies to those who benefit from them. Equally, it may be doubted whether religions, in the Durkheim sense of *a social institution*, or in Malinowski's of a force making for cultural integration are merely psychological excrescences of physiological urges or the inevitable results of infant disciplines. We may note variations among Mohammedans, Catholics, or Protestants, Buddhists, Jews, Shintoists or Animists depending on regional cultures. Religious psychology is not biologically or fatefully beyond good or evil.[145] It is highly probable that human defenses and uncertainties get established as modes of thought, emotion or action in the texture of whole cultures. But this applies to law, to economics, and to political structures as well as to the artistic and the religious. One has only to mention along with ritual compulsives and the work of imagination, hostile competitiveness, meaningless constrictions and taboos on positive or creative human expression, and the compulsive production and adherence to sterotypes. Where ritual interests are suffused with artistic or economic ones in cultures having little science and technology, or where shamanistic religions function in lieu of medicine and psychiatry, the anthropologist has little clear evidence of the projections being parataxic distortions. Perhaps this is why "primitives" have no Sundays or do have sincere and compelling forms of art connected with myth and ritual. Among them, it is frequently the large scale scientific and technical innovation that challenges religious forms.

On another level, that of emotional form and content in different cultures, the pan-human theory has further difficulties. When a certain number of Chinese schoolboys smile engagingly during a reprimand of the master, and mean by this the acme of respect and concern for their ineptitudes, there is some qualification upon the meaning of serious respect for all mortals. When an Apache Indian, in the white heat of uncontrolled anger, drops his voice to a scarcely audible whisper, he is about to convert verbal anger to serious assault. Dropping from a loud voice, or lowering the voice, means quite the opposite with us. When a tears-greeting in a third culture is accompanied by a copious flood of real tears, and the person doing the greeting falls weeping into the lap of a visitor, he is being assured of a hearty welcome, the utmost hospitality, and a positive attitude at his arrival. The language of emotions varies so markedly that a Masai warrior of standing will honor a young novice by spitting in his face. An Eskimo will show sincere concern and respect for the aged and infirm by abandoning them to die before they grow older. And a Siamese lady will show her breeding and respect for visitors by refraining from pointing her feet in their direction. Among the Tuaregs, noblewomen of the warrior caste frequently led men into battle or presided with the stringed instrument at medieval love courts; if the men, who wore the veils, accidentally showed their faces above or below the eyes, this was considered immodest in the extreme. Among the Japanese, where thwarted love led frequently to double suicides of the couple concerned, or where the chief item of classical fiction by the Lady Murasaki, *The Tale of Genji*, is a protracted account of courtly liaisons, assignations, and fervid letters of passion and feeling, the very notion of kissing in public is shameful and disgusting, whereas public nudity in town or village baths is a matter of no consequence. In Japanese hotels, even today, the most staid male guests are asked, with utmost decorum by equally staid chambermaids, if they wish to be undressed. Among the Ute Indians, female breasts have no sexual significance; and in another context of this culture the dead are best honored by Ute relatives forgetting them immediately. A visitor to Italian opera in the smaller locales of South Italy will witness an audience empathizing in a most emphatic and audible manner. And religious practitioners in a range of cultures do not worship supernaturals at a respectful distance; they control them, evoke them, imitate and incorporate them with pleadings, cajoling, commanding, and mimicry.

Just as there is no single language of appropriate emotions or the means to their expression, so no society is built, as Benedict implied in *Patterns of Culture*, out of one process of psychological selectivity from merely one range of emotional expression. Despite naive assumptions of wholly cooperative or wholly competitive cultures, none can be built forever on hostile, competitive lines, the Melanesian Dobuans to the contrary notwithstanding. In each culture, some unities and peer-group associations operate to facilitate creativity. It is interesting to read Benedict's picturing of the raw competitiveness of the Kwakiutl and in Middletown, and then to read Sapir's or Boas' account of the vast amount of cooperation within the *numaym* (bilateral kingroup) of the commoners in terms of whose labors the chief's potlatches (competitive give-aways) can only originate, or really ultimately benefit. In Boas' discussion, the background of these customs was in real warfare among coastal village sites. In Sapir's parallel descriptions of Northwest Coast social organization, the real economic privilege, along with the prestige symbols, is clearly described. Among the Nootka, *topati*, or prerogatives, are both real and tangible, as well as prestigeful. Under modern conditions, it is clear why both warfare has now ceased and yet group production and competition has continued. These social integrations of a cultural group are classified by the anthropologist, Radcliffe-Brown, who claimed them to be more beneficial in counteracting competitive and divisive incursions into social solidarity and mutual interest where they promote *closer* solidarity and cohesion. He regards them as being more important for human society in general where they become *wider* in effective extent.

This interest in the functional integration of social structures has become a dominant ideation of British social anthropology. When even a highly segmented social structure like the Japanese of the Meiji period (with authoritarian controls, fixed classes, an outcaste *eta* group and attendant or buttressing custom and etiquette) contained, as John Embree showed in *Suye Mura*, remarkable patterns of mutual aid, social solidarity, village cooperativeness, and family unity, then clearly one may speak of social integrations which are segmented on one level and cooperative on another.

In one experiment unfortunately visited on Japanese-Americans, the values of social solidarity, cooperativeness, family unity, and organizational ability were clearly shown among Japanese who came primarily from rural and fishing villages of Hiroshima and Wakayama provinces.[146] If the village level contains and defines these positive values, they may, for Japan as a whole, be widely represented in the common total of population.

In much the same way, when the anthropologist studies the folklore and arts of a people, he finds himself close to the channels of positive human expression as lived in a culture in its most enduring forms. When we turn next to the more negative components of cultures, we find that the destructiveness, in Rado's sense, rarely accounts for the whole cultural tradition. Stereotypes like passive-dependent Pueblo Indian, the paranoid Kwakiutl, and the hostile Dobuan fade from view. In the cultural life of people, a compulsive adherence to stereotypes, a substitution of myth and delusion for reality, or a Nazi transformation of people into godly paranoids are, respectively, hostile gestures, cultural distortions, social aggressions and deadly fears which last only as long as a willful turning away from realities of world history can last. When once they fall from the sheer weight of distortion, the social and cultural life of a people does not end, at least it has not as yet. In brief, whatever important qualities of character and temperament are characteristically developed in a cultural setting, they are found simultaneously on both levels of human action, the individual and the cultural. On the cultural level, most people in most cultures have the necessary modicum of functional good health. In cultures, as with individuals, only when this ceases to be the case are the dire predictions of a Toynbee then in order.

However, the analogy of culture and the individual must end here. The two phenomena are different. The tendency of R. H. Lowie in his *Social Organization* or of Malinowski in much of his writing to ascribe a biological need basis to culture points to a truth, but not the whole truth. Other human gregarious needs, beyond the confines of individual biology, are supplied by culture. The arts, science, religion, philosophy, relaxation and recreation supplement sexual, nutritive, shelter and protection requirements of man. The various social, religious, artistic and other organizations by which these are achieved constitute a first and additional step in analysis which goes beyond biological man and which immediately separates him from his primate brethren. When we proceed to the level of communication and expression in whole cultures, the latter become irreducible to individual personalities. More careful statistical methods of grouping and estimating personality variations are then necessitated.

In anthropology, the clinical model of a particular kind of personality disorder has too often provided a yardstick for assessing "culture and personality." Types of aberrancy common in Western European and American cultures erroneously provide "clues" to the understanding not merely of clinical typologies, but cultural ones as well. By claiming a close correspondence between the clinical model showing predisposition towards extreme forms of psychotic behavior and adult personality, the culture is so stereotyped.[147] Edward Sapir, who founded culture and personality research in anthropology, warned repeatedly against viewing cultures, by simple analogy, as being obsessive, hysterical, paranoid, and the like.[148] While the cross-cultural comparisons can probably never end in a purely relativistic set of conclusions, and the "normalcy" of one become the aberration of another, neither can they be reduced by analogy to a clinical model of a personality disorder. Comparisons of the prevalent psychopathology developed in cultural frameworks show these to differ, but here prevalence or incidence must not be assumed. The epidemiological yardstick is the number of persons of given biological and social characteristics becoming ill in a given period of time. Anthropologists interested in culture and personality must recognize this principle of the medical and health sciences.

In the same fashion, it is doubtful whether data on isolated cultures, or isolated humans in a non-representative series, can furnish the kind of information required to establish a science relating to the psychology of cultures and peoples. Epidemiological exactitude is one necessity, but cross-cultural comparison, controlling variables other than the cultural is likewise desirable. There is face validity to the proposition that humans, living in families and social groups of a culture, fall into a continuum from well to ill. Their interpersonal communications, with language or with other symbolic means commonly defined, add to the basic determinants of their biological natures and material culture all those elements of meaning and emotion, character and temperament which make them what they are. While it is common to speak of these cultural affairs as the traditional superstructure of social living, traditions change and "super-structure" need not connote remoteness.

Human organization and functioning, in social and cultural contexts, is more than bodily need and physical impulse. One has only to think of the Navajo who will starve rather than eat fish, or the broken taboo which in Polynesia should lead, and often does, to death. In exactly this sense of cultural complexity to regulate behavior by non-biological proscriptions and prescribed conduct, culture becomes irreducible to mechanisms of defense (the Freudian view), or to neat, patented resolutions of all conflict. For most persons, the invitation to all sorts of cultural activity is accepted unconsciously and easily, and the inevitable coin of the realm of behavior is cultural coin even without their examination of it. However, while personal meanings, conscious or unconscious, intrude into this well-populated area of social personality, they do not ordinarily alter or change the course of traditional, "normal" functioning. Still less, do the personal meanings disrupt or swerve a history built up by countless generations. An individual's "culture" or sub-culture may vary uniquely from these norms with hardly a ripple in the stream of history. Cultural analysis is always this first necessary and preliminary bow to the human scene at its most commonplace. When the generic cultural factors are established, there are then reference points or norms *against which personalized psychologies can be studied.* In such studies, the individual is observed in his actual human and social relationships within patterns that are never wholly of his making. If we are to know him at all, his meanings and those larger meanings which are cultural play as light and shadow, foreground and background, or as texture and form constituting the complete picture.

The chief limitation of the Freudian view is that it was not geared to these necessities of a larger perspective. Partly for this reason, as Kluckhohn has implied, cultural anthropology was most often associated with the modified, more recent wings of the psychoanalytic movement.[149] However, both fields historically established earlier relationships in subject matter and method. Psychoanalytic theory as first promulgated by Freud and his circle was in agreement with the basic position and even the data of Nineteenth Century anthropology. In both, originally, the conception of man's mind (and his culture *as consequence*) were envisaged as developing in a biologically predetermined evolution through stages from infancy to maturity. In both, the legacy of this childhood and of man's early social development were found in survivals to later stages. Spencerians spoke of savagery as the childhood of man, calling this early development a time of simple, undifferentiated impulse and biologically conditioned action. Psychoanalysis spoke of the neurotic as "regressed to primitive stages" of thought. In one early psychoanalytic system, *the* child was virtually caricatured as rehearsing the past of his "race" by virtue of a primordial "mass psyche" imbedded in him. In this fatefully pessimistic system, the savage, the child, and the neurotic were compared, as fantasy-ridden, a prey to physical impulse. Children and the adults of remote cultures were said to be emotionally and morally "undifferentiated," or in Spencerian terms, naively egoistic, irrational, uncooperative, and incapable of finer discriminations. The appropriateness of childhood fantasy in the development of a more adult statement of human insight and imagination, or the uses of childhood confusions in the absence of full, mature information; their spontaneous impulses in the presence of rapid growth and high energy utilization, all of these factors in child maturation were not fully appreciated in this humorless drive towards a system. In *The Problem of Lay Analysis*, Freud asks seriously whether the "soul-life" of present day children does not reflect "the same archaic moments" that prevailed "at the time of early civilizations." The answer from both psychology and anthropology has long been an emphatic negative.

Today, we see the simplicity of both schemes in anthropology and psychoanalysis as reflecting the success of Darwinism in the decade before. The popularity, in Freud's day, of such highly systematized and imaginative works as Andrew Lang and Atkinson's *Social Origins and Primal Law* are noted as a chief source of his own *Totem and Taboo* in their immistakable similarity. This work, by Andrew Lang and J. J. Atkinson, was published in 1903, and antedated by a dozen years Freud's *Totem and Taboo* which belongs to the period 1912-1913. In it, a "pre-totemic race" unaware of incest or exogamy is first posited along with the familiar promiscuous Cyclopean horde, the dominance of the older men, and the jealousy of a youthful band of classificatory kin-brothers. Next come the inevitable parricidal acts. With the functioning of guilt mechanisms and ritual displacements is born the totemistic injunction against killing and eating an ancestral animal and symbolic figure. Along with these guilts and rituals emerge incest regulation, exogamy, religion and ethics in the real functioning social world. No wonder J. C. Flügel, in his *Freudian Mechanisms as Factors in Moral Development*, could, with a sense of security about his anthropological data, incorporate this same theme of equating the primitive, the child, and the neurotic. As late as 1924, in his address before the Royal Anthropological Institute in London, Ernest Jones reiterated the same points.

In place of mental stages, biological and mental in essence, one today notes the important effects of culture upon individuals throughout the life course. Instead of an unvarying notion of child development, transcending cultures and world history back to an "archaic past," today we consider developmental needs of children in relation to cultural and social situations, unconnected to a hypostatized "primitive mind." Specific background factors and influences can be tested for their effects upon mental, emotional and ethical growth. Mind, as such, is in one sense mental functioning, to be sure, but it is even more crucially an *organization* of beliefs, attitudes, perceptions, meanings and emotions derived from social and interpersonal experiences in a particular setting. In place of defenses that mark *stages* of mental functioning, the anthropologist adds a broader category, namely the typical patterns of response and expressivity that individuals of a culture utilize in the most characteristic business of living. These, of course, include defenses. But in addition they include patterns of response to infant and child-rearing methods, to family and kinship organization, to parental roles and the handling of inter-generation conflict, and to the more subtle influences in any culture which promote or constrict the handling of emotions, impulses, or attitudes. Terms like education, physical or mental illness, sexual expression, or work and leisure, all connote mental processes. Since a culture, by its very nature, will provide characteristic modes of harnessing human energy and will relate typical problems to typical solutions, no meaningful life experiences within its boundaries, whether birth, growth, maturation, or death, are free from its affective charges. The latter, far from occurring only in an individual arena of unique "experience," are bound inevitably to human interrelationships, or in short, to the realities imposed upon individuals by group phenomena. Commonly defined meanings and sanctioned behavior favored by the group in its manner of maintaining itself or its members affect all mankind.

In this light, the expressive symbolism and folk art of a given culture has a function and type of expressivity impossible to disconnect from the realities, or "conditions," of the culture. To cite a single example, in hunting and gathering societies marked by marginal living (Australian,

African Bushman, South American Siriono, American Ute and Apache) the very nomadism means there will be no adjustment of means to remote ends. Ceremonies are often dramatic or mimetic of nature, and religion involves direct contacts with an animated (we say animistic), highly anthropomorphic set of supernaturals. All this John Dewey noted in his *Philosophy and Civilization* where he discussed such variations. The contrast to Indian Pueblos and their ceremonial of group formation with its air of sculptural inevitability and the *ethos* of restraint, cooperation and sobriety was noted both by Dewey and Ruth Benedict and applied by the latter to the whole society. These are people with priesthoods; not, as with the hunters and gatherers, people who act directly. Instead they plant, and wait, and pray. They live as a village with sanctions against competitiveness. And their cultures have no more in common with hunters and gatherers than they have in common with Italian, German, Irish, or Hungarian. They leave to those of the list labeled nomadic all the dramatic or vividly mimetic elements in religious ceremonies.

These comparisons and the typology implied in modern cultural anthropology are far from Freud's source of stages in work by Lang and Atkinson. In *Social Origins and Primal Law*, or in Freud's other sources, such as Frazer's *Golden Bough*, imaginative authors had postulated the existence of what they termed a Cyclopean, original "family" in earliest times. They did so not to describe a given known culture, but to categorize several. Dominant males in possession of the females, until vanquished and slain by younger males, do not characterize the male population of any known culture. The parallel of Nineteenth Century anthropology to the Oedipus myth or to *Totem and Taboo* is clear, but no psychology of any individual or any culture has been depicted. Even totemism as the thinly-veiled ritual projection of a life-drama does not describe any totemistic people. In the Freudian version, both parricide and incest occur, followed by poignant regret. Culture, religion, morality and a social sense flow from this more lurid and phylogenetic version of Oedipus. The account is poetic, and one anthropological reviewer, Goldenweiser, suggested Freud only poetically over-embroidered an imaginative elaboration. In some circles the same embroidering still continues, however. Culture has appeared on the scene as the merest epiphenomenon. It becomes a consequence of psychology, not a cause.

Others, like Rank and Róheim, saw Oedipal structure growing out of ontogenetic factors, birth-trauma or "resistance against" cellular fission processes in the embryo. Such bizarre psycho-biological theories signalized the danger of moving a theory of cultural behavior *away from* legitimate concerns of social psychiatry and *in the direction* of an ontological straightjacket. By the 1920's, when English translations of *Totem and Taboo* were being reviewed, Kroeber, accepting Freudian mechanisms like repression, regression, or sublimation, nevertheless pointed out that no known culture started on a sheer libidinal premise of dominant male strength. One might have added that in culture, with weapons and tools, all Goliaths have their Davids; others simply noted the frequently *fixed* monogamic marital forms in the simplest known peoples (whether Australians, or Andaman Islanders who lacked fire). While S. Zuckerman's studies of social functioning, in *The Social Life of Monkeys and Apes*, correspond to "primitive life" according to Freud or Lang and Atkinson, the simplest human cultures do not. Instead, the family and exogamy of one sort or another always prevail.

Totem and Taboo was translated during World War I. Freud, in the *Problem of Lay Analysis* could note that Theodore Reik and Géza Róheim, the ethnologist, "have taken up the line of thought . . . developed in *Totem and Taboo* and, in a series of important works have extended or corrected it." While Freud was right in the assertion that Rank, Róheim and others were extending his theories beyond *Totem and Taboo*, it was apparent that they were modifying these in a more clearly ethnological direction. Today *Totem and Taboo* can only be reviewed as poetic fantasy.

The deluge came in the 1920's. Besides the sharply critical reviews of *Totem and Taboo* by Kroeber and Goldenweiser, a third anthropologist, Malinowski, then in England, published a series of extended studies of a Melanesian people, the Trobriand Islanders. One of these volumes, *Sex and Repression*, was devoted to a masterful rebuttal of *Totem and Taboo*. In brief, as Kroeber had suggested, libidinal attachments and revulsions were not always charted as in the family of Oedipus Rex or Austrian Vienna. In the Trobriands, there was no father-authoritarian. The word for father there meant *tamakava*, "stranger in my village," a village under a matrilineal kinship system. While father was a cherishing companion for an infant, male or female, the mother's brother and his kin were feared from adolescence on by either girl or boy in an economy which centered in a maternal uncle's needs, demands and orders. The subsequent discussion of different kinds of family constellations the world over was a healthy revision of Freud's fixed stages, single origin point, and uniform psychodynamics throughout the world. Perhaps no discussion of culture was more prone to regard culture as an afterthought, an epiphenomenon, than Freud's in *Totem and Taboo* and none shattered as dramatically against the hard facts of cultural relativity.

However, Freud's discussion of the presence of emotional mechanisms connected with family structure (although of one type), of sex role identification, of child training or conditioning, and of the affective importance of one kind of family functioning were still of tremendous value. Even if the role of culture was hopelessly confused with a resultant of innate and inevitable psychological processes, and even though fixed, rigid modes of behavior were referred to "mass psyche" phylogenetically derived, the dynamic system soon proved flexible enough for useful modifications. While Karl Abraham enthused over the response of language (its emphasis on gender), to the Oedipal situation, anthropologists piled up evidence from a hundred languages (Algonquin, Athabaskan, Hungarian, and Bantu) to the effect that sex gender was often not the system of classification. While *Totem and Taboo* had set a dead stamp on all human behavior, later psychiatrists of a modified psychoanalytic persuasion, like James Clark Moloney, the Leightons, Joseph and Murray, were willing to go to other cultural scenes to study the actual and variable behavior of human beings.

Following critiques of *Totem and Taboo*, Freud revised his system in *The Ego and The Id*. This volume is of fundamental importance in the Freudian system because it explicitly stated a turning point, in which, to ego, id, and ego-ideal formulations was added the super-ego. The super-ego, the new element, was phrased ultimately as "the heir of the Oedipus complex, and represents ethical standards of mankind." This bowing out of Oedipus, and the substitution of an initial formulation on cultural value systems, was most important as an insight into personality backgrounds, even though it never came to be used for extending research perspectives self-consciously in the direction of social personality concepts.

In this new work, Freud's ego-ideal formulations are of interest as for example: "The tension between the demands of conscience and the actual attainments of the ego is experienced as a sense of guilt." In another place Freud asserts, "Social feelings rest on a foundation of identification with others, on the basis of an ego-ideal in *common* with them." What is common and shared? The answer is certainly cultural experience and values. No longer is this simply an individual psychology or individualized psychiatry. What Clara Thompson refers to in her book on psychoanalysis, where she marshals the trends toward what she calls the healthy"revisionists" of orthodox Freudianism by alluding to Horney, Fromm and Sullivan is exactly this type of theoretical revision. It is what Fromm develops in his concept of social character, or Sullivan in his frequent references to social relations.

In anthropology, the same trends have been noticeable. Culture, as generator and judge of the normal and abnormal in behavior, is no idle reification once we realize that real cultures, real sub-cultures and real people lie at the heart of the system. A personality, as Sapir once put it, "is carved out by the subtle interactions of those systems of ideas characteristic of a culture as a whole, as well as those systems of ideas which get established for the individual through more special types of participation with the physical and psychological needs of the individual organism." These Sapir calls "individual sub-cultures." They are Freud's egos. Sapir's culture as a whole is Freud's ego-ideal. Sapir goes on, we think to more crucial statements of what is involved in the interrelation of culture and mental illness. Rather than a one-to-one relationship, he writes as follows: "The personal meaning of the symbolisms of an individual's sub-culture are constantly being reaffirmed by society, or at least he likes to think they are. When they obviously cease to be, he loses his orientation—a system of sorts remains and causes his alienation from an impossible world."

What is needed to fill the framework of interdisciplinary

collaboration are two things beyond the uses of anthropology and psychiatry which Sapir implies. One is the necessity for psychiatry systematically to gather data on social and cultural backgrounds and systems of meaning which configure always in the background of real cases. The second is the necessity for anthropology to become sensitized not merely to the cultural backgrounds from which cases emerge, but to the typical modalities of mental functioning in human beings. The common ground we refer to, simply, as psychodynamics, requires, in other words, adequate medical psychiatric analysis of real people and real cases against a background of cultural understanding.

One final word. Anthropology speaks often of the "unconscious patterning of behavior in society" (the title of a famous paper of Sapir). A primitive is unconscious of the grammar of the language he speaks—though it is there; of kinship systems having symmetry, though they have; or of regularities in many realms of behavior. Besides the importance of unconscious processes—for both fields— there is the point that much of the content of culture, like the content of minds, is symbolic: the X that stands for functions, activities, movements, and expressions of human energy which are cultural in the first instance. The dream, the image, the belief, the action pattern are, in the individual, most often symbols in terms of which activity is expressed and lives are lived.

Obviously, defense mechanisms may figure in this study, but must be recognized as developing, if at all, within the framework of a larger conception of ego-organization which is culturally variable and corresponds roughly to the Sherif-Cantril psychology of ego-involvements. Cognitive *attitudes*, to judge by the enormous data of psychiatry, influence both cognition and perception on the level of the way in which persons of different culture interpret events, see objects or hear sounds within the normal range. In like manner, where distortions of events, or hallucinatory behavior occurs, as in the schizophrenias, cognitive attitudes have undergone distinctive changes. In the perception project of the Menninger Clinic, George S. Klein, Philip Holtzman and Diana Laskin write as follows:[150]

"... Much of our work assumes that ego organization (*id* becoming 'secondary,' M. K. O.) is in part a network of controls organized to modulate claims of drive and reality. In psychoanalytic theory, impulse control has been discussed mainly in terms of defense. It seemed important to investigate the possible function of cognitive controls observed in our laboratory situation for the delay and discharge of need-tension. The question is relevant also to the general issue of structural constraints upon the directive influence of needs. Thus a series of experiments demonstrate that the effects exerted by the need in perceptual-associative behavior are distinctly different where the cognitive attitudes and adaptive problems vary. These studies and others seem to suggest that a wide variety of controls, *of which defenses may only be one form* (My italics, M.K.O.) *condition the working of need and drive and behavior*. These studies have contributed to our attempts to establish more explicit links to the psychoanalytic framework. For instance, it does not seem likely that the concept of defense, even 'autonomous' defense in the psychoanalytic literature is wholly adequate to describe the regulative strategies that subjects have shown in our perceptual tasks."

While several authors, Heinz Hartmann,[151] Ernst Kris,[152] and David Rapaport,[153] in their writings on ego-autonomy and problems of human adaptation, have tended to speak of personality functions not exclusively related to conflicting drives, Klein and his associates have attacked problems in perception and cognition as being not merely autonomous, but as being "themselves idiosyncratically organized within peoples into 'styles' or regulative principles."

The problem may not be whether Italians or Irish become entangled in personal conflicts, or repress, but rather *what* and equally important, *how* they repress, *how* they convert energies or direct them, and *what* cognitive attitudes and outlooks motivate them. These regulatory and control functions, no matter how much they become internalized in individual personality, have, as outer limits the cultural backgrounds, themselves uniquely organized into "styles and regulative principles." Although there is no need to assume a one-to-one correlation between the regulative principles and styles of thought, attitude and emotion in a culture and among its component individuals, we can still seek in each individual, as indeed psychiatry does, the really constructive forces or the assets within him, and note where these provide a bridge back to culturally shared traits. At the same time, what Fromm has called the "culturally patterned defect," (the pathological *tendencies* which a combination of cultural and psychiatric method may bring to light even in the study of the so-called normal) represents one set of factors in terms of which goal-selection, role fulfillment, concepts and cognitive attitudes, and even styles of emotional expression will necessarily vary. Thus a culture which is, at the present point in history, widely predisposing to conditions that breed disturbances in one's relations to others, or in the self-identification, goal orientation, family and social roles of the sexes and status groups within its social matrices, will reap the consequences of widespread compulsions, almost obsessional fears, patterned hostilities, and conflicting sets of motives. When these operate from individual to individual, they become reflected in the variances of incidence and types of disorder we have seen exist historically in the annals of human maladjustment.

In a more positive sense, every people and culture bring their own gifted solutions, their own unifying philosophy, to each individual at any point in his history. A person may give to this life-way, or this world view, his own interpretation in its affective dimensions. But he can no more create it from the outset than any one individual can design from the whole cloth of personalized abstractions any cultural product. If he can synthesize and integrate ideas, perceptions and emotions at all, he must do so in a manner and with an interpretation culled from experience in a larger more or less systematic patterning of human reactions about him. These premises of behavior and human relations are not learned by rote, and it is fruitless to assume as Hsu has done,[154] that in one culture a mechanism like repression generally operates, while in another suppression alone is the touchstone of existence.

Rather the regulatory controls, the styles of expression, the ordained goals and social role behavior are defined within the definition of the situation (its meanings and communicated symbols) long before anyone of us is privileged to select and construct a life pattern, or indeed, add personal understanding and interpretation to it. These dominant conceptions and assumptions of a culture, its group aspirations, religious lore, science, technique, custom, and ethical code may be internalized through unconscious habit in consistent patterns, as presumed by Benedict in *Patterns of Culture*, or they may contain the very inconsistencies, conflicts, outlines and demarcations which make a strain towards consistency more difficult in the individual case. It is the latter which defines cultural psychopathology, the culturally patterned defect, not the existence of one clinically defined type of aberration, deposited in the culture initially and then discovered by a selective description. Culture and psychology do not stand in even relationship, as effect and cause, cause and effect. While the way of life of a people may achieve internal coherence and unconscious canons of choice develop within it, culture is still an instrument in the adjustment of man and nature which mediates to achieve control, solve the problems of social conduct, economy, politics, religion and philosophy, and regulate behavior.

Any concept of national character, like any other concept, is real only insofar as it investigates, understands and communicates the dynamic working of a kind, or kinds of phenomena. If the individual and his culture are more than "interacting," in the language of early Twentieth Century sociology, and it appears that they are, then the structure of a personality and that of the culture from which it emanates, are caught in the same contexts, face the same problems, and develop the same general patterns and modes of action as solutions. Basic to any discussion of psychodynamics in a person are the modalities, biological, psychological, and social, governing the workings of need, drive and behavior. Over-individualized psychological systems minimize such central tendencies. Central tendencies, whether biological, or psychological and social, govern the workings of need, drive and behavior on the interpersonal cultural level as well. Descriptions of cultural patterns, as simplified statements of sculptured, inevitable ways of life do not fully explore these tendencies. When the actual dynamics of groups forming a cultural system are studied in terms more closely corresponding to need, drive, behavior, and the regulation of conduct, a psychology of peoples and cultures then becomes possible.

4

Culture and Psychiatry

HAVING REVIEWED much of the relevant literature in social psychiatry, we are now in a position
to state simply some basic propositions of this emerging
interdisciplinary science. It is significant that its drive
and direction is towards a generalizing behavioral science
of man. As such, the classic interests of psychiatry in
diagnosis and treatment are linked with considerations of
the prevention or mitigation of mental disorders in socio-
cultural groups, and in improvements from an epidemiological point of view in the range of adjustment or adaptation of persons not functioning at optimum levels of health
and creativity.

As we have seen, enormous descriptive and analytic
problems concerning human behavior are involved. Only
recently has the attack upon these problems included
notions of man, not merely as a creature of biology and
physiology responsive to overtones of his psychological
existence, but as a social and cultural animal. As such,
humans are equally responsive to cultural evaluations and
attitudes as these impinge through family systems, art,
religion, science, work and leisure, or even politics. These
institutions of a culture or sub-culture are themselves
unconsciously patterned into typical ways of thinking,
acting and believing, but as custom and belief at its most
commonplace they are constant in their influence on conscious and unconscious functioning as well. In simplest
formulation, the texture of our conscious existence and the
fabric of unconscious motivation, our daily lives so to speak,
are constantly affected by larger patterns of behavior.

All humans therefore speak a necessary common language of survival and adaptation, viewing events as "beneficial," or "deleterious," or possibly "neutral," "inconsequential" and of no concern. The gregarious nature of the human primate, and his ability to communicate ordinarily in symbols which are cultural in the first instance, subject him immediately to all the conditions and consequences of such communication. As internal communication, in conflict *with himself*, the Freudian movement has brilliantly plotted a part of the course of personal entanglements, often with too little awareness of the relativity and the difference in symbols, attitudes, standards and evaluations which are measured differently from culture to culture. Therefore, even the internal conflicts, involving the regulatory and controlling tactics, and in Freudian language, "the defenses," are staged in quite different arenas of operation and expression.

Apart from these modifications of Freudian theory now in order, dispelling its fatalistic, narrow constriction into one culture scene, a second expansion of the theory long overdue is the relationship between internal conflicts in communication and the external world which influences them. The distinction here is not simply Jungian, the introvert and extravert dichotomies still centered in the individual; by pointing out the inevitable relationship between the inner and outer worlds of human beings, we involve ourselves in an analysis, on cultural and psychiatric grounds, of basic human values and the relative standards of normality which exist from culture to culture.

Consider, for a moment, the sense of communicating with others as discussed by Harry Stack Sullivan. These communications are not based solely, as he suggested, on an awareness of a common humanity in two or more persons, though of course this consciousness of humanity is of initial and prime importance. Self-object relations, or self-other conceptions require as an immediate part of external objectivity, a *specific* perception and cognitive evaluation of human *actions* or events without distortion and with reasonable possibility of the prediction of behavior in others. The contrary sense of isolation and loneliness reflect both this disturbed awareness, and the distortions in communication, certainly between inner and outer worlds. But schizoid withdrawal and its extreme isolation are no direct and accurate portrayals of the same state of communications, perceptions, and cognitive evaluations in the real world.

This fear of others, or of the consequences of one's own hostile motivations, stem from experiences which slowly and relentlessly destroy a sense of identity and of common humanity with others. Yet in cultures if the same sense of identity and humanity is tenuous, then the conditions within the culture help erect a towering barrier which can only connote the speeding of separation from others, or in Sullivan's language, the following of disjunctive relations. The helplessness of hostile motility disturbances in extreme fear and anger, or the individual reintegrations on new fantasy levels are not built unaided in family settings alone. They may be aimed at what seem to be the capacities for internal objectivity and self-esteem, or may be antisocial or asocial, depending on the discrete or specific symptomatology. But nevertheless, when we say such disordered and ill persons are no longer acting and thinking in terms of positive cultural values or normative human attributes, we mean fundamentally that not only have communications broken down in the individual or in the family, but that cultural norm and social group also allowed the sphere of their operations to become wholly internalized and incoherent. Thus the person partly is removed from *both* the contact with sustaining *cultural realities* and deprived of the ability *to adjust to gross environ-*

ment with perceptions and cognitive attitudes dedicated to healthy survival.

The curious thing about cultural realities, which vary within types or limits and never achieve abnormal integration wholly is that they affect individual conditioning processes. Basic human cognitive, perceptual and attitudinal equipment varies. Both this equipment and the norms of most cultures are inclined towards survival and healthy adjustment and are ordinarily, in the normative conduct of most people, so intended. Even the most violently anti-social symptomatology, like sociopathic disorder and extreme forms of paranoid schizophrenia in our own culture, or *amok* in Malaysia, rarely point to total genuine regressions and complete loss of contact or communication. Such individuals have, indeed, lost a cultural coloring, or broken completely from a pattern of certain kinds of self-other conceptualizations. But in a negative sense, they reflect the cultural stress system. It is likely in the passive forms of illness (the automatic obedience disorders, marked by lack of will, weak ego-organization, echolalia or echopraxia, *latah*, or "Arctic hysteria"), that each of these wide ranges of disorder are frantic attempts to organize autistic behaviour patterns and methods of communication and symbolization as a typical resort of certain cultural stress systems. All such illnesses do, in reality, reflect cultural demoralization. The distinction between health, on the one hand, and one typical form or another of illness in a culture is not merely between those who communicate, and those who do not, or those who fulfill needs, and those who have been thwarted. In each case, though quite opposite paths of symbolization, adjustment, and communication have been utilized, *both have derived from different aspects of the cultural realities.* In the one case, the adjustment of internal necessities and external conditions has been mediated by regulative principles, defenses, modes of communication, and cultural symbols and values pressed in the service of healthy adjustment.   In the other, with the same modes of communication at his disposal and the same range of symbols to draw from, the values, cognitive attitudes, regulative principles, percepts and defenses have been critically affected by the stresses inherent in the cultural scene.   In the most serious illnesses, we see an individual drawn finally into lines of conflict that are internal to be sure, but mark a warfare between the self and "those others" now dimly perceived, distorted, misunderstood and hated as values and standards attenuate, grow weak, and lose their persuasive quality.   We may thus speak not only of weaknesses in individuals and in families, but in cultural values.

The fear, in social science and psychiatry, of dealing with values-systematizations, as if man were merely the prey of irrational and psychological forces is a sign of our culture and our times.   Many have been taught to feel helpless before impersonal mechanistic forces.   Wars have not mitigated these feelings.   In our mass-production, highly-specialized, anonymous, and distantly regulated mode of life (all of which David Riesman in *The Lonely Crowd* designates as "other directed" standards of living), we cannot see the interpenetration of particular kinds of essentially human values with the potentialities of a richer social and cultural life.   We sense a sameness in social and cultural experience for all men, when, indeed, either history or travel would convince us of change and diversity.   Our problems and solutions in human psychology are not always repeatable in history nor reduplicated across the earth's surface.

These differing incidence rates of mental disorder and psychosomatic illness are not matters of group biological characteristics like race.   Essential hypertension in malignant form is rare among unacculturated Negro peoples of Africa, but relatively common among American Negroes. A variation by historical period has also been noted in mental illnesses like the Dancing Manias of the Middle Ages which are rare today. Different *forms* of schizophrenic illness are characteristic of different parts of the world. We have suggested that varying culture standards, values and ways of life are responsible for this regional and group differentiation. In so doing, we have combined certain brilliant insights of the Freudian movement with clinical and social data stemming from post-Freudian anthropological and psychiatric movements. Our position has been close to that of Wegrocki who states,[155] "Obviously abnormal behavior is *called* abnormal because it deviates from the behavior of the general group." However, it is not the fact of deviation from a norm, but a causal background in the breakdown of adaptive functioning and regulatory principles *in reactions to stress*. Wegrocki does not call Plains Indian visions abnormal, for instance, but calls those of the schizophrenic in whatever culture by this term, stating that the two behaviors may *seem analogous*, but that they are *not homologous*. The essential difference Wegrocki sees in a tendency of abnormal behavior "to choose a type of reaction which represents an escape from a conflict-producing situation." Thus, it is not "a mechanism that is abnormal; it is its function which determines its abnormality." One could add that the kinds of conflict typical in a given society and family system will favor the functioning of certain mechanisms. Apparently, total personality function in the totality of a cultural context is the point at which to locate the difference between normal and aberrant.

If a mechanism like withdrawal (and repression of a sense of indentification with others, as a human being) is so basic a response pattern in a prevalent illness, it will reduce cultural contacts to the barest minimum. To note that a process of abnormality is in motion seems unnecessary. Any society may contain, in this sense, its noncultural, aberrant types. But not all societies and cultures show withdrawal symptomatology in such abundance. These persons, to be statistically significant at all in the meaning of deviancy "from the behavior of the general group" must be responding according to reaction *patterns* (not identities) which force certain kinds of dislocation of need, drive, behavior, and impulsivity-regulation to the fore, in which for the ultimate forms of disorder, cognitive attitude and adaptive behavior undergo distortion under the pressures of a wide number of traumatic agents: anxiety, hostility, and a sense of alienation among them. In another society, brief confusional states may be the more classical defense mechanism.

What LaBarre has called the ability of man "to be spectacularly wrong and wrong over long spans of space and time" has led him in his recent work, *The Human Animal*, into a style of thinking identical with that of Ruth Benedict. There is no discernible difference, writes LaBarre, in the content of a culture and a psychosis.[156] While the number of respective "communicants" in the normative case may be fifty million, and in the other aberrant situation of a mental disorder showing withdrawal it is always one, LaBarre notes quixotically that both are qualitatively based on symbol-systems. So is culture based upon the most positive characteristics of human beings without all cultures at all times evidencing this. Granted the same array of symbols "at disposal," the adaptive means and functions are forced into patterns destructive of enduring human relationships only in psychotics. To group one aspect of cause (the culture) with its consequence, the prevailing form of disorder, is highly misleading. Yet LaBarre presumes both culture and psychosis allay anxiety. The only difference he discerns is that the schizophrenic is "oriented relatively to the 'inside'," an amazing oversimplification, whereas the scientist, for example, is oriented "to the 'outside' of his organism." LaBarre's noncultural and nonpsychological usages of words like "know," "orient," and "symbol" suggest that the system cannot discover the actual contexts of normal and aberrant behavior since it has no reference to scientifically viable concepts of conditioning, motivation or function in either an anthropological or psychiatric sense. The reduction of culture to psychosis follows, as it does in so many systems because it is not based on acceptable scientific proof of obvious differences between the two phenomena.

The actual fact about the culture-personality interrelation is that the relationship is valid only if normal behavior can be related to the positive values of a culture and the disordered *in* a culture to its stress system. This requires properly weighting the enormous effects of culture in its relationship to individual members of a society. One contemporary American philosopher, Feibleman, has spoken of cultures as "wholes like organisms, *at least in the sense that they consist in something more* than the sum of their parts."[157] In this sense of larger, over-arching values or value orientations, Kluckhohn has stated a value-orientation may be defined as a "generalized and organized conception, influencing behavior, of nature, of man's place in it, of man's relation to man, and of the desirable and nondesirable as they may relate to man-environment and interhuman relations."[158] Therefore, the values of a culture have come to be almost synonymous with the conditions and psychological consequences of that culture, seen in detail as well as in general contours. But we must recognize that social action is not, in any culture, a duplication of its stated values. The link back to personal behavior of this cultural equipment is, nevertheless, very close indeed. Cassirer, in *An Essay on Man*, reports recent research on the psychopathology of language: "Patients suffering from aphasia or other kindred diseases have not only lost the use of words but have undergone corresponding changes in personality." Work by K. Goldstein and A. Gelb suggest that the loss or impairment of speech caused by brain injury is never "an isolated phenomenon," since such a defect alters the whole character of human behavior particularly where abstractions are required in cognitive thinking. Cassirer continues: "Without symbolism the life of man would be like that of the prisoners in the cave of Plato's famous simile. Man's life would be confined within the limits of his biological needs and his practical interests."[159] No person, not even the most constricted hebephrenic, lives wholly in Plato's cave. So with values. Perfection in them is rare from society to society and no one yet inhabits, with other millions, the perfect culture.

The chief linkages of values themselves are to symbols as culturally defined. Even here, there is a difference between ideal culture values and the reality situation. Disturbances which disorient a patient as to time, place, or the reality of actual circumstances about him may center, even in masked and disguised form, chiefly in disturbed relationships with others in one's immediate network of relationships and associations. Yet characteristic styles of interpersonal relationships in a society can color family functioning as readily as one's experience in a family can color his social relations. Few psychiatrists have escaped becoming at one time or another, father figures, or mother figures or sibling figures as the case might be. This kind of thought is peculiarly dependent upon cultural systems and symbols. If common symbols, such as these, become fraught with fear and uncertainty, or are colored and distorted with hostilities, they become problematic areas for the pursuit of rational thinking or even emotionalizing. But even dependency, hostility and fear can be injected into families. Affects appear disproportionately out of range where they are fostered with intensity in a whole culture. Over- and under-reactions become possible. A Thematic Apperception Test, or Rorschach evocation will produce father-male or mother-female symbolizations (in their relation to ego) as having unusual attributes in a culture where such attributes are nurtured. Yet no area of interest, economy, sex, religion, philosophy, or indeed, aging, authority, death, prestige, or illness, is, in any psychiatric or cultural theory, immune from such distortion.

Aberrant systems of thought and action or delusions which are always departures from "reality," are not made from whole cloth in an entirely private pattern. They refer to areas of stress, confusion, or outright aberration in the culture itself. Rather than culture *and* its symbols, being indistinguishable from psychosis, as in La Barre's theory, the symbols and value-orientations are so patterned and stylized as to provide the typical points of reference between the individual and "the reality he tests," if indeed he still can do so. While a cultural *insistence* upon a range of conduct is no burden on one whose symbol-usage is unimpaired, the entire matter of whether inadequate and self-destructive defenses are used, or whether sheer immaturity blocks growth, is dependent upon the nature of these cultural insistences in the first place.

Cultural values may be scrutinized for their universality or the chance they provide for alternatives. They may also be considered for their characteristic tendency to promote or thwart healthy development.

While it has been fashionable in psychoanalytic circles to attempt to define parental conduct or marital relationships which "produce aberration" or reduce it, it is likely that the social roles of mothers and of fathers in a given setting, the nature of the marital institution, and the various social and economic qualifications upon human relationships in general constitute the real conditions of emotional existence. These conditions are visited upon individuals in all stages of the life cycle, become determinative of individual role and are perpetuated or reduplicated by tradition.

A recent study by Louise J. Despert among adolescent and pre-adolescent children in the urban United States has pointed to severe withdrawal, constriction and fear among children suffering from obsessive-compulsive disorder, but greater fantasy, hostility, and weak, amorphous ego-organization among schizophrenic children. The crucial factor for the psychotic children is that reality-testing more generally fails and contact is more thoroughly lost. In this light, the compulsions of the obsessive group appear often as symbolic acts in *relation to reality*, and in terms of which intellectual functioning and reality-testing are retained for the present. However tyrannically they are used and distorted in symbolization, compulsions link to reality. The relative *loss* of reality contact in the schizophrenias, though rarely complete, shows at the very least, an inadequate reality-testing. In the schizo-affective disorders, the emotional imbalance and loss of realistic intellectual functioning go hand in hand as they do in the schizophrenias generally. The point of referring to this phrasing of the progression from psychoneurotic to psychotic states is to indicate that the partial loss of reality-contact does not mean the irrelevancy to the patient of the *kind* of reality experienced. Clinics and hospitals, since the time of Adolf Meyer, or even before, are aware of the importance of the patient's current environmental setting. In the same way, the kinds of communication a patient is utilizing habitually and subtleties in the relationship of physician and adjunctive personnel to these patients least able to cope with negative features of their environment are significant features of modern therapy.[160] There can be no doubt that even the most disturbed patients continue to read and interpret a socio-cultural environmental map.

Frieda Fromm-Reichman has written pointedly of the cultural factor as utilized by patients:[161]

"There are great differences of opinion, however, among various schools of psychoanalytic thinking in regard to the genetic frame of reference in which interpretation is done and about the patient's selection of content matter for repression and dissociation. The genetic frame of reference of psychoanalysts is oriented upon Freud's basic teachings of the fundamental significance of the developmental history in infancy and childhood. However, there is a difference in the interpretation of the events and emotional experience of the patient's early history, as determined by the psychosexual concepts of Freud *versus* the interpersonal interpretations of H. S. Sullivan. The patient's selection of subject matter for repression and dissociation, according to my thinking, is determined by the existing cultural standards governing his life. His medium of adherence to these standards is their acceptance by the significant people in his immediate environment and in his group."

We are indebted to Fromm-Reichman for putting the entire matter of patients' reaction-patterns in the framework of a functional and dynamic culture and personality scheme. Societies and cultures, no less than the normal and abnormal persons who constitute them, have their more or less patterned ways of doing things. Notions of proper behavior, styles of thought, and reactions to situations are governed by cultural standards designed to cope with the most usual problems of human conduct. While each individual handles these problems in his "own way,"

giving them his particular interpretation and personal
stamp of approval, he neither creates the problems of his
culture, nor in any but the most strained and unrealistic
sense, singlehandedly accounts for their permanent solution.   We are, especially in our Western culture so convinced of our uniqueness and variation from a nuclear
pattern of behavior in common with others that we fail
to see points of dependency upon those others who are
constantly impinging upon, and often positively influencing, our development.   This myth of absolute uniqueness
is nowhere seen more clearly than in the schizophrenic
with paranoid reaction who marks his departure from a
pattern no longer acceptable by a personal denial of its
reality.   Here indeed there occurs a substitution of a
highly individualized set of meanings.   Few have seen in
this, one type of reflection of a cultural standard.   To one
unaccustomed to the existence of patterns in culture and
in behavior, these bizarre variations from a sense of identity with others are discussed as if only infantile regression
were occurring.   In the mildly narcissistic the same value
system will often escape notice and go unobserved.   What
we often forget in these neurotic cases, as in the most
bizarrely organized systems, is that there has been a
highly influential social pattern to draw upon and even
to vary, and that only experience within a cultural framework, no matter how unsatisfactory or painful in personal
history, can cause this deviation.

Where personal experience within a cultural framework
has taught one to vary or even to misconstrue its standards
and values, we learn that patients can learn to fear them,
hate them, or anxiously reject them.   The cultural patterns of feeling, thought and action may include such me-
chanics as repression and guilt for sin and sex.   But beyond
that which is repressed as forbidden, or the degree to which
shame or guilt are used in cultures, there are standards

fragmentized and dissociated from other affective areas of thought and action. It is hackneyed to speak of nonacceptance or rejection by others, chiefly parental figures or their surrogates, as marking the first arousals of this sense of expected disapproval and consequent anxiety. How often, in our culture, is women's social and economic role stereotyped and condemned? The fact, even in mental hospitals, is that the arousals, unless skilfully avoided, can blend with other areas of resentment concerning male and female roles since they have long since become patterned behavior. The personality failures of individuals are often to a large extent failures in the social ethics and cultural system in which they operate.

This relationship between the individual and his sociocultural environment is the crux of the matter. The anthropologist, by studying the affectively-charged patterns of behavior of groups of people, both in terms of range and at their most typical or commonplace, can provide data on what Fromm-Reichman calls "the anxiety-provoking character of culturally unacceptable experiences." Not only do patients bar culturally unacceptable experiences from conscious awareness but they may be conditioned to do so either through dissociative or repressive mechanisms. One culture may promote fantasy projections in one area of living and another foster emotional abreactions of an activity sort in the same context. At the same time, if the inconsistencies and points of antagonism in the culture are studied, they may be seen to have direct effect on those rigidly adhering to its normative standards and becoming more directly involved in the cultural stress system. Among Western cultural traits producing unacceptable kinds of human experience and behavior, Fromm-Reichman has listed the growing extent and cruelty of war, the curbing of personal friendliness and its overt expression, the overdependency of adults, and the overpossessiveness or ideas of grandeur and magical thinking which Western cultures of our time actively promote.

The psychiatrist, who studies these patterns of reaction as developed in extreme forms within the total contours of a personality, still requires in his study of conspicuously deviant persons, a clearer statement of the standards or norms from which patients are recoiling. Here students of cultural values cannot take for granted that a coherent social environment, necessary for ego-integration, was available for the patient, or indeed, that unique traumatic events account for him alone. Before we can assess the degree of individual damage, it is necessary to plot not only a personal case history, but one in conjunction with the cultural standards and values to which the patient was exposed and to which he has reacted in some characteristic fashion. The individualization of a patient's treatment need not end when he is seen as being, in part, a product of his culture. Quite the contrary, in most cases it can only then begin.

The psychiatrist who makes cross-cultural corrections for standards and values guards against his own culturally-induced limitations, and adds to his insight and wisdom about human affairs. For some, according to Fromm-Reichman, such limitations interfere with the ability to see matters in a therapeutically valid perspective.[162] These attitudes about value concepts, even when they are not dogmatized, or given over to the extortion of "confessions" of a patient can be so closely adhered to that they amount to the therapist's insistence upon his own conventions or prejudices. Where the minimal task or first objective, quite often in therapy, is to develop in these patients the beginnings of self-esteem and the ability to live their own lives, standards and values must be provided to promote a sense of coherence and prevent chaotic disintegration. Even spontaneous self-expression has standards.

There are balances, in therapy, between over-relating and under-relating, between minimal expectations and the maximum elaboration of the most personalized choices and classifications of what is true or good. In some schools of psychoanalytic thinking, insight into a patient's *particular* history and *specific* cultural background is subordinated to a valuational scheme which insists on one course of development, or ontogenesis, from "polymorphous perversity" of the infant on out. A more positive and less fatalistic system was propounded by Otto Rank who noted that abnormality is by no means synonymous with maladjustment. In some societies, and even in some individual ethical systems, certain kinds of deviation from the norm are allowed and the abnormal individual is not necessarily maladjusted in his cultural setting. Such a typology of normal (adjusted), the ill or aberrant, and the creative artist, allows Rankians (and some interpreters of Erich Fromm) to describe as "normal" those who are said to have uncritically surrendered their individual wills and accepted the "will" of the group. The neurotic deviant is then described as one who cannot conform to the will of the group, and yet is not free to assert his own will, or individuality, in defiance of his group. Rank's third type, the artist, affirms his own will and is therefore free to assert or express truly constructive elements within himself whether these are contrary to standards or not. However, group standards in the systems of Rank or Fromm are defined in advance as being dull average.

Yet the anthropologist fears that those who are "tough" about cultural values are really the worst sentimentalists. Beyond the obvious yardstick of those things which are most beneficial to most people, or which the Benthamite would say produce health and happiness for the greatest number, the anthropologist does not see why all values must be declared at the start as existing in some hypothetical individual when they *emerge* in clearest form in actual group living. Why must they be abstracted from one person's behavior, when they are implicit and varying in any enduring interpersonal relations? Why must they be incorporated in absolute codes apart from science, when all science is concerned, directly or indirectly, with human values? Why must they be unchanging when human situations change? The fact that man is not the equal of his body, that by virtue of his exploratory mental capacity, he "condescends" to live in it, does not mean, as some philosophers have put it, that the locus of behavior is wholly biological and internal, or psychological, or cultural, or merely individual at any one time. A Beethoven is never so individualistic, or in a social sense, cultural as when he presses an arbitrary cultural framework, the sonata form, with its given aesthetic potentialities for balance or proportion, to the limits of emotional expression in a language most people understand. Yet the necessity to speak the language of emotions and individual interpretation of set, given forms was so characteristic in Beethoven's day that it stands in contrast to the unemotional experiments in sound and orchestral color which come later. The subtle and quiet understatement of Japanese painting of the Kamakura period, as influenced by Zen Buddhist emphasis on "universal truths" which lie beyond the individual, are a second example of values which are not centered in the individual. Any reader of Elizabethan literature knows that the English were once more emotionally demonstrative about personal affairs than they now are. Max Mueller, in the Nineteenth Century, was told it was frivolous for males to play the piano. We may be sure from anthropological studies of music, literature and graphic or plastic arts that there are norms over and beyond individual variation which affect such variation. While there is no such thing as an Italian race, there are variations, individual and regional, of an Italian language; and the same is true of Italian regional variants in character and expression.

In the study of mental disorder, we are not dealing with such positive emphases of the culture at all. The schizophrenic's elaborated fantasy life, denial of reality, and strange emotional and motility patterns lose something of this spirit of cultural epitomization, cultural enlargement, or even cultural adherence. Both the neurotic and the psychotic toning down of identity and emotional communication with others, and their distortion or destruction of viable cultural symbols stand in opposition to the creative artist certainly, but they stand also in defiance of the average more positive interpretation of the values, standards and life patterns of the culture at its best. As stated earlier, aberration is not innovation and psychosis is not culture. But neither is creative innovation a wilful turning away from the interests and concerns of other people. Artists using one or another "language" or form of emotional communication, do of course express constructive elements within themselves, but they do so by expressing humanistic aspects of the culture within patterns which can reach others. If there are no satisfactory outlets for such constructive expression, an individual can repress or distort his sense of identity with others only at a wasteful cost of guilt and anxiety, or he can maintain the marginal "will" and adjustment of one who has lost in growth and development or is petrified by the thought of anything but the most rigid adherence.

Ernst Cassirer, in his *Essay on Man*, states that the difference between man and the infra-human Primates lies in the difference between a human, propositional language, based on symbols culturally defined, and an emotional language which animals possess as an affective system of signs and signals. Charles Morris and Leslie White, in philosophy and anthropology respectively, have noted that signals belong to the physical world of vertebrate being, and symbols to the human world of meaning. In this sense, Charles Morris suggests that symbols are "designators" which in combination may themselves define what is thought to be distinctive, desirable, proper behavior influencing choice, or in short, matters *of value*, or of things *existent*. The combination and blending in man of the two languages, propositional and affective, has influenced some scholars in denying what Cassirer calls "a creative or constructive imagination" in animals beyond the practical, biological level. Such writers unhesitantly bestow on man a "symbolic imagination and intelligence." However, these symbols, and hence the degrees of intelligence and imagination they connote, derive from culture as an adaptive or adjustive means in establishing controls in the world of nature or the world of understanding (science, myth, philosophy). The world of interpersonal relations is uniquely dependent on them. That cultures are unconsciously patterned like languages and styles of art need not surprize us; for even the component personalities of a culture are dependent on *systems* of meanings understandable for other individuals, and likewise unconsciously patterned. Sapir has suggested that this patterning of cultures, to be genuine, must be expressive of real human needs and aspirations. We may add that individuals, to be healthy, must also express these crucial aspects of their culture.

The best in art, science and philosophy never fails in human quality. For these reasons, the complicated content of a values-system is always larger than the reach of discrete individuals. It is measured, in ultimate form, again by human needs and aspirations, but translated now into terms consistent with cultural situations and possibilities. Thus, realistic values in a group and in a person can function to narrow the distance between the real and ideal so far as these same needs and aspirations are concerned. In this sense, Cassirer is right that human cultures taken individually are systems of value, and taken as a whole the cultural process may well be the process of "man's progressive self-liberation." The process is not automatic however. The tensions and frictions in cultures and in mankind cannot be overlooked in philosophically viewing this panorama of achievement. It is dubious whether, in any real ethical sense of values, most people of the modern world enter fully into this domain of progress and self-liberation.

In their recent volume, *Social Science in Medicine*, Leo W. Simmons and Harold G. Wolff have commented on a wide range of sociocultural stresses which evoke "protective patterns" and promote or exacerbate illness and retard treatment. The social structure of a hospital and its functional organization, if related to such pre-existing patterns in the patient, may contain elements complicating or delaying recovery. Knowledge of sociocultural backgrounds along with the patient's adaptive or adjustive assets and liabilities which stem from long-established or recent methods of coping with stress are indispensable tools in reducing or eliminating "the very stressed-charged elements" that earlier provoked inept responses.[163] While it is likely that patients in general do not shed their sociocultural attributes with the onset of illness, it is equally true, as these authors point out, that little account is ordinarily taken in hospital centers of these pervasive and potent factors.

In psychiatry, however, the problem has been different. Here attention has long been paid to the problem of reaction formation and even to protective reaction patterns which are occasionally beneficial in the light of total personality assets and liabilities. Here again, the observation of personality patterns, in their total contours, is made with concern for character and temperament, individual assets and liabilities and the structure of psychopathology as it operates, or has operated, in the course of an entire life. Nor have family characteristics, or personality balances within them, been ignored. What we may say is that while there are known connections between family background and personality, persons responding ineptly to sociocultural stresses are viewed *on the symptom level of personalized disturbance without portraying inadequacies in the cultural value system.* A great deal of what is loosely charged to national "temperament" or personal "character" is really nothing, on scrutiny, but the effect of traditional patterns of conduct.

In a culture, for instance, that looks critically on informal demonstrativeness, the spontaneous human tendency known from children to display emotion spontaneously becomes more than normally inhibited. Since all human conduct is culturally modified, the task becomes one of looking more closely at those, like the Irish, which set greater store by fantasy, the "omnipotence of thought," the power of the word, and the oral expression of strivings and status aspirations. Such patterns may be more a matter of history, economy and family organization than a matter of nursing and weaning. Redlich, writing of normality and values, has written that: [164]

> "The normative approach is specific for a given culture. Although psychiatrists are just beginning to think in cultural anthropological terms . . . there is much less acceptance of the fact that most normative propositions are specific for a subculture . . . Kingsley Davis showed that our notions on mental hygiene are ideas of the middle class. There can be no doubt that culture to a large extent determines the scope of normality."

If again, the culture promotes the acting out of emotional

feeling directly, especially in given areas of life adjustment as in South Italy, can it be doubted that this will be felt in the actual operations of the family of orientation (into which one is born) and the family of procreation (in which one later functions)?

The statistical approach, denoting both typical conduct and the range of variation, is helpful at this point. Edward Sapir, who studied perceptively the formal structure and the particular quality or "genius" of a language, or of language stocks and families, noted the general harmony or consistency of these systems of expressive symbolism. Yet he concluded that the central tendencies of any language system are imperfect in containing expressivity: "all grammars leak." It is possible, therefore, that a combined cultural and clinical approach to the normal-abnormal continuum will add to statistical knowledge on central tendency and variation some further picture of the roots of repression and dissociation among those who vary from a norm. We need special notice of the actual contexts in which affect becomes disturbed or circumstantiality and denial operate. Before hostility can be combatted, we must plot its course. Or before the imbalances of identification and distortion of reality become "necessary," we must know why they become necessary. To accomplish this, we need no new definitions of words like wish, hope, attitudes, disparagement or dependency, nor novel definitions of mental health other than those already provided. We must, however, have the temerity to question the "perfection" and suitability of various styles of cultural values, after searching them for operational imperfections, for inconsistencies, for elements of confusion and aberration, and for inadequacies in promoting "man's progressive self-liberation."

A. Edel, a philosopher, has recently put the matter similarly. Writing of the search for unity in value phenomena, he notes the prevalent tendency today to seek this unity in the exclusive terms of biological or psychological theory. Here he adds:[165]

> ". . . It is arbitrary postulation to assert that because man is an organism and all activity has a biological basis, therefore all aesthetic, political, religious, moral valuations *must* have biological *import* which only lack of knowledge prevents us from tracing . . . The hard-won lessons of the sciences of man concerning the relations of levels should not be surrendered in value theory."

Concerning Freudian psychology with its similar drive for exclusiveness, Edel states: " . . . It does not seem likely" that psychological unity will be achieved "without bringing social factors so far inside the structure as to make it no longer a purely psychological framework." Besides a possible cultural basis for a unitary value concept, "suggested by the anthropological concept of a culture pattern," Edel writes of an intercultural or cross-cultural, historical unity relating to the career of mankind in the world. He suggests with less exclusiveness and more interdisciplinary good sense that a final synthesis may come to represent "the growing unity of a knowledge of man."

To designate nearer goals or interpretations, and less distant consequences, we may say that in mental disorder the simplest human values, the possession of will power, decisiveness, the ability to control impulses while remaining spontaneous and socially considerate are denied many people of Western cultures. These are cultures with varying emphases on self-display and status, with the need for superiority and competitiveness in our own culture marking an extreme emphasis. The capacities for dispassionate detachment and self-analysis as any Buddhist well knows are no achievement of the Western world. Even insight into one's own emotional reactions and their bases suffer.

In Morita-therapy, in Japan, the latter emphases come naturally. It is not enough to chart these different cultural courses generally. The ability to live reasonably ordered lives, socially and culturally rewarding, with proper responsibilities and free from insecurities is statistically and qualitatively not characteristic of American sub-cultures. Allport's criteria of maturity, containing such character traits as objectivity, detachment, self-content, or even humor, or Leon Saul's of emotional development including high adaptability, low tendencies to regression, and minimal vulnerability, are not combined in most individuals. Obviously, the millenium is not here, but worse still it will not even be envisaged until the full force of behavioral and social sciences begin to challenge processes destructive of human happiness.

III
Research Designs

5

Theory and Direction in Research Designs

CULTURAL EVOLUTION AND THE PSYCHOLOGY OF PEOPLES

E VOLUTION is a process by which specific kinds of integration, of matter, of life, or of culture, undergo transformations from one type to another. In each realm, physical, organic, or cultural, we speak of this process as a generic one. We do not, for example, refer to various *evolutions* in the organic world from Paramecium to Aunt Polly. Nor do we confuse the process that produced Aunt Polly with the process that produced the physical world she inhabits, or the cultural world she may, more or less, participate in as she lives her life. Thus we do not talk of various kinds of cultural evolutions to explain social and behavioral developments along the human pathway from hunting and gathering to atomic energy. The process is one.

The focus in each type of evolution is upon regularities of this general process. In a science of culture, it is recognized that each kind of integration and change is dependent upon the general nature of culture itself. If the stories of cultures are to become a general science of culture, general principles of integration and change must be established. It is true, also, that this generic process may have particular aspects. That is to say, culture has such aspects as the material, the social, the ideational, and the behavioral. White has commented on anthropologists' attitudes, especially in America, toward generalizing *versus* particularizing.[166] It is no doubt true, in science as it is in logic, that an expansion of the scope of science occurs when wider generalizations are attempted and evolutionary principles established.

In American anthropology, as we shall see, a recent tendency has been to particularize about given cultures or geographical areas. However, this tendency has not constituted the major difficulty standing in the way of analysis of general cultural process. If our views of specific cultures, areas, or traditions in each case analyzed a kind of integration or a type of change accurately, we would undoubtedly find analyses of the general process in culture emerging naturally and somewhat inductively from these data. But few sciences are built in this fashion, and anthropology has been no exception. An exclusive preoccupation with specific cultures is a deterrent to generalization. Yet a more basic difficulty standing in the way of analysis of general process is seen when we ask not only *why,* but *how,* American anthropologists have tended to particularize. While most have avoided analyses of general process beyond single cultural or traditional boundaries, this has been done by confusing questions of integration and change with psychological interpretations. Of this confusion, White said: "Psychology and culturology deal therefore with biological and extra-somatic aspects respectively of one and the same set of events. Both sciences are essential to a comprehensive interpretation of human behavior. It is necessary, however, in order to avoid confusion, to know and respect the proper boundaries of each."[167]

However, one aspect of culture is cultural behavior; and moreover, psychology deals not only with biological aspects of human adaptation (or "adjustment"), but with cultural or extra-somatic aspects of human behavior as well. The confusion lies in failure to link the psychological *with* cultural interpretations, and to recognize that psychology (that is, the psychology of peoples) is a result of such cultural influences as the material conditions under which a culture operates. Further, the way in which society is organized directly influences behavior. In this sense, cultural existence functions as *the* human psychological environment. The "psychologies of peoples," rather than being causal in the cultural equation, actually result from both the extra-somatic as well as the biological events White discusses. The real confusion lies not only in particularizing or in avoiding analyses beyond one cultural or traditional boundary, but in the confusions of integration and change which occur with *assumptively causal psychological explanations*.

In other words, cultural integration and cultural change, both key concepts in any evolutionary process, are often themselves blurred in American anthropology because of further basic confusions as to the role of psychology. The explanations of integration, ordinarily based on particular cultures, are usually psychological in character. Yet, as we shall see, these explanations are usually proposed as causal statements of cultural change or dynamics. Psychological approaches to given cultures are used to account for both cultural stability or cultural change. Recently in American and British anthropology, such approaches have frequently been offered as alternatives to cultural evolution. Finally, psychological approaches to cultural integration replace principles of evolution by proposing that culture is, in essence, psychological in character.

This difficulty may be resolved by noting that while cultural behavior is by definition psychological, *the psychology of peoples is cultural*. The psychology of a culture becomes understandable only in the light of its being one aspect of the culture as a whole. It is a part or an aspect of culture. A generalized psychology of peoples therefore depends upon the evolution of the culture and is illumined by the material conditions of existence in that culture. Psychology is, then, a result of environmental influences in which culture and the conditions of cultural existence always operate. There is no doubt *an evolu-*

tion of behavior, not as Spencer saw it, apart from and causal to cultural developments, but as an ingredient and as a *consequence* of those developments.

The fact is that integration and change, which are Spencerian concepts, figure in evolution which includes behavior as well as social forms. A kind of integration presupposes a type of change, whether we are speaking of social organization or behavior. Actually, all cultural integrations appear to be based on two essential types of phenomena: first, a material base of culture acting upon the conditions of existence within that traditional setting and changing traditions with changes in the material base; second, the manner in which these conditions of existence are socially organized. The first factor is obviously a basic motive power or causal element in cultural change. The second, affecting any actual process of transformation, is not merely epiphenomenal, although it is a result of the first factor. Rather it is present and contributes to the aim and direction of an evolutionary process.

This does not mean, in the triad of material conditions, social organization, and behavior, that behavior or psychological phenomena can mysteriously determine the direction of change; nor can they singlehandedly produce a type of cultural integration. There is no such thing as a psychology of peoples apart from the conditions of existence, but there are, indeed, such generalized psychologies connected both with material conditions and social milieu. Some have proposed that evolution in culture occurs regardless of a psychological process. To the contrary, the causal chain goes from a material base and the manner in which these conditions of existence are socially organized, to a *resultant* behavior, or psychology, of peoples. To be sure, there is no such thing as "psychology" predetermining the material base or social organization, since a generalized psychology of a people is the result of the vicissitudes of the evolutionary process. However, this does not relegate psychology to a negligible or wholly unimportant role in the actual lives of actual people. As a dependent or resultant variable, as a particular aspect of culture and evolution, as a potent force in specific human lives, and as a means of interpreting the meanings in culture, we prefer not to rule psychology out of court. In fact, uniformities in behavior and the psychology of peoples are the very stuff of culture, best studied as uniformities and typical relations in the cultural process; a generalized psychology is either a part of given integrations or of specific changes. This essay examines these positions in terms of a series of propositions and precepts stated by various teachers and colleagues with whom the author has been associated in the last three decades.

For example, one teacher, Ruth Benedict, wrote in *Patterns of Culture* of a final operating principle of "psychological selectivity" and "unconscious canons of choice" residing in each cultural pattern. This unique stamp she placed upon a cultural integration determined the formation or development of the pattern itself, according to her view. Her *Chrysanthemum and the Sword,* on patterns of Japanese culture, was attacked repeatedly for its nondynamic view; that is, for its failure to note class and regional variations and the various differences between pre- or post-Meiji Japan. More crucial, and less noticed, was the theory of cultural dynamics which she implied. According to both books, the development of total patterns is no more mysterious than the emergence of a style in art, or a type of emotional expression.[168]

Benedict forgot, of course, in this analogy, that most of the affective expressions in a culture can express only the culture itself, or aspects of its organization. She failed to note, therefore, that her idea of cultural development was descriptive rather than analytic. In logic, such proofs or demonstrations are called circular. Her explanation begs the question: What in turn determines the principles of psychological selectivity which shape the culture pattern?

Benedict did not stand alone in this recourse to psychological "explanations" of cultural forms. Another of the author's teachers, Ralph Linton, wrote of a cultural basis of personality development, but this too referred merely to psychological descriptions of peoples, sometimes with historical overtones.[169] Linton provided his one exception to psychological reductionism in an analysis of shifts in Tanala culture subsequent to new modes of rice production. Otherwise, Linton implied, the tree of culture merely grew. In *The Study of Man*,[170] his most influential work, there are triumphant announcements, running counter to the Tanala case, of technology and economic institutions reflecting a people's culture. For example, rank and status in one Polynesian culture are said to have modified the form of High Council chambers to a circular form accommodating many statuses! No doubt, the psychological bent in a culture affects technique and economy on occasion, but Linton adduced very flimsy evidence in one case to account for cultures in general. His cultural universals and alternatives, when examined, are really deep in the realm of attitude and motivational system. Thus the "tree of culture" grows, again as a shape or style, with periods, moods, regional and physiographic roots, and with an occasional impetus from a strong leader. Nothing could really explain culture. The "tree" simply puts down roots here and there in most of the world.[171]

Benedict alludes to Dilthey as sharing her view. But among her contemporaries who also stress psychological types in cultures, she might have referred equally to Sorokin's sensate and ideational cultures, or Kroeber's cultural climaxes as bearing a general resemblance to her own principle of psychological selection. Toynbee, too, prefers striking psychological examples. All these, and a host of others, postulate a history and prehistory in which forms are described and discussed in psychological terms. Sorokin's liking for medieval attitudes, Kroeber's interest in style and climax of historical patterns, and Benedict's predilection for describing polar psychological types are each emphases on given cultural systems of affect. They are intended to stand for theories of kinds of cultural development or dynamics. Sorokin so entitled his work,[172] and Benedict entitled her first essay on the patterns in the American Southwest "psychological types," implying at the same time emergent, developing styles in culture.[173]

Another teacher, Leslie A. White, has been more concerned with the theoretical distinctions between psychological and cultural phenomena. He has held that cultural evolution is best studied apart from psychological considerations—*as if* the individual and his psychology did not exist. Kroeber's doctrine of levels of organization provided a superorganic realm separate from psychology to be investigated by a separate science of culture. White studies culture as a thing of its own type, and in accordance with principles and techniques appropriate to such an entity. To understand this difference and the clash of doctrines adequately, we may allude next to the central position in the main stream in recent American anthropology, from which, as a matter of fact, Benedict's and Linton's work stemmed only as variations.

A fourth teacher, Franz Boas, represents this dominant position in twentieth-century American anthropology. Because of Boas' influence, and that of certain of his associates, American anthropologists came to be suspicious by and large of all general theories of cultural development. This applied equally to Graebnerian *Kulturkreislehre,* Spencerian evolutionism stressing laws of progress, or Lewis H. Morgan's anthropology, with its developing "germs of thought" and its theory of technological indicators and the influence of productive systems in cultural change. Boas advocated detailed descriptive studies of particular cultures and specific historical influences. Regarding dynamic questions, one spokesman of this school, Goldenweiser, repeatedly noted that his colleagues studied the place and function of various aspects of cultures in terms of psychological meanings to participants in these cultural systems. Thus, the American School of historical ethnology, as he termed it, disregarded general theories of development.[174] It was psychological rather than evolutionary, descriptive rather than generalizing or analytical, and devoted to the study of particular cultures and regional diffusions, rather than to the analysis of the cultural process in general. It was in this sense that Benedict and Linton, despite their modernizing tendencies here and there, represented movements well within the orbit of a nongeneralizing, particularistic, and psychological American anthropology.

This position or approach obviously applies better to questions of particular cultural integrations than to questions of integration in general. It is far distant, as a research design, from investigations of questions of general cultural evolution. To typify it theoretically, we may use the analogy of the common nursery game played by children in Japan. As in our children's game of matching digits of a hand, two Japanese children may symbolize any one of four objects by hand gestures. The objects symbolized are, for example, Scissors (two fingers), Paper (flat hand), Rock (fist), and Match (one finger). According to rules of the game, each object relates to another. Scissors can cut Paper and Match burns it. Rock blunts Scissors and breaks Match. But paper conceivably can be used to wrap a rock, so Paper stands highest in this single relationship. In other words, the possible connections of items in the series may be tested empirically. But consider the standard rule or convention by which no single item is always more effective in all relationships than any other. Science constantly seeks to isolate such selectively weighted and significant items which are constant in their effects in a total process. It explores dual relationships and connections of an item in larger configurations, to be sure, but it goes beyond this point to the elucidation of larger total processes and constant effects. One might call the Scissors-Match approach classificatory, descriptive, and historical, even though it weights one factor, in each instance differently, since it proceeds according to simple, nondynamic rules to classify and describe phenomena as they "seem" to occur. The similarities and differences in phenomena, or how "they hang together," will appeal to a descriptive classifier, like Linnaeus, or to one who is essentially an epitomizing poetic artist, like Benedict. One is essentially *describing* random relationships, not seeking invariant relations or causes. These approaches will set the descriptive tasks of a science far ahead. But the urge to describe and classify is not all of any science. Each science also seeks invariable relationships, regular processes, and laws or principles governing uniformities or similarities in a general process. Defining relations in given configurations is but a first short step toward locating regular processes in nature. Biology had its Linnaeus, but also, fortunately, its Darwin.

In American anthropology, from Boas to Benedict and Linton, static or functional relationships and historical inferences were most important, as if these led, somehow, to dynamic understanding of developmental process, or replaced it. The descriptive tasks of the science, the careful accumulation and classifying of data, *were* set far ahead. But the game continued, seemingly without end and without better-defined scientific purpose or goal. In a descriptive nongeneralizing or particularistic science, there are no parameters or set outer limits for determining probabilities and causal relationships, no search for invariant factors which are always significant, and consequently no discoveries of *regularities* in process. With Benedict, as we have seen, anthropologists were set a new descriptive task; the institutional relationships, she stated, were less important than the configuration itself.[175] But in each such instance, as in her Southwestern studies, a psychological touchstone was sought to "explain" the emergent pattern.[176] Linton's portrayal of specific cultures broadened at best to a larger historical delineation of particular traditions or geographic areas. But the tree of culture, even in the symbol selected to represent it—the banyan—in its growth and development, sent out aerial roots which only occasionally rooted in soil.

Edward Sapir, another gifted American anthropologist, summarized frankly and clearly in a work on *Time Perspective in Aboriginal American Culture* the bases for historical inference in continental areas. Sapir's chief contribution, aside from this monograph, was a volume called *Language*. Here, and elsewhere, Sapir sought to establish a theory of linguistic change which he appropriately called language "drift." Inspection of this theory indicates that it applied, somewhat coincidentally with Benedict's work on culture, the configurational approach to language structures, attempting to denote a genius, or special flair, or form-quality in whole families of languages. The word "drift" simply implied that qualitative or psychological tendencies in a language structure might become further adumbrated as the language changed slowly over time. It is obvious that Sapir's work just as that of Benedict or Linton falls within the orbit of the historical, particularistic, and psychological tradition of American anthropology, though it stressed, at the same time, greater historical synthesis than Linton attempted. Sapir also paid much attention to psychological meanings in language as did Benedict's configurational approach in cultures. That the psychological theory of culture remained a matter of "unconscious patterning" was also made explicit by Sapir.[177] He attacked Kroeber's superorganic as an extraneous, unnecessary addition.[178] Impressed by the subtlety and almost endless creativity of Man the Artificer, Sapir felt there could be no set limits for determining cultural regularities.[179] In culture-personality theory, he spoke of "outlines, significances and demarcations" of conduct developed in specific cultural traditions, but such meanings or personalized interpretations required psychiatric, more than social, analysis.[180] There was never the slightest hint in his work that any one item in a configuration weighed more heavily than all the rest. Again one finds description of psychological meanings within cultures, languages, and other forms of behavior, but these are largely categorized as unconscious patterings of conduct in society. Most crucial in understanding this penetrating and sensitive, but always elusive and nongeneralizing, quality in Sapir's work on language, culture, and personality is his feeling that human affairs are not underwitten by law or principle at all. They lend themselves only to historical and psychological description. Observing in one essay that the laws of crystallography, for example, applied to phenomena that are unchanging, Sapir contrasted human affairs as being unpredictable in advance or unceasingly changing in retrospect.[181] This, again, is the position of the descriptive historian, not the social and cultural analyst. Despite the complexity of all systems of nature, scientists assume that the tools of analysis may be shaped to investigate any materials at hand. If, indeed, culture changes, then investigate its change. However, Sapir's talent was never so employed. In anthropological linguistics, in culture, and in personality study, or in ethnology, he developed only the descriptive and particularistic aspect of science which appealed to more pedestrian colleagues.

It is fitting that someone as perceptive as Sapir should have noticed the fact of cultural change, society's dynamism, as being a basic characteristic of culture even if this fundamental proposition about change were used in so curious or limiting a fashion. For crystallography, his "science with laws" is the epitome of a descriptive, nongeneralizing, and particularistic science, however much it is related to more dynamic disciplines. In science, moreover, we have learned that all systems of nature have their complications and time enters into all of them. To suppose a timeless, ideal type of understanding is to go back to Plato and away from a philosophy of science, or naturalism. Even in respect to atoms of a given type, we now know ordinary predictions and laws of probability give way to stochastic or somewhat less determinate rules and measures, in order better to investigate hidden probabilities, varying time values, and dynamic change. Most positively, the laws of crystals will differ from the analysis of stochastic principles applied to the radium atom, or from cultural laws in form and content. But to suppose that causal inquiry and some kind of probability, or science itself, will stop at a cultural boundary in the universe is arbitrary and quixotic in the extreme.

If one searches the positions which Goldenweiser termed the American School, one finds no variation in this point of view. Two British anthropologists, after distinguished careers in England, came to the United States where they were influential in the early 1930s. Each man, Bronislaw Malinowski and A. R. Radcliffe-Brown, adopted the term *functionalism*. In both positions, the familiar point was made that an aspect of culture interpenetrates with or relates to another, and for both men such functional interrelations overshadowed an interest in historical questions. This stress on function and integration is seen clearly in Malinowski's view of the institutional parts of culture: religion, social organization, and economy, for examples. As in the Scissors-Match game, ultimately this method stressed an integration in which the parts of a culture functioned or "interrelated" with perfect equality. This lifelong preoccupation with a merry-go-round view of single cultures, with "integration" as Malinowski had described it painstakingly for the Trobriand Islands, was repeated in a series of volumes from 1927 to 1935.[182] Malinowski held that no part of culture is basic to its final integration. Where a general theory, say of magic, is developed, it is based wholly on psychological attitudes within a cultural setting (for example, the point at which uncertainty and fear may enter in).

A. R. Radcliffe-Brown, while developing a theory favoring the study of cultural integration, was somewhat anomalous in his distaste for approaches emphasizing psychological factors to account for this phenomenon.[183] He was also at odds with the general current of opinion favoring historical reconstruction. To him, "synchronic" research, as he called it, was the study of social organization and kinship system, and was basic to any understanding of integration. This must precede "diachronic" research, the analysis of change. Although he presumed he followed Durkheim, the only intrusion of the latter's extensive theorizing on a doctrine of cultural conditioning appeared in Radcliffe-Brown's descriptive listing of social sanctions, ritual, punitive, or collective in character. In such a system the basis for behavior is seen as social, and this conceptual system is descriptive rather than dynamic. It contrasts with the historical-descriptive theories of Boas and his followers, but yet it agrees with them that no general theories of development account for any culture or cultures in the plural. The Boasian group might study limited influences and diffusions, such as the diffusion of traits in the Sun Dance or the influence of the horse in Plains Indian cultures, but Radcliffe-Brown insisted on static, cross-sectional studies of social organization, ritual, or penal and legalistic matters, as a basis of comparative analysis. While Radcliffe-Brown rounded out his system with vague allusions, à la Spencer, to types of integration which were narrow or wide in extent, and close or loose in Durkheimian social solidarity, neither he nor the Boasian group can be safely credited with a dynamic or a generalizing position in anthropology, since both advocated studies of specific integrations.

The historical-descriptive theory of Boas and his associates was even more popular in American anthropology than Radcliffe-Brown's parallel emphasis on integration when Leslie White took up the cudgels for cultural evolutionism. There has been much discussion, entirely behind the scenes, as to whether cudgels preceded careful exposition of the evolutionary position. Of all those mentioned above, White agreed only with Radcliffe-Brown and Kroeber in separating psychological from cultural study; but at the same time his interest is focused on process, and he stresses cultural change and evolution, whereas Radcliffe-Brown's interest was static or "synchronic." The author, having studied with White, Boas, Benedict, Linton, and others, and having had, in his formative years, extensive correspondence with Malinowski and Sapir, cannot be accused of simple partisanship. In searching for a fruitful and creative synthesis in anthropology, one must especially consider scientific theories in relationship to the purposes and methods of science in general.

A science systematically extends its exploration of an aspect of nature usually after a first descriptive-observational or classificatory phase. The theories we have reviewed in anthropology, with the exception of White's, mark such an initial period, since the main effort is to observe, describe, and classify cultural phenomena. It is instructive, therefore, to consider movements in the history of science which followed similar initial descriptive tendencies.

The Copernican revolution in astronomy and its strengthening by Galileo occurred in a setting of observation and description in which earlier confusions in the analysis of process required major correction by sound evolutionary principles. The warfare between evolution in astronomy and theological dogma was still being waged in the nineteenth century when geologists demonstrated that not only had a solar system evolved, but the earth too had developed according to definite processes. The battles of Darwin and Huxley came next, though Linnaean classification preceded them by a full century. An order of evolutionary discoveries, from the remote astronomic to the earth and life sciences in the sixteenth to nineteenth centuries, witnessed extensions of developmental principles much as our own century has begun to see them applied occasionally in psychological and social sciences. In biology, psychiatry, psychology, and anthropology, the descriptive phases preceded analytic ones.

Just as in geology, where its descriptive-exploratory schools came first, so in biology, descriptive-classificatory or taxonomic movements preceded Darwinism. In psychiatry, one thinks of early German descriptive schools and Kraepelinean classifications making their appearance. The analogies between a nonanalytic behaviorism in psychology and an equally nonanalytic functionalism in anthropology are not chance phenomena in the philosophy of science; nor are the configuration-Gestaltist movements, the clinical Freudian emphases on genetic history, or ideas of stimulus-diffusion in both the psychological and anthropological fields. For some, culture-personality theory in anthropology has meant the simplest kind of merger between descriptive psychology and descriptive anthropology, marked by the use of Freudian clinical models of the effects of child-hood disciplines. Descriptive-historical positions run parallel, but these are followed by analytic and dynamic approaches in each discipline as it matures.[184]

In the development of analytic and dynamic approaches in maturing disciplines, science integration and cross-fertilization may even give rise to new interdisciplinary fields as inventories and observational phases are at some point supplemented by such general analytic formulations. One thinks of astrophysics, biophysics, and biochemistry, geochronological and biochrono-logical methods in archaeology, serological and genetic studies in physical anthropology, or ethnopsychiatry and comparative social psychology. While evolution operates in the physical, biological, and cultural systems of nature, it is obvious today that the Spencerian theory of an organic and psychological evolution governing social and cultural development is defi-nitely not the key. A refinement in technique, such as geo-chronological dating derived from physics, has not added or detracted one bit from evolutionary principle though it has made history more accurate.

However, comparative social psychology and ethnopsychiatry can throw light on aspects of cultural evolution precisely be-cause they deal with symbolization processes and the psychology of peoples. Rather than return to Spencerian formulations, based on ignorance, we suggest that emergent evolution is closer to the mark in that wholly new *systems* appear in nature, and require analysis, even though the novel appearances are based upon successive transformations affecting life forms. As White has noted, man's evolution from earlier primates has given rise to new forms in behavior or psychological functioning. It is his work on the importance of symbol-using in human behavior, or in culture, that points to a functional difference in the psychology of humans as the Pandora's Box of cultural emergence. Man as a social and political animal depends upon energy harnessed within specific cultures for the type of social structure which develops.

Alfred North Whitehead's idea of separate systems of evolution and organization in nature, operating on different levels, is similar to White's, as are his warnings against the fallacy of reductionism, of reducing the terms of one system (like the cultural) to those of another (like the psychological). This does not mean behavioral variations are not linked to cultural evolution, or that ethnopsychiatry is not, rightly, a part of anthropology. Such reductionism to sometimes vague and repetitious "First Principles" plagued Spencer's *Principles of Sociology*. It still plagues a good many anthropologists who castigate Spencer for what they call his ethnocentric Victorian racism, but who nevertheless "explain" whole cultures or even cultural "dynamics," as we have seen, by some bald and unadorned psychogenetic principles.

Whitehead also spoke of a fallacy of misplaced concreteness which is relevant at this point. It is not that a people's psychological functioning is unrelated to their cultural forms, Radcliffe-Brown notwithstanding, but that behavior in a most active and everyday sense is the very stuff of cultural forms. However, the approach through the individual is not, statistically, the study of normative culture or necessarily a study of its characteristic ranges of behavior. Even more important, in anthropology, the material conditions under which a culture operates constitute the setting and *binding conditions* affecting this *range* of behavior. To put the matter otherwise, that culture limits itself (and not people) is a prime example of misplaced concreteness. One fallacy lies in explaining material conditions under which a culture operates by psychological resultants; another fallacy consists in mistaking individualized affects, as in consequences of early childhood training, for group psychological norms which may or may not be consistent with them. Of all Benedict's papers on the psychology of peoples, the most useful one runs counter to ideas of psychological epitomizations of whole cultures, and is on continuities and discontinuities in *cultural* conditioning. In this paper, Benedict deals with cultural forces and conflicts influencing psychology, not the opposite, as in most of her work.[185]

Sapir[186] and Linton[187] were more consistent in seeking a cultural basis for personality development. However, in the Linton collaborations with Kardiner,[188] this position is fairly negated by portrayals of cultural systems as stemming from systems of child-care. Sapir's concern with why cultural anthropology needed "the psychiatrist" is certainly ambivalent, if not contradictory, in reducing cultures to the status of mere epiphenomena, while proclaiming elsewhere the formative influence of culture. Neither Linton nor Sapir hints that the material conditions under which a culture operates, and which affect social structure, the value system, or religion, will inevitably affect the unconscious patterning of personality as well. For both men, the cultural emphases in discussions of normative personality development remained on descriptive, nongeneralizing planes, applicable only to specific cultures.

We have already noted that these theories of culture and personality apply better to discussions of particular cultural integrations than to questions of integration in general. No doubt, this delimitation troubled many anthropologists seeking psychological explanations of cultural forms. Though violently opposed by Sapir and Linton, the tendency of those attempting wider generalizations was to confuse culture and clinic, and to find in Freudian explanations of clinical phenomena the universal explications for any human behavior.[189] The difficulty with these last generalizing, analytic formulations is that they did not concern culture. When Benedict indicated that "abnormals" of one culture might be the "normals" of another, she displayed considerable ignorance of clinical psychiatry. When, on the other hand, Róheim[190] and others claimed to have found psychopathology a chief characteristic in most nonliterate cultures they discussed, they entirely missed the adaptive and creative features of such societies, imputing statistical significance to shreds and patches of psychiatric evidence before they established the norms and the clinical proofs from which pathology could be inferred. Since it is our position that a general and analytic concept of integration and reintegration or change mediates between cultural evolution and the psychology of peoples, the remainder of this essay will be devoted to these relationships.

Although culture is, as Tolstoi said, "what men live by," its presence in all human groups is not haphazard or random. White has noted that energy-utilizations and symbolizations constitute its chief mechanisms, and these permit tool-specializations, productive systems, and growth of knowledge or control over nature, which, together with symbol-using, are peculiar to *Homo sapiens*. None of the categories in the above listing is immutable by its very nature. There may even be retrogression in one part of the world or another without basic interference with the evolution of culture as a whole. Two grimly destructive world wars in the twentieth century illustrate this. With progress and retrogression, with recurrent debasement of humans over continents and in remote island territories, this century has been thus far a period of contradiction, of steps forward and stumblings down blind paths of reaction. Over wide areas, advances in technological application of physical sciences have been achieved, while social science has been applied very little. The twentieth century has been to the present a century of engineering and of dangerous drifts, of speed in communication and of towering barriers, of remarkable discoveries and deepening fears.[191] Nor is the contention of a Toynbee, that a dozen civilizations have come and gone, really reassuring. The anthropologist, with easier access to the solace of centuries, is also the most aware of the passing of social isolation in the remotest regions of the modern world. For him, the species is one under different cultural banners. As cultural processes converge in modern history, it becomes more important than ever to understand cultural process in general.

In this setting of modern times, anthropology was born with great promise. It boldly explored social relationships between the wars, and captured with some success and prodigious labor the many patterns of culture fast being caught in the current flow of intercultural communication. If culture is what men live by, science is today their chief weapon. The older social sciences could not deal adequately with man's course since they were, after all, not holistic in their approach and geographically delimited in perspective. Anthropology spanned the range of social relationships and ambitiously covered the world. It was concerned with revealing the nature of all social phenomena which are fundamentally human and cultural. Such revelations required an ever wider integration of facts, but more important, the tactic of ordering data. Such an organization of data, as we have seen, came under descriptive, particularistic, and psychological rubrics, and not under general analytic principles of cultural process. Consequently, the progress that was made was from essentially idle antiquarianism to cultural history, from the comparative method of tearing traits and complexes out of context to fit preconceptions to studies of given cultural integrations, and from isolation to active collaboration with other behavioral sciences. However, descriptions were not analysis, and this much was done without benefit of dynamic or analytic principles. It did not, for example, challenge Malinowski's merry-go-round view of culture in which nothing is basic or formative in any given integration.

To understand why anthropology turned its back on analytic tasks and exhibited studied preoccupation with data-gathering and description, one must realize that the new science, or series of sciences dealing with man and culture, developed in a period of conflict. As Lancelot Hogben has pointed out, scientific knowledge, even in its more puristic mathematical forms, reflects the organization and problems of the real world. Twentieth-century culture and society—in a half-century of contradiction—has been caught between the necessity of a science of man and culture and the very conflicts affecting science and ethics. The fear of formulating general principles may be noted in such classic essays as Boas' "Limitations of the Comparative Method of Anthropology,"[192] stating hesitantly that laws and principles of cultural development may someday be found, and again in his "Aims of Anthropological Research," thirty-six years later,[193] which despaired of any such possibility. The contrast with White's sense of urgency in this respect and his pleas for a science of man and culture, founded on principles, is all the more noticeable when we review the meanings of anthropology in early, more hopeful periods.

From Aristotle on, the term anthropology is used. To Aristotle, despite his generous use of the organic analogy, culture was a thing *sui generis,* requiring separate study along with man, equally a product of a separate evolution. While encyclopedists of the Enlightenment stressed traditional aspects of human experience in the same scientific spirit, the data of anthropology from the sixteenth to eighteenth centuries lent themselves to speculative, if not wholly imaginative, outlooks. Yet to Rousseau, the men of the Enlightenment, and the naturalistic materialists must go credit for seeking rewarding values and meaningful ways of life in other cultural milieus.

Increasingly, however, scientists required data from cultures the world over. As American anthropology came on the scene, with men like Jefferson, Gallatin, and Morgan, the inflated myths about "primitive man" had already become fantastic and baseless. Concerted efforts of anthropology served to lay the ghosts of the "primitive mind," the White Man's "burdens," and the popular prejudgments. Regional studies and monographs revealed a wide range of customs across continents, both ethnographically and archaeologically. The visit of Humboldt to America in 1804, the linguistic classification of Amerinds by Albert Gallatin in 1836, the monumental fieldwork and publication of Lewis H. Morgan from 1850 to 1881, the founding of the Bureau of American Ethnology by J. W. Powell and William H. Holmes in the last quarter of the century, and of the Peabody Museum, largely through the efforts of Frederic Putnam in the quarter before, indicate the tempo of anthropological development in the United States. It appeared, at first, that there was no one drama of the human life cycle, no single model of cultural adaptation to the world, no universal touchstone of belief for achieving rapport with the universe, and no fixity in art style or philosophy.

In 1886, Daniel G. Brinton founded the first department of anthropology at the University of Pennsylvania, his title stressing linguistics and archaeology. Before the turn of the century, the general trend of anthropology in America was not far different from the European tradition built up from Linnaeus and Blumenbach to emphases on physical anthropology, archaeology, and broader conceptual trends implied in the names of Tylor, Bastian, and Waitz. To match Tylor and Waitz in European cultural anthropology, America had its Lewis H. Morgan.

These great synthesizers, European and American, augmented the search for facts and the organization of fast-accumulating data by an even greater concern for their context long before the fashion for functionalism. Social science, like all science, was the discovery and denoting of general regularities in *processes*, particularly in such social and cultural phenomena as were found to be essentially dynamic. There were then limits to such data. But sparse as the facts were, they were analyzed according to logical and realistically conceived method. This early trend toward a generalizing science of culture proved that anthropology was too advanced in data, methods, and perspective by 1900 to be called a product of the twentieth century. Since then, its sustained and current impact on the social sciences gives it its particular claim to modernity. Other social sciences have neither the tools nor, at times, the inclination to analyze whole cultures, intercultural relations, or cultural process. For this reason, philosophers like Cassirer have at times assumed the title of anthropologist. Historians like Toynbee, Turner, or Beard have attempted to blend historical description with cultural analysis; and psychologists, psychiatrists, and sociologists have turned to anthropology for cross-cultural perspective.

However, general dynamic analyses of culture gave way to relatively simple propositions such as the claim that major social segments of any culture are structured and have definable functions, or that man's characteristic psychodynamic tendencies in any group are also structured and reflect the interpenetrations of culture and personality. Such theories of integration are themselves formal. They are solipsismal in that they are limited to current deductions about single traditions, and incapable of further dynamic generalization. Cultures do not exist in traditional immutability, and the society embodying a tradition cannot remain static any more than its individual culture-carriers can. In this sense, a society is more or less structured, and its definable functions are merely a current balance of forces, social in origin and expression. Even psychodynamic tendencies in individuals and groups exist only as balances of forces which men like Freud saw as being often in opposition, or in the polite diplomacy of truce.

A cultural integration, far from being a sculptured, fixed, and inevitable arrangement of constants, psychological in nature, such as Benedict and others sought to describe, is constantly in a state of flux. It is only a more or less stable set of conditions for social existence found among specified groups of mankind and operating for limited spans of time. Thus cultural integrations contain within themselves the seeds of reintegration or change. Just as all grammatical structures or morphological systems of language are imperfect, or as Sapir bluntly put it, "all grammars leak," so social structures and kinship systems are merely outlines and general indicators of conduct and custom. Social organization is ordinarily most responsive to the steady and inevitable impact of material conditions of existence. Since a culture contains the traditional modes of coping with both physical and human nature, its economy and social organization will of necessity be related. When this relationship becomes tenuous through changes in economy, either the old society and cultural traditions change in a process of reintegration, or the cracks and fissures multiply and the culture dies. The past is strewn with both instances: reintegration and forward development in some traditions as society and culture develop, or disintegration, death, and decay in others. Benedict and others have written that necessity is *not* the mother of invention, either in economic or social affairs. Perhaps not, so far as the slow but rapidly increasing tempo of economic and scientific inventions goes. At any rate, on the social and cultural side, material inventions become the mother of necessity; and either necessary social changes are made or the society goes under.

At one time, anthropology had such perspectives. As early as 1844 in the United States, Gallatin, as founder and president of the American Ethnological Society, wrote into the constitution of that body, "The object of this society shall comprise inquiries into the origin, progress and characteristics of . . . man." Jenks, writing with Rivers and Morley by request of the Carnegie Institution of Washington, also stated in 1913 that "the anthropologist . . . makes his studies of both the past and the present with an eye to the future, in order that those things which vitiated or benefited the evolutionary process in the past, and which vitiate and benefit it today, may serve as guides for future generations."[194] Sir Edward Tylor's closing passage of his great work, *Anthropology*, put this matter clearly as early as 1881: "Mankind is passing from the age of unconscious to that of conscious progress. . . . The study of man and civilization passes at once into the practical business of life." Either anthropology today accepts this challenge to formulate a dynamic science of culture, or we blindly and emotionally renounce the practical aspects of human existence.

Having already noted that questions of particular cultural integrations are different from the question of integration in general, we are faced with an old problem of whether mankind should be studied in unity or diversity. In biology, one thinks of Claude Bernard's famous aphorism: "The life of the animal is only a fragment of the total life of the universe." In cultures, which grow and change not only through internal inventions and accretions, but through contact and diffusions, the life of a single culture is but an instance in the story of culture in general. In Raoul Allier's badly-titled *The Mind of the Savage*,[195] the anthropological tradition of the fundamental unity of the human species is presented, especially as it emerged in French social thought. The position of Fontenelle, so characteristic of the eighteenth century, was that culture alone made men diverse, while psychological equality and the even distribution of natural gifts argued for a fundamental unity of mankind. With Helvetius and Montesquieu, comparisons of humanity in general with men in Europe (termed "savages" by Voltaire) led to the idealization of nonliterate peoples. The classic statement of Baron de Lahontan, "They know nothing of thine and mine, have no class distinctions, but live in the state of equality nature intended," is an attempt at such dignifying, which Comte rephrased in opposition to Rousseau as evidence merely of higher potentialities always present in man.

In anthropology, early periods of discovery and first formulations provided more than descriptive data and methodological cautions. In general approaches to man and culture, anthropologists were busy laying the ghosts of exploration and conquest. Racial mentality was recognized as the empty echo of self-interested minds. Human nature was seen undergoing transformations in the crucibles of culture. What was added to eighteenth-century romanticism, however, was mainly the first clause in the dictum: "Cultures are many, though man is one." Even before Boas, the second clause had been recognized in the anti-racistic emphases of the French Enlightenment, the naturalistic materialists, the schools of fundamental human unity, and the more penetrating evolutionists like Tylor and Morgan.

At this point, a reference to Theodor Waitz is instructive. Waitz, in his *Anthropologie der Naturvölker*,[196] proceeds immediately from a position assuming fundamental unity of man to an analysis of what "human nature" basically includes. Here we are reminded much more pointedly of White than Boas. Culture, as a superorganic adaptation to man's need for food, shelter, and protection, as a mode of regulating human relations, and as expressed in religion, art, recreation, and knowledge, is despite manifold forms and exemplifications a generic *process* coexistent with mankind. By page 272 of the first volume, the bases of all human or cultural behavior are isolated in the ability to make tools and to symbolize, especially by means of that "specific human peculiarity, language." To be sure, in Waitz as in Boas, the shibboleth of the "primitive mind" is assaulted vigorously, but while Boas is led to present the data of cultures piecemeal and in separate and supposedly unique circumstances, the method of Waitz is synthesizing and generalizing. One is reminded here of Kroeber's critique of Boas in the essay "History and Science in Anthropology":

> From physics Boas brought into anthropology a sense of definiteness of problem, of exact rigor of method, and of highly critical objectivity. In brief, one may define the Boas

position as . . . being aware of the requirements of cultural or human material: the need for all possible context, the strong element of uniqueness in all the phenomena, and extreme caution of generalizations savoring of the universal. All these are criteria of sound historical method; and because he observes them, Boas is right in insisting over and over again that he uses historical method. Only he does not *do* history. And that does make some difference.[197]

Obviously, one cannot *do* history, much less generalizations on processes in culture, until one notes similarities as well as differences. How far Kroeber was correct in intimating that a doctrine of cultural diversity led Boas to historical atomism may be seen in further examination of the latter's paper, "The Aims of Anthropological Research."[198] After indicating certain obvious correlations between population size and food supply, Boas attacks materialistic explanations:

> We do not see how art styles, the form of ritual or the special form of religious belief could possibly be derived from economic forces. . . . Economics and the rest of culture interact as cause and effect, as effect and cause. Every attempt to deduce cultural forms from a single cause is doomed to failure, for the various expressions of culture are closely interrelated and one cannot be altered without having an effect on all the others. . . . It seems justifiable to question whether any general conclusions may be expected that will be applicable everywhere and that will reduce the data of anthropology to a formula which may be applied to every case, explaining its past and predicting the future.[199]

This tendency of history to describe the unique event led Boas to conclude that anthropology "must be a historical science . . . the interest of which centers in the attempt to understand the individual phenomena rather than the establishment of general laws." If this were history, wrote Boas, then psychology would consist in seeing "how many of our lines of behavior that we believe to be founded deep in human nature are actually expressions of our culture and subject to modification with changing culture. . . . By a study of the universality and variety of cultures, anthropology may help us to shape the future course of mankind.''[200]

How this generous light could be shed without knowledge of the laws and principles governing cultural change and development was not considered. What art, social organization, ritual, and religion contributed to the psychic economy of individuals and the social economy of cultures was not explained. Of particular interest here is the amazing claim that close interrelation of the expressions of a culture blurs cause and effect relationships. On the contrary, it should make these all the more apparent. Obviously, this is again the merry-go-round view of single cultures. But more important for our thesis, we find that it is not a fruitful theory of integration for a single culture and even less a theory of cultural integration in general. Again, the Scissors-Match game is proclaimed to be the final aim of anthropology. It is suggested, to correct such aberrations, that if the amazingly complex material universe may be approached by formulae—not one, but several—then cultural phenomena, especially in terms of the relations of institutional aspects in change, may also be so expressed.

While, indeed, history may describe the unique event, science does not stop there. Anthropology is not mere descriptive history, but the science of man and culture. Therefore, a useful theory of cultural integration, one which explains and analyzes rather than merely describes cultures, must have general as well as specific reference.

Turning to Boas' second proposition, the notion that human psychology is merely an expression of a *particular* cultural content, how then can one explain, as Boas was fond of doing, any independent inventions? How account for such forms as clans, states, nomadic bands, totemism, shamanism, priestly cults, or, indeed, any of a variety of phenomena found across continents and in remote island territories? A. A. Golden-weiser attempted in a paper called "The Principle of Limited Possibilities . . ."[201] to set formal limits within which human creativity operates. Yet within such limits, the many minor variations on basic themes seem unrestricted, and human creativeness is certainly not at fault. Boas' statement that a change in *any* one aspect of culture changes all the rest appears unlikely in the light of survivals, cultural persistence, and traditions which resist change. Boas erroneously applied equal weight to all aspects of culture.

A notion of interests—economic, sexual, and artistic—might be helpful here, provided we rid ourselves of the extravagant idea that "anything" can happen in culture. In the human species, man must first seek food, shelter, and protection to survive, and all social systems emphasize some form or elaborated versions of these simple economic functions. There is no society which does not regulate, or formalize, social and sexual relationships. All develop ideas and practices for achieving some type of relationship or rapport with the universe. They contain in all instances forms of artistic expression and types of recreation. But in no instance are the psychological capabilities and biological or social needs separate from the meanings of a culture to its carriers. There is no formal, psychological limitation to human invention, imagination, or culture, except the material conditions under which a culture exists, and its systems for regulating conduct. Economic and technical aspects of a culture set the limits and constitute the bases of culture, and even these change. The formal similarities noted by Goldenweiser, both in technique and in the social superstructure of cultures, generally are due to similarities if not identities, as he found them, in the evolutionary process the world over.

Our review of tendencies in American anthropology reveals a series of common pitfalls. Perhaps the most common, illustrated by Benedict, Sapir, and Linton, is to treat psychology of peoples or the results of cultural conditioning and milieu as a causal explanation of particular cultures or cultural traditions. Of the three, Sapir was closest to doctrines of the importance of cultural meanings and unconscious patternings of behavior in psychiatry. Nevertheless, he was ultimately as far as Benedict or Linton from the more important point in social psychiatry that psychology reflects culture, and not the opposite. In Goldenweiser's attempt to explain away cultural similarities and generic patterns, we find the epitome of this recourse to a formal psychological principle "explaining away" cultural dynamisms. Boas' historical atomism, Radcliffe-Brown's notion of synchronic kinship studies preceding diachronic ones, and Malinowski's descriptive, nonanalytic integrations are all related as essentially static systems. It is proposed to restore ethnological theory and the psychological content of culture to their proper relationship. This the author has earlier attempted to do.[202]

Anthropology today requires a generalizing analysis of the complete process of cultural evolution—material, social, and behavioral. Only within this framework are particular analyses of given cultural integrations and reintegrations meaningful. While cultures are many and diverse, the unity of mankind and generic similarity of human psychological processes make each society part of a larger process. The psychological content of specific cultures, while having importance in individual lives, is one resultant of the particular conditions under which one culture operates. Anthropology has other tasks: it preserves a rich account of culture; it notes where the toll in individual lives, both biologically and psychologically, has been too great; and hopefully, it may apply principles discovered in the larger evolutionary settings to specific cultural integrations. Already in American anthropology there is every indication that a dynamically oriented, analytic, and generalizing science of culture is on the way.

ANTHROPOLOGICAL AND CROSS-CULTURAL ASPECTS OF HOMOSEXUALITY

This discusion of homosexuality pivots upon a combined behavioral and social-science view of man's fate. This combination of sciences, however, provides no ready-made answers about the fate of sexual impulses. The anthropological view does not ignore biological and physiological factors and is particularly receptive to psychological ones. At the same time, however, it insists that social and cultural forces not be neglected and that cross-cultural differences be given recognition in any analysis of human behavior.[203] This interdisciplinary view is the minimal requirement of an anthropological approach. But how the biological, psychological, social, and cultural factors are presumed to mesh and operate depends on the scientific synthesis. I shall attempt such a synthesis with regard to the problem of homosexuality.

Let me begin with a psychological point of view, the Freudian. In his analysis of the Schreber case,[204] Freud's insights into Schreber's Oedipal struggles led to the formulation that homosexual trends are a defense against immature infantile desires of males for mothers and females for fathers. Homosexuality was seen as a defensive structuring of unresolved conflicts in this realm. The infantile urges might first be denied with compulsive thought or conduct. But if compulsive, hysterical, displacing, and repressive defenses wore thin, wish projections and distortions might be tried in the Oedipal struggle. The problem of homosexual trends was thus seen as a root problem in paranoid schizophrenia.

The key to this approach is, of course, the theory that psychosexual development is the prime behavioral unfolding that determines all else. As Charles Brenner[205] and other accurate commentators have pointed out, the point of view is one of psychic determinism with a psychosexual emphasis. But the biologist or physiologist asks, "What of biological and hormonal sexual variations?" The sociologist notes that the Daughters of Bilitis have their own organized press. The epidemiologist points to quantitative variations in the appearance of overt homosexual behavior by class, culture, nation, and perhaps historical epoch. The anthropologist points out that there are cultures in which homosexuality exists and others in which it does not, occasions on which it has behavioral organization and sanction and others on which it exists surreptitiously, and societies in which the raw stuff of Oedipal striving, castration fears, or the Greek or Nazi versions of male solidarity hardly can exist. The suggestion is that what Freud perceptively observed was one set of psychological hazards, behavioral evolution, and conditions of existence (middle-class Viennese society).

What Freud discovered, using one set of factors in one general type of culture in one historical period, hardly could be used in the framework of cultural relativity for different cultures. Yet the matter can be put more fairly to give credit to the factors he did discover. Perhaps most of all, in emphasizing the psychological factors, Freud located one paramount sequence of causality. We shall claim that it is only one part of the causal change or nexus, but this claim does not diminish the importance of the discovery. The principle he established was that biological functioning in humans is subject to profound social and cultural inhibitions and that, in this sense, psychological factors have primacy and control over organic ones. This emphasis, of course, had a tremendous impact on the organicist tradition of German medicine, and Freud was attacked and berated as a sexmonger and sensualist, almost the opposite, of course, of what he really was. A doctrine that stresses the necessity of ego controls and the formative dominant position of the superego in all development is a form of psychic determinism, to be sure, but hardly argues for unilinear and one-sided sexual determinism. In *The Ego and the Id*,[206] Freud called "culture" the "heir of the Oedipus complex"—in just so many words—and, though he lacked the anthropological training and data to know what to do with culture as a prime factor in establishing "ego" and "superego" supremacy over the id, nevertheless he proclaimed it the principle by which individuals are normatively controlled.

In *Totem and Taboo*,[207] however, Freud's lack of anthropological training and data led him to create a fantasy about the nature of primitive societies and cultural evolution, using the aboriginal tribes of Australia as his prime example. Let us consider the Australian tribe that practices subincision of the male penis in coming-of-age ceremonies used as the *rite de passage* for adolescent boys. The casual reader who learns about incisions with stone knives up to the urethra, the laying flat of the whole cylindrical organ, and the binding with leaves for a painful healing after a painful operation without anesthesia and then discovers that the older men (fathers, grandfathers, and paternal uncles) are the mutilators might presume that this operation climaxes or arouses extremely severe castration anxieties in a society in which males and females live nude. Does this ceremony then lead, as it is claimed in Freud's *Totem and Taboo*, to castration anxieties, the primal parricidal myth, and the symbolic injunction against eating the ancestral totem animal (pseudo-"anticannibalism," in the tortured explanation)? Nothing could be further from the truth! The pain is suffered willingly, even proudly, by lads learning tribal lore and religion from patrilineal elder kinsmen. The latter are models of concern and sympathy and, more than that, are sharing precious rites and tribal lore with the novices. Indeed, these boys have seen male and female nudity, know animal anatomy in addition, and are well versed in sexual and reproductive functions far beyond the children and adolescents of our "modern" cultures. Any vestige of castration anxieties—could they even exist—are nullified by the ceremonial ritual in which the penis mutilation occurs, a ritual imbued with the religious sanctity of becoming an adult in the society and coming into the possession of sacred lore, adult prerogatives, and adult fellowship.

The point about these societies and other nonliterate hunting and gathering societies is that homosexuality is generally rare and, in some instances, virtually nonexistent. In the first tribes this author ever studied under field conditions, the Mescalero and Chiricahua Apache, this rarity stands in marked contrast to modern urban American or English culture. The standard work on Chiricahua, *An Apache Life-Way*, by Morris E. Opler,[208] notes that homosexuality is forbidden among them and considered to be a form of witchcraft. Informants had heard about boys, but not adult men, experimenting homosexually. One berdache, or transvestite, who engaged in women's pursuits (but apparently not in homosexuality) was reported to have died before 1880. A few Lesbians dated back to days of detention at Fort Sill in Oklahoma. Some women had masculine interests. But other than these scattered and historical instances, in which, incidentally, no organic findings were available, homosexuality was notable for its rarity. Later, in fieldwork among Ute Indians of Colorado,[209] this author's check on such topics yielded amusement, disbelief, and counterquestioning on American urban culture.

The reactions of nonliterate peoples, on the simplistic hunting and gathering levels of economic development, help to answer the question whether rates of homosexual behavior vary among different societies. Driver, in *Indians of North America*,[210] discusses typical examples of Plains Indian berdaches, or male transvestites. He notes that relations with women were symbols of male prestige in these cultures and that the general social dominance of men over women was probably stronger here than in any area north of Mexico, except the Northwest Coast. In this setting, some men with strong aversions to the ultramasculine role donned women's clothing, did women's work, and sometimes (apparently a minority) lived homosexually in actual fact.

Writers on South American Indians offer equally sparse examples. Steward and Faron, in *Native Peoples of South America*,[211] mention examples only for the Calamari, among whom there was a special class of male inverts, as well as one of women prostitutes, who went from village to village selling sexual services, and for the Nata townsmen, among whom there was a class of homosexual male slaves who did women's work.

Margaret Mead, in various writings but notably in her book *Male and Female*,[212] goes beyond the bare bones of such reporting to suggest that human societies evince two polarities in regard to sexual arousal. One is a tendency toward erotic specificity, so that sexual arousal depends upon particular conditions. The nape of the female neck in Japanese lore of the past century is one instance of cultural specificity, whereas intersexual bathing and nudity are alleged to have had no such connotations. Among the Ute Indians, whom this author has studied, it is claimed that female breasts are devoid of sexual meaning. On the other hand, positive sexual arousal, including homosexual arousal, has been described as being stimulated by a wide and diverse range of nonspecific sources. It is possible, however, that such description derives from generalizations from cross-cultural data such as those of Ford and Beach in their *Patterns of Sexual Behavior*,[213] which stress complex patterns of cultural learning. The Ford and Beach survey lists cultures in which virtually all males engage in homosexual practices at times and other cultures in which such practices are interdicted and relatively rare. Unfortunately, most studies of the survey sort tear information out of context, so that one is quite uncertain whether the investigator is concerned with the normative sexual experiments of preadolescents or with adult homosexuality. By contrast, Rado, in his *Psychoanalysis of Behavior*,[214] distinguishes the "situational homosexuality" of prisoners and sailors isolated from opposite sex mates; the "incidental homosexuality" of some adolescents and preadolescents or of sociopaths; the "chaotic sexuality" of certain impulse-ridden schizophrenics; and the "reparative homosexuality" of some neurotics traumatized from heterosexual contacts.

In my book *Culture and Mental Health*,[215] I have reported briefly on Bogoras' fascinating work, *The Chukchee*,[216] which deals with a well-studied tribe of Northeastern Siberia. The developmental course of Chukchee transvestitism practices is carefully described. Bogoras relates the Chukchee practice of insisting on a bride price, or *kalym*, which often takes a man seven years to amass, to high rates of aberrancy. Bogoras also describes the floating population of perennially unmarried laborers. The problems of building the nucleus of one's own reindeer herd or of a son's protracted adolescent status in relation to a long-lived property-owning father indicate two ways in which rigid patriarchal controls over property inheritance may operate. Bogoras describes the frustrations of delayed marriages, the development of fantasy outlets, and the social sanctions for transvestite shamans to practice as a kind of escapism. The pathology he describes, such as notions of wandering out over the tundra, are direct expressions of the escapist theme. That members of the floating populations of laborers, youths, or sons-in-law "serving time" may receive this "call" to respectable livelihoods as shamans is entirely expected, and the relatives are enjoined to be duly respectful of the sanctity of this profession and watchful of the developing shamans' safety. Not all shamans take the route of transvestitism, however. Apparently only a few do go to such lengths, but the cultural sanctions accord the transformed shaman particular compensations in *religious* potency.

Animal studies are not in the least analogous to such rich

cultural accounts, but they do give some notion of how extreme discomforts can lead to chaotic sexuality. Harlow's well-known studies[217] of rhesus monkeys deprived of mothering and further isolated from reparative peer-group contacts show breakdowns of normative heterosexual behavior in both males and females. Calhoun's studies of Norway rats[218] showed that those subjected to adverse environmental conditions in the crowded settings he calls "behavioral sinks" developed failures in nest building, interruptions in normal transport of young, and both homosexual and infant-rat sexual approaches. In the "pansexuality" that developed, both male and female rats were increasingly bitten on the scruff of the neck during mounting, although female rats sustained these aggressive attacks in greater number. Carefully developed mammalian studies have demonstrated that disturbances in sexual behavior are accompanied by concomitant disturbances in social behavior and other functions. Indeed, Harlow's study appears to demonstrate that proper peer-group contacts can help to heal wounds occasioned by faulty mothering.

As most persons familiar with anthropological literature know, heterosexual experimentation often has greater social sanction in primitive societies than in Western or European cultures. The Andamanese, described by Radcliffe-Brown in *The Andaman Islanders,*[219] practiced strict monogamy, prohibited and punished adultery, but allowed both boys and girls to participate freely before marriage in sexual experimentation that frequently led to "trial marriages." The Ute Indians of Colorado are in no sense connected historically to the Andamanese, but they practiced precisely the same sexual customs. The Tahitians of Polynesia furnish a third example of a people among whom the years between puberty and marriage are expected to constitute a period for experimental love affairs. Yet these societies, which are permissive in their heterosexual customs, accord homosexuality a most aberrant status. Actually, no society, save perhaps ancient Greece, pre-Meiji

Japan, certain top echelons in Nazi Germany, and the scattered examples of such special status groups as the berdaches, Nata slaves, and one category of Chukchee shamans, has lent sanction in any real sense to homosexuality. Regardless of what may be said concerning all the factors—social, legal, and psychodynamic—entering into homosexual behavior, one thing is clear: In the absence of an organic or hormonal basis, homosexuality in practically all cultures is regarded as a deviation from the majority values and norms of conduct.

On the other hand, while most cultures recognize the normative character of heterosexual bonds of one type or another, most also place enormous psychological emphasis on such matters as the social control of sexual behavior. Even the Andaman, Ute, and Tahitian peoples limit heterosexual experimentation to a particular life period. While all three are fairly egalitarian and permissive about divorce, the fact remains that cultural norms and rules still function as social definitions of sexual conduct. The heterosexual norm and its social control in all cultures suggest that the problem of relative incidence of homosexuality is not a function of organic and hormonal variations in humans but of differences in the cultures themselves.

As we have seen, the psychosexual developmental theme of Freudian psychology has extended the causal nexus of experiences influencing organic functioning to include culture, which in turn influences experience. For this reason, mammalian animal studies, while instructive, cannot reach the level of Rado's classification of "incidental, situational or reparative homosexuality" in humans. If we ask whether there may be homosexual subculture groups, particularly in modern urban and industrial societies, as there are in the scattered primitive instances, the answer is, of course, yes. These subcultural groups are also special responses to strains in the normatively heterosexual cultures and not simply individual psychodynamic phenomena.

As culture is a prime means of human adaptation and in this sense aids individuals in adapting to the world of nature and of social relationships, cultures define norms of sexual conduct in the same settings or patterns that they define social, educational, economic, and political relationships. A cultural point of view on any aspect of human behavior therefore stresses *social* identification, as well as *sexual-* and *self*-identification. There are, in all cultures, *social* definitions of conduct linked with *sexual* definitions and with notions of proper *personal* behavior. In fact, such linking is how cultures aid man in adaptations to the world of nature, to the "cosmos," and to others, male and female, in the society. The norms that define sexual conduct are of the same substance as those defining social and personal conduct. Freud discovered parts of these connections in the causal nexus, in particular the connections between sexual and personal functioning. Social functioning was subsumed under such concepts as "sublimation of libidinal energies" or "specific consciences" or "superego" to invoke the notion of human striving beyond the pleasure principle. Because, cross-culturally and biologically, the weight is thrown on the side of heterosexual standards of conduct, it is tempting to assume a fixed biological proclivity in this direction. Yet a biological deviance in hormones and sexual structures such as occasionally occurs in sexual maturation does not always produce so flagrant or florid a form of homosexuality in humans as does mere confusion in social, sexual, and self-identification. Indeed, this point is foreshadowed on the animal level in studies of the Norway rat and rhesus monkey, among which behavior is a function of social, group, and interanimal contacts rather than of biological endowment. In the same sense, biological deviance is only one factor among many in human *gender-role* definition. Indeed, social expectations and self-conceptions may transform the biological deviant into a model male or female from the cultural point of view. Studies of hermaphrodites have indicated that social and familial expectations can shape the outcome toward male or female gender roles, regardless of the actual genetic sex involved.

Not that culture does not ideally stress the existence of usual, normative, and common standards of a male or a female type. The point is simply that this highlighting is done culturally. A Navajo Indian may be a he-man, a gambler, and a philanderer while dressing in bright blouses adorned with jeweled belts, necklaces, and bracelets. French courtiers in the retinues of effete monarchs were equally philanderers, though rouged, powdered, and bedecked with fine lace. The Andaman Islanders like to have the man sit on his wife's lap in fond greetings, and friends and relatives, of the same or opposite sex, greet one another in the same manner after absences, crying in the affected manner of the mid-Victorian woman. Like the Ute, they value premarital sexual experimentation and sexual prowess and technique in any later life period. Obviously, the style of social and sexual behavior is something of an amalgam and is culturally influenced.

The formula of social, sexual, and self-identification combinations, in addition, is useful in defining homosexuality. In our culture, with its tendency toward sex segregation in the latency period, preadolescent and adolescent sexual experimentation is often labeled "homosexual" no matter how rare, intermittent, or experimental the behavior actually is. Such rules of thumb, deriving from the theory of psychosexual dominance, often do considerable harm to an individual's later self-evaluations or are viewed with undue apprehension by physicians. Goldman, in his monograph on *The Cubeo, Indians of the Northwest Amazon*,[220] labels as "homosexual," for lack of a clearer or better term, what appears to me to be limited sexual experimentation on essentially the maturing adolescent masturbation level. Among the Cubeo, in a rare instance of rigid sexual controls that contrast with Ute, Andamanese, and similar customs, adolescents may reach the age of marriage without having had sexual relations with an eligible marriage partner. Instead, young people are limited to semipublic "homosexual" play, in which girls may stroke one another's nipples to produce erection or boys may indulge in mutual masturbation. The alternative to this activity is clandestine incestuous (between sib, not familial, brother and sister) experimentation in which actual intromission is regarded as *really* constituting incest and is avoided, so that the act consists only of external genital rubbing. True coitus or intromission would be punishable by death and, as true incest, would be followed by the offenders' souls becoming animal souls unfit for human association. As Goldman recognizes, *true* homosexuality among the Cubeo is rare if not absent, for he learned of no cases of persistent male homosexuality and of only one organically abnormal "woman" who developed strong male characteristics including, eventually, a penis. The Cubeo premarital limits are balanced by later widespread adultery and by female aggressiveness in enticing sexual intercourse—which continues even after menopause. Cultures in which female sexual aggressiveness exceeds that of the male, such as those of the Cubeo and upper-class Tuareg female courtiers and troubadours, are often those in which males are the social custodians of morality to such an extent that our Western European notions of biological, male-linked, sexual aggressiveness have to be modified. This difference is present not only in sexual but in social and ego-adaptive areas as well.

For those who give psychosexual development primacy, it is well to remember that among the Cubeo it is a common male complaint that wives are too ardent, whereas among the upper-class Tuareg the male would blush furiously in the love court of female troubadours if his veil were to slip (the men rather than the women are veiled). These cultural conditions are by no means common, nor do they negate other normal biological proclivities. Goldman notes, for example, that Cubeo women, no matter how sexually forward, prefer to be vigorously subdued in actual sexual intercourse. The Imashek of the Tuareg, like women in most Sahara cultures, are likewise interested in strong male sexual prowess. What we are describing are profound cultural *modifications* of biological sex but not its obliteration.

In most anthropological theory, the notion that biological needs or drives are modifiable by cultural necessity holds sway. If we were to discuss the matter more philosophically, there might be a tendency to claim that moral or legal sanctions mold behavior in some direction. This formulation, indeed, is one way in which concepts of superego, or conscience, have been used. In Freudian formulations, however, moral or legal sanctions are viewed as part of cultural constriction and as inhibitory rather than formative. Idealistic positions in philosophy might hold, by contrast, that ideas rather than environmental experiences determine conduct. We hold with the Freudian position that moral and legal sanctions are part of the culture pattern, but we should add to Freud's inhibitory notions that cultural patterns of sexual or other biological behavior may be not only restrictive and prohibiting but also prescriptive and positively determining. For example, Cubeo adolescent experimentations are publicly displayed as sexual modalities for children and youth, and masturbation is conducted without shame. Similar prescriptive patterns are observable (in balance with proscriptive ones) in such cultures as those of the Ute, the Andamanese, or the Tahitians, which we have used as examples of predominantly permissive systems. Homosexuality is rare in such permissive but organized and directive systems. Such societies are, of course, culturally homogeneous, well understood by their members, and in aboriginal times so socially and economically integrated that little cognitive mapping was required to give moral and legal sanctions to kinds of sexual behavior. Far from agreeing with Benedict's *Patterns of Culture*[221] that a process of "psychological selectivity" is at work deriving ethos and outlook from an endless arc of possibilities, we believe the *conditions of existence* in a culture (economic and social, primarily) are determinative of the themes that may be selected. Sexual and self-identification themes are only a part of such an ethos. There is a vast difference between the view that "anything can happen" in a culture and the position that parts of the pattern are more determinative of its details than are other parts. Our concept of pattern excludes the former brand of psychic determinism but includes the latter form of psychosocial determinism, according to the *conditions of cultural existence.*

Although culture is, by and large, a generalized and extra-somatic agency for serving all manner of human needs, it does not follow that the needs themselves are entirely supra-individual or nonsomatic. Economics, for example, may aid in the organized procurement and even development of "needs"— some of which may be somatic and some not. It is conceivable that Navajo practices of male adornment may be distantly related to primate tendencies to bedeck and adorn, such as those observable among monkeys and apes, which are not culturally determined. Economics touches, however, upon basic conditions of existence in a culture, and, because of human appetites, economics is enormously and repetitively concerned with daily somatic needs. The Kinsey reports on male and female sexual behavior in American society, even if we disregard the improper and sometimes even curious modes of sampling that they employed, clearly bring out essential class differences in sexual conduct (although the unit of analysis is not conduct but biological orgasm). Similarly, even a psychoanalytic popularizer like Edmund Bergler cannot fail to note in his writings that homosexual symptoms are part of wider personality disorders, are susceptible to educational campaigns and organized medical countermeasures, and have social as well as individual contexts, creeds, and organizations. Few writers on the problem of homosexuality in modern society have failed to notice profound differences in social-class patterns of homosexual behavior analogous to the widely known social-class differences in normative heterosexual behavior. Besides sexual needs, other forces—"needs" for prestige, social desires, and even factors bolstering self-esteem become important. The chief's yam-houses with their rotting yams among the Trobriand Islanders and the burning candlefish oil and broken copper plates of a potlatch, or give-away ceremony, among the Kwakiutl Indians of British Columbia are two well-worn examples of elaborations on simple economic patterns.[222] Sexual customs are similarly elaborated, as in the Trobriander's myth of no physical paternity or the Cubeo's claim of female sexuality increasing to the menopausal years. At the same time, the Trobrianders, even those from the rich garden districts of Kiriwina, do not omit garden magic; the Kwakiutl do not neglect the basic subsistence economy contained in fishing and timber; and the Cubeo formulate sexual restrictions until mar-riage—all for good reasons. To presume that an economic system can be based on prestige ideology alone, that sexuality does not have social definition and regulation, or that the cul-tural ethos does not attach to elements important in the daily round of the culture is poor anthropology indeed.

We begin with economics and the cultural pattern as ex-amples because, in most discussions of the psychic economy, it has so often been assumed that the sexual factor is not only pre-eminent but that it operates alone. To our way of thinking, these conceptions of a psychic (and organic) *primum mobile* acting alone are inadequate in explaining the amazing adjust-ments sometimes achieved by the organically inadequate and the variations in both type and quantity of abnormal conduct in cultures in which the physical human organisms are essen-tially normal in biological endowment. Similarly, zonal theories of development, such as that of Erikson in *Childhood and Society*,[223] are negated as *primum mobile* theories when we contrast his warlike Sioux Indians with the peaceful Ute of Colorado.[224] The Sioux roamed the plains and showed cruelty to women occasionally, not because of cradleboard inhibitions to movement or nursing past the stage of tooth eruption, but because Sioux culture is essentially patrilineal and nomadic in its hunting of buffalo. The Ute, who did not roam the plains and were egalitarian in sexual codes, used a similar cradleboard and nursed infants and children even longer, but Ute culture was organized differently in its social and economic aspects. Neither do purely individual sexual ideologies determine sexual conduct and proclivities. We have never encountered a purely individual ideology about sex. Although the psychosexual factor has tremendous importance in the total development of individual behavior, it is doubtful that we can abstract sexual development from concomitant social and self-identification processes. The basic error of the *primum mobile* theory of psychosexual development is that it tears sexual development from its meaningful context and ceases to weigh it together with other connected developments in human growth.

In nonliterate societies, social groupings by kinship, age group, clans, sibs, and associates in various functional relationships far outweigh social groupings by sex. In fact, Lowie[225] was one of the few modern theorists to discuss groupings by sex at all, and he used such pallid distinctions as those among bachelors, spinsters, and married persons. Although most kinship distinctions include sexual criteria, some do not, and, in general, most kinship groups have not one but several criteria for admission. Clubs and societies have on occasion been sex limited, as in Melanesia, but there is no reason to believe that this limitation has promoted homosexual behavior in these social, economic, or sometimes ritual settings—or indeed that such behavior exists at all in such instances.

Holmberg, in his monograph *Nomads of the Long Bow*,[226] about the Siriono of Eastern Bolivia, has noted that, in the hand-to-mouth existence of these South American Indians, anxieties about food gathering and sharing occur regularly but seem to be divorced from sexual matters. The Siriono practice nudity, chiefs have many wives, and there is no question that young males see "mothers" and are aware of menstrual functions. Although, in our modern Western European cultures, both male and female paranoid schizophrenics typically show evidence of both overt and "latent" homosexuality, if the theory were transculturally valid, the paradigm of incomplete Oedipal repressions followed by male castration fears and female fears of seduction would have a flying start among the Siriono. In actuality, the Freudian anxiety of Oedipal origins, the projective conversion of "I love him" to "I hate him," and its later defensive generalization to paranoid persecutions do not find ready analogues in Siriono culture. We suspect that what have been left out of account are other massive processes of social and self-identification.

In our belief, not only do self- , social- , and sexual-identification processes co-exist and interweave, but also, with self-identification chronologically consolidated in the first stages, social identification doubtless impinges on the cognitive processes associated with language. In this manner, areas labeled "social" and "learned" have a curious way of invading the other two from the outer cultural and family environments. Only a total life-cycle perspective would ever give weight to social-identification processes as such. Piaget,[227] Sullivan,[228] and Fromm[229] have initiated trends in this direction from child studies, life-cycle, and social-identity theory respectively. The epidemiological interests of social psychiatry have already proved this point on a different frontier in a multitude of studies on variations in every form of mental disorder by age-sex or class-cultural analyses. To suppose, against this massive evidence, that we have one model of human development, male or female, or one process of ego adaptation to describe is to set the scene only for psychologically based theories of sexual adaptation or self-identification. Both exist but not alone. *Their existence is essentially meaningless unless social identification is immediately added as a concomitant in the life cycle.*

SOCIOCULTURAL ROOTS
OF EMOTIONAL ILLNESS

We are discussing anxiety and depression presumably because they are sick states the physician is called upon to treat. Whether the doctor regards this as his primary charge as a psychiatrist, or whether he is an internist who encounters such complications, the fact is that modern communities contain many persons who suffer from emotional illness in one form or another. As a principal investigator of the Cornell Department of Psychiatry's Midtown Manhattan Community Mental Health Research Study, I can report that 80 per cent of a population in the largest city in the United States suffered from some degree of impairment in life functioning which might be called "Emotional Disability." These impairments ranged in a continuum from mild and moderate disabilities on the one hand ("mild symptom formation" in 36.3 per cent of the population, and "moderate symptom formation" in 21.8 per cent) to the astoundingly high percentage of 23.4 per cent showing marked, severe, or incapacitating impairments. This last figure doubles previous estimates, using less exacting methods, in Boston and Baltimore surveys.

Our study in New York City evoked front-page headlines in such papers as *The New York Times* and *Herald Tribune* when our first volume of the three-volume series of books appeared. The first book, *Mental Health in the Metropolis (The Midtown Manhattan Study)*,[230] is less full of surprises than one might expect if one considered the fact that half of all hospital beds in the United States have for some time been devoted to psychiatric patients. Or looked at another way, we would expect in an epidemiological survey of a total population such grand totals as 80 per cent if a survey of all nonpsychological *organic* impairments were attempted. As it is for organic impairments from mild ones to totally incapacitating ones, so it is, apparently, for emotional illness in its various dimensions. As to whether one wishes to use an 80 per cent figure, or the still shocking figure of 23.4 per cent, this depends on whether one is concerned about mild impairments as well as those labeled "marked symptom formation," "severe impairments" or "incapacitating" ones. While some newspapers chose to emphasize that one person out of every five was designated as "mentally well" and went on to report the social and cultural distributions of illness, others chose the comparable 80 per cent rate, that is comparable to a figure for all organic ailments, as a rate of some degree of disability. An earlier paper which I published under the title "Epidemiological Studies of Mental Illness"[231] in the U.S. government's Walter Reed Army Institute *Symposium on Preventive and Social Psychiatry* stressed that *total* epidemiology is important in assessing the range of emotional impairments. If one wished to stop at those who are impaired but in treatment, one could do a study of the simple sort of prevalence, the prevalence of those in treatment such as was done by Hollingshead and Redlich. If one wished to designate the impaired in the community, both those in treatment and those never treated, one could use the 23.4 per cent figure. But if one wished to face up to the total preventive and social tasks of medicine and psychiatry, no doubt the 80 per cent figure is our most honest and humane estimate.

In this account of the Midtown findings in epidemiology, we have used two concepts that are central to our approach. The first is the notion of a continuum from well, through mild and moderate disturbances, reaching finally to "marked symptom formation," "severely impaired" and finally, "incapacitated." In New York City, we found people who had never been known to psychiatry or psychological medicine who were as utterly incapacitated as any I have ever seen in chronic wards. Further, the rates for impairment in general, and for extreme degrees of impairment also, were not randomly distributed in the population. Both lower class and certain poorly established ethnic communities, the Puerto Rican and the Hungarian specifically, had greater impairments in general, or extent of therapy-need, and more than their proportionate share of the serious categories of disturbance in addition. In the 23.4 per cent figure, we pointed out that 13.2 per cent showed marked symptom formation, 7.5 per cent exhibited severe symptom formation, and 2.7 per cent were virtually incapacitated. Such total proportions for the community as a whole are raised, not lowered, when one considers the combination of lower social class and certain ethnic groupings such as Puerto Rican and Hungarian. In his studies of hospital admissions by class and ethnic group, Dr. Benjamin Malzberg reaches the same conclusions when, for example, he finds that Puerto Ricans have higher representation than their numbers warrant in the population of New York State for hospital admissions labeled schizophrenic. While hospital admissions data have their limitations, our epidemiological survey of community samples supports Malzberg's contentions.

In medical sociology, as a matter of fact, ethnic and social class variations are being constantly discovered in organic illnesses which no one claims are psychological in origin. A colleague of mine in Buffalo, writing on "Social Factors in Relation to the Chronic Illnesses," in the *Handbook of Medical Sociology*[232] comments chiefly on studies of cancer and of hypertension to this effect. Dr. Saxon Graham[233] notes class and ethnic variations in such instances. In other words, social conditionings affecting behavior may involve cultural group or class group in biologically pathogenic functioning. One could say, all the more, that in illnesses which are emotional and have a psychological intervening variable between culture on the one hand and personality functioning on the other, the illnesses are bound to have social and cultural roots in the final analysis. In the Midtown Manhattan studies, 75 per cent of the total population showed high ratings on an anxiety scale or dimension. We hasten to add that this is a global assessment which technically does not discriminate between such clinical types as anxiety neurosis and depressive states in which anxiety is prominent. However, when we did gather data on such clearly defined clinical entities as psychosomatic disorders, class and cultural variables were again prominent.

In the Midtown Manhattan Study, conducted with the late Dr. T. A. C. Rennie at the Cornell University Medical College Department of Psychiatry, we reviewed with each community respondent a series of ten somatic disorders often assigned a psychogenic basis. These included rheumatoid arthritis, asthma, colitis, allergies, stomach ulcer, essential hypertension, and diabetes. While Hilleboe and Larimore report that over 2 per cent of American adults are afflicted with diabetes, our own findings for population strata from ages 20 to 59 was only one per cent, with percentages of 19.4 for arthritis, 9.4 for essential hypertension, 5.3 for colitis, 4.5 for stomach ulcer, and 4.4 for asthma. The pattern of prevalence for diabetes, however, was interesting, since it increased with progressively lower social strata. Social status was analyzed from the points of view of education, housing and parental occupation and income. The pattern for diabetes of finding the disorder most frequently in low-status groups, shared with essential hypertension and rheumatoid arthritis, accorded well with the belief that diabetes relates to certain ways of handling life stress. The prevalence of colitis, on the other hand, decreased with progressively lower social status, while asthma was found most prevalent at the extremes of social level. However, diabetics and ulcer patients had only medium-high scores on tension-anxiety scales relating to restlessness, nervousness, sleep disturbances and overt worries that get one "down physically," suggesting relatively passive adaptations. This they shared with ulcer patients. By contrast, asthmatics and victims of hypertension had low tension-anxiety scores suggestive of a conversion or hysteriform mechanism, whereas skin disorders, colitis, and rheumatoid arthritis correlated well with high scores on tension-anxiety scales and implied a group with more direct somatization of their problems.

When we commented on the Midtown Manhattan Study, and noted that diabetes increases in prevalence with progressively lower social strata, we might have added that such strata derived predominantly from immigrant and second-generation Italian, Czech, Hungarian, German, and Irish communities, and that some, like the Italian for example, were mainly second generation. One has then a class component made up of ethnic components. As early as 1945, Calabresi found differences in the prevalence rates of diabetes in various ethnic groups—as a matter of fact—among Italians, Poles, Germans, and Irish, in the United States. Refining this approach in a study of several generations of much the same ethnic groups in Butler County, Pennsylvania, Graham found that diabetes (and exactly as in Midtown Manhattan, also rheumatoid arthritis and essential hypertension) showed relatively low rates in the first or immigrant generation, but sharp increases among their descendants of the second generation, this being followed by declines in rates in third and sequential generation levels. These rates of diabetes were, respectively, 12 per 1,000 for the first or immigrant generation level, 22.2 per 1,000 for the second, which is almost a doubling of rate, and 12.3 per 1,000 for generations third or over. Such rates were, of course, for a standardized age and sex composition. Graham's conclusions are like ours for the Midtown Manhattan Study; namely, that immigrant generations will themselves show better mental health status, including psychosomatic rates, than their children of the second generation. The latter are involved, as we hypothesized for Midtown Manhattan, in sociocultural strains enveloping personal stresses since parental and child values (the parental versus those of a peer group of age mates) stand in conflict.

The concept of a continuum from well to ill in every society and culture means that "impairment in life functioning" will vary as to types of disease and quantity of impairment in each cultural group. In 1956, in *Culture, Psychiatry and Human Values*,[234] the two conceptions of "impairment in life functioning" and a cultural theory of its epidemiology were developed. In that book, the present author surveyed mental health epidemiology through several reports from cultures around the world. Mental illnesses were found to vary both in type and in amount, or in prevalence and incidence of the disturbances, on every continent for which there were clear data. Not only that, but in Western European psychiatry, diseases had changed in type and in amount. The result was that the book postulated a *relational theory* of social psychiatry stating that both the forms of mental illness and the amount of disturbance vary with the cultural milieu both historically in our own tradition, and cross-culturally when we compare one culture with another.

In 1959, however, I published another volume called *Culture and Mental Health: Cross-Cultural Studies*[235] for which I furnished only two cultural studies, but for which, as editor, we gathered full contemporary studies from every continent. The strategy was to see whether the relational theory of 1956 held good according to the work of contemporary scholars, persons in behavioral sciences who were professional psychiatrists, epidemiologists, anthropologists, sociologists, and psychologists. The relational theory—that is, the hypothesis that culture determines form of emotional illness and its quantity—was again confirmed, in this instance by twenty-three authors representing the above disciplines and for the most part working independently and in different continental settings.

This theory, now partly confirmed, stands in sharp contrast to the ideas of Thomas Szasz in his book, *The Myth of Mental Illness*.[236] Further, the Midtown Manhattan Study first volume, published in 1962, fully supports the relational theory. Both the theory and the Midtown Study state that mental illnesses, far from being a myth or a game played by practitioners and actors, are realities, in fact widespread and probably increasing realities. Szasz holds that sympathy arousal is the essence of the illness game or myth. In reality, we find that illness is the kind of malfunctioning and actual impairment in life functioning that destroys freedom and spontaneity. In 1956, further, in our first formulation of this opposite theory to that of Dr. Szasz, we predicted that such disorders as afflict modern man are probably on the increase. We pointed out that people in preliterate cultures suffering from conversion hysterias are frequently helped by the shaman and by an abundance of community supports in emotional crises; but that modern man, freed for the most part from conversion hysteria and simple "nuclear" forms of the schizophrenias, was now open to psychosomatic disorders, deep-set schizophrenias with paranoid reaction, or equally devastating affective disorders. These observations on changes in types of disorders, taken together with Midtown Manhattan epidemiology, should disabuse us of the false notion that mental illness is a myth—a professionally kept secret. My opposing formulation is that mental illness, now proven to be more widespread than we ever imagined before, is a *social reality*. As such, it becomes a moral problem that Dr. Szasz theoretically avoids or dismisses. The probable increases in psychosomatic disorders and in more profound forms of schizophenias stand in contrast to such small counts of mental illnesses as Dr. M. E. Spiro divulged for the Micronesian culture of Ifaluk in my book *Culture and Mental Health*.[237] The statistics on mental health in such cross-cultural surveys contrast markedly to very serious disorders in our Midtown Manhattan survey. The issue is no longer whether culture influences mental health epidemiology, but rather, *how* does culture help or harm in each milieu. Freud's phrase for being "thrust into conflict" in his work on group psychology may now be rephrased into the question: What are the conditions for being thrust into conflict, or how does personality impairment and disintegration occur? We are today closer to the answers. Obviously, what Freud phrased as the "conditions for conflict," we must, in social psychiatry, rephrase as the social conditions for conflict, for impairment, or for personality disintegration.

In these formulations of social psychiatry, much has been published since 1955 in our *International Journal of Social Psychiatry* rounding out the picture of such *conditions of existence*. Our position is obviously evolutionist on a social level, as Freud's was on an individual maturational level. As evolutionists, we do not believe in an absolute relativism, but rather, that human adaptations are to social and cultural scenes. The hope is that change in the future, informed by the findings of social psychiatry, can restore freedom and spontaneity to the probable half of all those with illnesses today having psychological and social roots.

SOCIAL PSYCHIATRY—
EVOLUTIONARY, EXISTENTIALIST, AND
TRANSCULTURAL FINDINGS

In theory, or better yet in active research, social psychiatry is the study of the etiology and dynamics of mental illnesses seen in their social and cultural environments. In practice, it mobilizes or combines all useful elements of the environment, including positive assets of the patient, as crucially helpful parts of therapy. Because I believe social psychiatry to be the future form of this behavioral science, its leading principles are listed below. It is international and cross-cultural in its concerns and efforts. It is multidisciplinary. It is not amiss to say in the century of Darwin that it is evolutionary, accepting general principles of evolution both for individual maturation and for the evolution of social and cultural forms. Finally, in this relational theory, a theory I presented in 1956,[238] the social and cultural evolution is the binding and controlling form affecting family and group functioning. It affects the epidemiology of mental ills so that they have changed both in form and in amount (i.e., incidence or prevalence) in the history of particular cultures like our own, and vary in amount and form in cultural examples taken from various evolutional levels of progress around the world.[239] In short, a basic tenet of this international and multidisciplinary science is that social and cultural environments produce, and could mitigate, the kinds and amounts of mental illness existing in the world.

It is worth adding that social psychiatry is optimistic in both theory and practice. At least it is not nihilistic in either direction. It is also obviously antireductionist. Speaking of levels of scientific analysis and the fallacy of reductionism in a relational theory which links behavior to environment, the fallacy would be to explain culture by principles of individual psychology, rather than the reverse, or to explain (as the Nazis did) individual and group psychology by organicist, racist causation. It is reductionist, in short, to explain the environing level by that which is environed or influenced. Culture and society are the setting and context of individual and group psychology, and the wider sphere influences quite conclusively the narrower, unless there is sheer organic deficit. Similarly, psychology influences organic functioning, as we have known ever since the work of Cannon, Selye, and others. This does not mean a disinterest in the gamut of naturalistic and scientific applications to therapy. *The International Journal of Social Psychiatry* has printed articles on the use of LSD and other forms of chemotherapy, and has been deeply interested in contributions of biochemistry and neurochemistry, as in physiological concomitants of emotional states. But this is like saying that sociocultural effects reach deeply and are so devastating in some of their results that not only is psychology touched much more than lightly, but the blows to *psyche* reach *soma*. Indeed, they almost always must—to give human cruelty its just due. What we are saying is that the causal chain is weighted, barring organic deficit or toxic intrusion, and no human behavior exists without influence from social and cultural milieu acting upon *psyche* and consequently upon *soma*.

The great discoveries of Pavlov, on mammalian conditioning or learning, are in the same direction of environmental influence, but one would add to the fallacy of reductionism the fallacy of misplaced concreteness if we mistook the dog for man. Similarly, the chimpanzees at Yale learning to use the chimpomat can learn by signals. But the use of symbols, the unique psychological ability of man, is absent in lower forms. Indeed, we are conditioned by signals, and with other mammals that swells the world of meanings. But our ability to use (or be conditioned by) symbols underlies sociocultural capacities, swells the world of meanings enormously, as any anthropologist knows, and allows the world of mental ills to vary according to cultural systems of meaning, as well as through the impact of sheer meanings. It is in cultural communication, as a matter of fact, that the meanings are applied.

These are simple things which I felt, many years ago, that neither Pavlovian learning theorists nor existentialists fully understood. Do the former realize that gorillas and chimpanzees, who might make good football and soccer players respectively, cannot invent the rules of the game? Do the existentialists, who are more exclusively interested in human experiences and meanings, realize the force of culture? Why the reductionism of interest to wholly individualized meanings? I have pointed out that the most personalized meanings have sociocultural roots and points of reference.[240] While no one is more interested in the organized, cultural systems of meaning than the anthropologist, is it not an equivocation, or at least a confusion to dwell on existential "truth" without being altogether certain that it is, or could be, different from such objective realities? This straining away from objectivity led Binswanger[241] to decide in *ex cathedra* fashion that Ellen West's suicide confirmed her "existential self" and consequently he seems to acquiesce to it. Heidegger has been accused of similar follies. (One is tempted to say *folie a deux*.) In a somewhat more sensitive work on schizophrenia, the existentialist R. D. Laing [242] describes an ontologically insecure person in terms of the self-description as "the ghost in the weed garden." But Freudians and neo-Freudians have written about disturbances in the sense of self, or identity, as present in various forms of psychopathology including feelings of worthlessness and death. In fact, we should be able to understand the self not simply as an ontological system, but one in which the experiences of the self, socially and culturally, are understood. These are the objective realities coloring experience, not the inner emanations of which existentialists are so fond. Cognition, emotion, and even proclivities toward certain perceptions are known to be deeply affected by sociocultural settings, giving meaning to experience.

Our problems of classification of illnesses and their prevention are similarly faced with the need for emphasis on group, culture, and milieu. Half of the hospital beds in the United States are occupied by patients with psychiatric disorders. Community survey of psychiatric therapy needs in New York City, a survey which we conducted with Dr. Thomas A. C. Rennie and others under the name of Midtown (Yorkville) Community Mental Health Research Study, indicated that over 80 per cent of the people in one of the largest cities of the world had psychiatric disabilities which could benefit from therapy. In 1956, while working with Dr. Rennie on this first urban epidemiological survey in North America, I decided to survey the extent of such epidemiological problems in mental health, cross-culturally and continent by continent. The resulting volume[243] shows the problem is not limited to North America. In fact, as new and formerly isolated regions with lower rates of mental illness undergo contacts with modern nations and experience forms of exploitation, their problems begin to approximate those of the modern world both in type and in extent. Carothers' African survey hinted at this. In a series of recent studies which I gathered for all continents and some island areas, the point is made repeatedly both in surveys of more primitive civilizations and modern ones.[244] Again we find, as in Midtown of New York City, that there are social and cultural variables affecting the etiology of mental illnesses. At the same time, these variables, located outside the individual in the sense that they affect whole groups, relate to the extent as well as the types of mental disorders.

If psychiatry wishes to communicate this knowledge of striking variations, both in extent and in typology, it must broaden perspective beyond one cultural tradition. Our classifications developed largely in a Western European setting in the late nineteenth century, with Kraepelin, and were readapted without an evolutionary perspective, that is for cultural evolution, by Freud, Bleuler, and Meyer. Freud alone attempted a typology for individual emotional maturation, and though he developed it within the framework of Western and Northern European family functioning, it is to his lasting credit that an evolutionary typology of maturation was outlined. Of all the rest, therefore, he and his colleagues and co-workers went beyond the first task of science which is ordinarily to collect data, to describe, and to classify. Of these various systems, the Freudian and neo-Freudian alone were interested in *process and dynamics*. These are the Darwins, not the Linnaeus-classifiers.

It is fair to add, in the process of facing present-day needs, that Freud's evolution of the individual needs correction, or expansion, beyond Western Europe, and that the system is inadequate for the broader framework.[245] The Freudian emphasis on individual evolution is a specific evolution, a particular form of adaptation, or for his time, a current adjustment. That it is based on a hydraulic analogy allows some to say it is mechanistic, and perhaps Newtonian. I can see the point of all these criticisms. But I can also see that the system is based on clear perception of the importance of symbol-using for humans. It is, after all, a stride forward in naturalism. It is fully as interested in linking mind and body (or the subject-object relationship of the phenomenologists and existentialists), to be sure, as is any existentialist. It has depicted and indeed discovered the notion of mental balance and imbalance, or the countless mechanisms like repression, denial, projection, and dissociation. And finally, we must recognize that Newton was not wrong, but a step toward relativity. The analogy appeals to us because Freud was the great innovator of an interest in process in psychology (psychodynamics), and if his heavens were the narrow ones of Western Europe, let us by all means invoke the larger world. The right question we should ask is: How is the system extended and revised in the light of transcultural evolution? I myself am already convinced that the Einsteinian breakthrough to the wider heavens lies in the direction of a relational theory involving the effects of cultural evolution on what Freud might have termed individual evolution. And so I come to the fifth principle of social psychiatry. Besides the fact that it is international, multidisciplinary, weights or notes the effects of sociocultural environment, and is opposed to reductionism in the opposite direction, it is interested in process or evolution throughout. It is interested in the evolution of the illness, but also of the cultural setting. This refers to general evolutionary principles, to adaptability, or to process in a relational theory.

I am further convinced that next steps in psychiatry, as Dr. Joshua Bierer[246] has often predicted, will be on organizational levels as well as these levels of the analysis of relational process. If cultural evolution is connected with the evolution of mental functioning, there is no need for therapeutic organization to go through the devious stages (and mistakes) of the past under conditions formulated as acculturation, culture contact, and the like. No biologist, believing in evolution, thinks that the amoeba must become a whale before he can be a man. Actually, this analogy is highly misleading since nonliterate and egalitarian societies furnish many supports on social levels to the individual that we have entirely lost in our society;[247] and the whole sense of group and community involvement in the problems of mental illness has a sophistication that we largely lack. I am proposing that as we leave behind our present emphases, we discard the purely *descriptive classifactory* nomenclature and develop new *cross-cultural diagnostic categories* more interested in process. As we do this, the newer experimental therapeutic processes can themselves, in turn, develop. Dr. Bierer has felt that the institutionalization of psychiatry in brick buildings, formerly locked, was a meaningless anachronism. The shift hospital, the community clinic, the therapeutic group, the therapeutic club are all next steps in the modern milieu; and all are important innovations. It is important to add that other societies may have other bases for building therapeutic systems, and it has been notoriously the case that not only have the forms and extent of illness changed, but the modes of therapy have also had sociocultural roots.

In the United States, the Hollingshead-Redlich study of New Haven, as reported in *Social Class and Mental Illness,* is a prevalence study of those in psychiatric treatment only, in public and private facilities or receiving treatment elsewhere. As in our New York-Midtown Study which added a random community sample to locate those requiring psychiatric treatment, but often not as yet receiving it, both studies—that in New Haven and that in New York City—find that the social groups most in need of treatment from the point of view of extent of disorder or its seriousness have the least access to psychotherapy. Institutional studies, like that of Kahn and Pollack at Hillside Hospital, found much the same thing going on inside brick walls. Ethnic or cultural distance, combined with lower class status, insulates the lower class from the needed forms of psychotherapeutic care. Obviously, these are class and cultural conditions which do not respond magically to the open door or chemotherapeutic aids. In fact, as Duncan Macmillan has pointed out for his country, and we might report for ours, the open door, while it helps, has led not only to higher rates of remission in its way, but to higher and almost equivalent rates of re-admission. It is rightly now called the "revolving door." And even so, as all know, it is most effective when the community truly participates in the staggering problem of mental illness, for it is then that the door truly opens in a psychological sense. At the same time, we have all too little community interest in the group approach, and certainly little start with the contribution of social psychiatry to preventive psychiatry. In the United States, consequently, the Joint Commission on Mental Illness and Health studies, in which I participated, when reporting on manpower trends or American views on mental health, have mainly a story to tell of needs, lack of mobilization of effective resources, and the like. In the light of the Midtown Study and its figure of over 80 per cent who would benefit in a modern city like New York, it seems clear that organizational and theoretical models could both benefit from the findings of social psychiatry.[248]

We have said that human responses are symbolic responses and are never reducible to objectively-defined stimuli, but that their actual coloring, affective force and use in the psychic economy arise always from individual experience in groups, in interpersonal transactions, and in a social and cultural milieu or background. These differentiations, testable in groups, mean much in the etiology and dynamics of illness forms such as schizophrenias. Considerations of the existing literature led to formulations concerning the differences in schizophrenias as they occurred in primitive cultures.[249] Forms like catatonic confusions, with high rates of remission, led us to speak of these as nuclear forms of schizophrenias, distinguishable from chronic and paranoid types, and containing such variants as imu, latah, amok, Eskimo Pibloktoq, and others. In the same year, 1956, we began publication on the more solidly structured and more serious schizophrenias of modern ethnic subcultures, one comparison of which may be seen in a recent publication.[250] Such differentiations among Italian and Irish, Germans and Puerto Ricans, and more recently Polish and Austrians, are etiological variations studied as to given cultural groups. The task of such a relational science of personality and its ills is to account for cross-cultural differences in mental illnesses with as few general constructs as possible. Purely individualistic or existentialist theories ignore such areas of meanings and values as the anthropologist uses in discussing environment. Theories of psychogenic evolution which presume a single type of society cannot like social psychiatry become interested in what I called in 1959 "the larger vista of people around the world and even in remote places as a massive laboratory for the study of the relations of culture to mental health and illness according to various designs for living."[251] As further stated recently:

> Whatever the generic similarities, no two cases are exactly the same and this very subtlety of each case is exactly what the classical nomenclature has missed. Such existentialist categories as *individual* subject-object patternings of experience are equally disappointing, however, since they produce their own reductionism. Yet in these same samples, particularly if one works to control variables by research design, one notes the cases fall into *deterministically generic patterns in terms of social and cultural variables.* . . .

> In preventive and social psychiatry, consequently, the relevant scientific specialisms must be mobilized to operate together. In modern societies undergoing rapid social change, it is important to realize that such primary groups as families, peers and neighborhoods, while they have significant roles in maintaining the potentialities for growth, maturation and mental health are the very groups often least able to function most effectively in promoting useful balances, adequate social controls or healthy ethical norms. A society in which these

groups show pathology is one which requires local analysis and mobilization of scientific resources to prevent further disintegration.[252]

The same may be said for efforts to promote positive mental health.

6

Studies in Culture and Personality

CULTURAL PERSPECTIVES IN
RESEARCH ON SCHIZOPHRENIAS

A GROUP of disorders known as the schizophrenias has long perplexed psychiatry. The French psychiatrist, Morel, called them dementia praecox, meaning a serious pathological state beginning early in life. Equally fatalistic, Kahlbaum's descriptions in German distinguished certain types in 1863 and 1874, each one having an insidious and disastrous course. Before the end of the nineteenth century, Kraepelin had published his famous classification of 1896 in which he argued that each type of schizophrenia was an organic or endogenous illness and one not due to external causes. At first, Kraepelin felt that this organic pathology was centered in the brain, but later he observed striking differences in the forms and frequencies of the illnesses occurring in Java, Malaya, and elsewhere. By this time, Bleuler had influenced Kraepelin to add a fourth type, simple schizophrenia, to the three types of illness originally named by the latter. But Kraepelin's more important concession to environmental explanations was to shift to discussions of metabolic disorders as accounting for the different forms and frequencies of the schizophrenias in various populations of the world.

Bleuler's classic, *Dementia Praecox or the Group of Schizophrenias*, appeared in 1911.[253] Where Kraepelin had contrasted populations from far-flung regions of the world, hinting at

racial and constitutional differences, Bleuler focused on a narrower range of peoples—from Holland, Thuringia, Upper
Bavaria, Saxony, and even the people of Berne and Zurich.
The latter were certainly similar in physique, but they had
"different reactions." Bleuler mentioned Irish and English
differences in the state of illness. He adduced the work of
Kraepelin and Ziehen where they had observed epidemiological
variance in several populations. Bleuler not only noted differences among peoples of similar racial type and discarded
Kraepelin's metabolic explanation, but he described various
psychological processes where Kraepelin had discussed *symptoms* and had ascribed them to organic causes. Bleuler, therefore, noted that a psychological process can underlie a cluster
or pattern of symptoms and their accompanying organic states.
In such illness states, patients were responsive to the impact of
environmental conditions. Their individual reactions could be
deflected, arrested, or channeled into new courses, depending
on the treatment applied. Bleuler's assertion that certain types
were responsive to given treatments was strengthened by his
observation of spontaneous remissions in others. He introduced
the hope that the schizophrenias were open to treatment and
voiced his belief that factors of group background "and external circumstances should be found."

While Bleuler was interested in the epidemiology of the
schizophrenias, the passages in his great book are tantalizingly
brief on this subject. One must look further to find a public
health, or preventive, approach to this problem. Even before
Bleuler, however, the reformist setting of post-revolutionary
France had provided the answer. Pinel's student, Jean-Etienne
D. Esquirol (1772–1840) wished to sharpen the acuity of
clinical observations with a more psychological, as well as
quantitative, approach to the emotional life. In a reaction
against the rationalists of the Enlightenment in France, Esquirol charged that they were preoccupied with intellectual
aspects of mental disease and with the pigeonholes of classi-

fication. Instead, he said, one must stress the roles played by emotions and values in human relations. Realizing that information of such a type was difficult to perceive and to accumulate systematically, Esquirol favored the gathering of statistical or epidemiological data with a view to preventive techniques in even the most serious schizophrenic disorders.

The convergence of these psychological, environmental, and preventive approaches was developed on the American scene by Adolf Meyer (1866–1950). At the Henry Phipps Psychiatric Clinic of the Johns Hopkins Hospital, Meyer and his colleagues built solidly on these earlier foundations. Preventive psychiatry was emphasized in the term "mental hygiene," which Meyer found in the earlier literature but succeeded in popularizing. His system, called "psychobiology," recognized each patient's problem as a complex of biological, psychological, and environmental influences reflected into his total personality. This encompassing view was called "a distributive analysis of relevant factors," but it led to the first massive epidemiological study of mental illness in urban surroundings, that made in the Eastern Health District of Baltimore. This striking research, including the schizophrenias, was carried out by Lemkau, Tietze, Cooper, and others in an interdisciplinary team of behavioral scientists.

Meyer not only stimulated epidemiological research, but, like Bleuler, he stressed the existence of several types of schizophrenia and differences in their prognoses or probable courses of illness. The responses to environment in every phase of their development or treatment were influenced by the psychological and cultural factors entering into a patient's self-conception or self-deceptions.

Contemporaneously with Bleuler in Switzerland and Meyer in America, the Freudian movement became interested in treatment of milder neurotic disorders. Meyer's notion of conflicts growing "realistically" out of experience and promoting habitual incapacities was replaced with conflicts dependent upon deeply rooted unconscious drives. Meyer's concept of the larger environment and its life-long impact was shrunk to the narrow proportions of early parent-child and sibling relationships almost exclusively. Despite this, the Freudian system contributed heavily to an understanding of schizophrenia. Pierre Janet had earlier spoken of "the loss of a sense of reality." Bleuler had described "conflictual ambivalence," a concept borrowed from Freud, as leading to the withdrawn or shut-in "autism" characterizing certain kinds of schizophrenia. In the Freudian system, the loss of reality contact was linked to the flooding of impulses from unconscious dynamic or symbolic sources, often poorly controlled and little understood by the patient. There was a defensive substitution of a world of one's own where reality failed. While the focus was upon the defensive mechanisms themselves, obviously an environmentalist revision of the system could point out that they were used against the stresses of life experiences and within social settings. If such defensive mechanisms distorted reality, how could they become habitual unless growth was blocked or reality appeared to be threatening?

It is clear that psychiatry had succeeded in typifying the general nature of the schizophrenias, while remaining largely preoccupied with the cause and course of these diseases in individuals rather than in groups. Today, more is known about the particular needs of a given case than about general detection or prevention in the community. Psychiatry has delineated types and discovered processes in the schizophrenias, but has only occasionally considered epidemiological backgrounds, or promoted a general understanding of the nature of the schizophrenias. In quite another field of science, anthropology has busied itself with the aspects of human existence that distinguish one group from another. It has located, in cultures, compelling and pervasive meanings which influence behavior. In brief, psychiatry as a medical science perfected knowledge of patterned behavior in individuals and in pathological states studied in Western European cultures. Social science studied patterned behavior in groups, with emphasis on ranges and contrasts in conduct, both normative or "normal" and aberrant—and located throughout the world.

Recently, social psychiatry has been developed to bridge the gap between such constantly converging fields. For example, the World Health Organization commissioned a British psychiatrist, J. C. Carothers, to gather data on mental illnesses in Africa. This resulted in a monograph in 1953, bristling with regional variations. The present author, in the same year, began a more comprehensive survey of the distribution of various types of mental illness among the peoples of the world. This work was published in 1956.[254] Again, wherever reliably reported, epidemiological and acculturation studies showed various symptom pictures and led to consideration of their differing etiologies.

For one thing, it appeared that mental illnesses differed from the organic deficiency diseases, or from germ-specific ailments,in several ways. In the schizophrenias, for example, they drastically and dramatically involved the total personality. Second, they often implied the instability and disturbance experienced by groups of individuals in their cultural environment. Third, and reflecting upon the recent overoptimism about "tranquilizers" and "wonder drugs," these serious illnesses had for decades defied the search for easy solutions and, instead, had required a whole process of re-education over a stretch of time. Because of their insidious nature, because of the total personality involvement, and, in particular, because of environmental influence, it seemed, especially in the schizophrenias, that attention was being focused upon the discrete individual all too exclusively. Most conceptions of schizophrenia implied—despite Bleuler, Meyer and Freud—only the private aberrations of essentially deranged minds.

It seemed, however, that typical strategies of research in public health and preventive medicine might be applied in this situation. In organic illnesses, such methods had proved valuable. Haven Emerson, in 1913, had found ethnic, or cultural, differences in measles, diphtheria, and scarlet fever rates which proved important in understanding the transmission of these communicable diseases. The year following, Clifford Abbott used the same methods to explain endemic developments of simple goiter. W. L. Aycock and J. W. Hawkins surveyed regional, cultural, and family relationships in leprosy, and R. D. Friedlander did so for pernicious anemia. In New York State, M. Calabresi had found different rates for diabetes, heart disease, pneumonia, and tuberculosis among persons of Italian, Irish, German, Polish, and British extraction. Following the Bigelow and Lombard studies in 1933 on the different frequencies of cancer at certain sites, H. F. Dorn and M. E. Patno each, in 1954, revived the case for ethnic differences in cancer development. F. R. Smith, in 1941, and E. L. Kennaway, in 1948, discussed cultural background differences in cervical and uterine cancers. A social scientist, Saxon Graham, reported a county in Pennsylvania where rheumatism, arthritis, high blood pressure, and diabetes showed low rates in the first generation of some ethnic groups, with an increase in the second generation and leveling off in subsequent generations.

A few of these illnesses had been asserted for some time to be psychosomatic in character. H. Blotner and R. W. Hyde noted in 1943 the high incidence of certain forms of diabetes in the Irish and Jewish male populations. Others noted high rates among Italians. Alcoholism was found among Irish to be a common accompaniment of more fundamental personality disorders. On the other hand, Diethelm's book on chronic alcoholism[255] notes that certain groups, like the Chinese in New York, are free of this symptom for a variety of social and cultural reasons. Haggard and Jellinek specify almost equally low rates of alcoholism for Italian and Jewish populations.

Klopfer, in the *Psychiatric Quarterly* of 1944, and Malzberg even earlier reported finding different frequencies in major mental illnesses among such groups as Italian, Irish, and German immigrants. In the same year as Klopfer's report, R. W. Hyde and associates found striking variations in Selective Service rejectees from the Boston area. Again such groups as persons of Chinese, Irish, Italian, Jewish, and Portuguese derivation were compared, although unfortunately such gross diagnostic categories as psychoses, neuroses, mental deficiency, psychopathic personality, and chronic alcoholism were used. Only studies by E. Stainbrook in the Bahian region of Brazil[256] or J. C. Carothers' compendium of African data discussed schizophrenia centrally, and even these authors discerned diagnostic variations more than differences in the etiology and developmental course of the diseases. When one turned to the *Diagnostic and Statistical Manual on Mental Disorders,* developed by a committee of the American Psychiatric Association, there was no clue to a cultural etiology. Nine headings were utilized for schizophrenic illnesses, exclusive of such personality disorders as "schizoid personality." Kraepelin's subtypes, like the hebephrenic or catatonic, were preserved to emphasize certain clusters of symptoms, but the symptoms themselves were overlapping; and the older terminology of autism, hallucinations, and disturbances of thought and affect was recurrent throughout the list.

The crucial point is that the correct weighting and profiling of symptoms makes etiological sense about why one specific illness has developed and not another. Only this can provide a differential diagnosis. Extensions of our knowledge of the psychotherapy of the schizophrenias, by Sullivan, Diethelm, Hill, Fromm-Reichmann and others, have suggested that interpersonal relations and stresses implicit in various cultural backgrounds are basic, perhaps, to different disease processes.

The author had explored this hypothesis earlier. In the period from 1938 to 1943, he studied small samples of schizophrenics at Morningside Hospital in Portland, Oregon, and noted differences in patients who were Eskimo, Aleut, Tlingit, or Tsimshian in cultural background, and further differences in those who were Alaskan whites. The hospital was a federal institution for persons from Alaska and surrounding regions. Unfortunately, the samples were inadequate and represented only persons hospitalized in the five-year period. However, they did bring differences in cultural background and acculturation processes into focus. Along with these factors went distinctions in disease development and indications, useful for the psychiatrist, as to possible treatment.

It appeared that the schizophrenias are not a collection of airtight entities since different cultural backgrounds defined variations in family and social structures that were reflected in pathology. In this way, the schizophrenias could highlight, rather than obscure, severely emotionalized conflicts rooted in culture. It was the latter element which had provided the family or the individual with systems of value, habits of thought, patterns of action, and even the attitudes toward interpersonal relations which proved to be so fundamental.

In 1954 and 1955, following studies of eight ethnic groups, it was decided to study hospitalized schizophrenic samples of certain cultural backgrounds. The backgrounds of the community groups from a section of New York City were of Irish, Italian, German, Hungarian, Czech, Slovakian, Puerto Rican, and older American types. The schizophrenic samples from the same area that are reported on here were of Italian or Irish background. Besides the aim of exploring culture differences in the schizophrenias, it was hoped to provide a check on data that had been obtained from random samples of persons residing in each functioning ethnic community. For each study, the normative community in New York, with its functioning picture of family life, good and bad, provided all the hypotheses necessary for understanding the schizophrenic illnesses in each specific group.

In the community, anthropological field surveys were used; questionnaires were applied to a random sample of adults; and intensive family studies of subsamples were made. In the hospital, it was possible to amplify these methods of community research with anthropological interviews and observations of patients; with psychiatric records and conferences; and with an independently operated battery of 13 psychological tests. The psychological test battery was devised by clinical psychologists of the Franklin D. Roosevelt Veterans Administration Hospital, and in particular by Dr. J. L. Singer and his staff at the hospital. The project as a whole was designed by the author, who assumed responsibility for assembling the anthropological data. He worked with patients, with the psychiatric staff, with preliminary records of psychiatrists, social workers, nurses, and occupational therapists to develop a complete account running parallel to the psychological tests. When the data were completed on the entire samples of Italian and Irish patients, the author and Dr. J. L. Singer intercompared their independently gathered data on each sample.[257]

The samples resulted from a complete census of four contiguous hospital buildings conducted by the author. All female schizophrenics of Irish or Italian background had previously been studied to determine—besides the community studies—differences in male and female roles in illness states. These samples of female patients were inadequate statistically, but interesting on psychodynamic grounds. The male patient census of four buildings drew samples of 40 Irish and 37 Italian male patients, each clearly diagnosed as schizophrenic. These represented the field study area. Patients were accepted for the sample only if without record of cerebral damage and if they had not been involved in psychosurgery. Practically all had received shock therapy. Other than this, no organic causation nor treatment beyond the usual barbiturates had been recorded.

The patients, entirely by chance, were limited to the first, or immigrant, generation; the second, or that of children of immigrants; and the third. When all 77 subjects had been studied intensively by anthropological interviews, psychiatric methods, and complete hospital records, each was referred to the clinical psychology staff composed of Dr. Singer and colleagues. Among the psychological instruments, reported on elsewhere, it was decided to use the Rorschach, Barron's Movement-Threshold Inkblots, the Porteus Maze, the Thematic Apperception Test, Time Estimation and Motor Inhibition Tests, the Lane Sentence Completions, and other behavioral ratings. These instruments, plus anthropological interviewing and ward observations, provided independent ratings of functioning to which the patient's history and consultation with psychiatrists could be added. Ten Irish and seven Italian patients were too ill to complete the test battery and were studied independently by the combination of anthropological and psychiatric means. They are not included in the tables which follow, since psychological tests were incomplete. However, they conform closely to the differential pattern of their ethnic groups as hypothesized and as found in matched samples of 60 patients, 30 Irish and 30 Italian, studied by all three methods—psychiatric, anthropological, and psychological.

In the matched samples of 60 patients, the mean age of the Irish was 32 years as compared with the mean for Italians of 30.5. (Age limits for both groups were 18 to 45 at the beginning of the study, when the census was taken; it had shifted, of course, to 20 to 47 two years later when the study was completed.) For the last grade of education, an Irish mean of 10.5 grades matched the Italian of 10.9. The intelligence potential, computed in Wechsler IQ averages, and again by means, disclosed an Irish sample of 108.4, closely matching the Italian 105.5. Length of hospitalization was hardly different, with a mean for the first year of 1949.8 (or .8 of a year after 1949) for Irish and 1949.5 for the Italian. In marital status, by actual count, 25 Irish and 22 Italians were unmarried; and none of the comparatively few marriages of the remaining patients could be counted distinct successes when studied. The variables matched or controlled for both samples were, therefore, age, sex, educational level, intelligence, first year of hospitalization, marital status, absence of organic or chronic conditions, and origin in the field study area. Only marital status showed, for the Irish, a slight and possibly culturally-influenced excess of bachelorhood. Yet illness and its particular pathology had made both groups primarily celibate, as will be seen.

Regional differences are important in Italian culture, less so among the Irish. As concerns this variable, the writers were again fortunate in eliminating it along with those just compared. All Italians but one could trace ancestral lines from the extreme south of Italy (Naples southward) or from Sicily. Luckily, all the Irish traced their ancestry to "southwest" Irish counties and villages. The one lone north Italian who occurred in the census and came into the sample consequently proved to be an interesting exception to the Italian group in both his psychodynamic and cultural patterns.

The table which follows summarizes seven variables in a total of ten that were found to be significant in distinguishing Irish and Italian male schizophrenic patients. Earlier, at the outset of the research, it was hypothesized that these differences accounted for two patterns, highly contrasting, in the etiology of each type of schizophrenia. The discussion of them may begin by an explanation of the differential terms used in accounting for each variable.

For reasons to be given, it was hypothesized that members of neither group would have clearly male sexual identifications in the illness state. Schizophrenics are notoriously troubled by homosexual strivings. However, it is of great importance in the total balance, or imbalance, of personality, how such sexual strivings are shaped and whether they are latent or overt in character. Certainly, Italians stress even more forcefully than the Irish the importance of masculinity for the male and femininity for the female. However, the Italians also emphasize the expression of sexuality, as they do that of any other human emotion or passion. In males who are schizophrenically ill and in whom both self-identity and sexual identification become impossible, the Italian model hypothesized was overt homosexuality, or a confused and active bisexuality which refused to pattern directly after the clearly male image of dominant and authoritarian fathers and elder brothers. Most of the Italian patients in this series were, indeed, younger siblings who had moved quickly and impulsively, judging by their life histories, through a confused latent phase of sexual repulsion from a male role and into overt manifestations of homosexual behavior.

The Irish by contrast, both in hypothesis and in fact, were fearful of a male role but repressive of homosexual trends, reactions based primarily on anxious attitudes toward mothers and other female images. One Irish patient who escaped this latent homosexual trend lost his mother at the age of three but was still fearful of domineering women. Another solved the problem by passively attaching himself to a woman exactly twice his age whom he exploited economically in her confused senility. The vast majority of Irish male patients were latent homosexuals who avoided the female world, but repressed overt manifestations.

In keeping with these characteristics, the majority of the Irish patients struggled with sin and with preoccupations of guilt concerning sexuality, whereas the Italians had no sin or guilt preoccupations in this area. Instead, the Italians' case histories and their current ward behavior showed disorders in the realms of poorly controlled impulses, weak personal attachments and widely fluctuating—or flighty—affects. The attitudes toward authority in the two groups diverged in parallel fashion, the Italians having been verbally rejecting or actively flouting of authority, as shown in tests or case history, while the Irish were hypothesized to be compliant for the most part, with only the most passive forms of outward resistance in evidence.

The delusions, based on compensatory imagination in schizophrenics, it was hypothesized, would become fixed in Irish patients, and assume the typical paranoid forms of omnipotence, or suspiciousness and persecution. While delusions are ordinarily developed in many forms of schizophrenia, it was hypothesized—on the contrary—that they would be largely absent among the Italians, or, if present, would rarely be systematized or maintained with great fixity. As hypothesized, practically none of the Italians had the highly systematized and elaborated delusions found frequently in the Irish patients, so that the table deals only with the other factor of fixity.

On the other hand, for reasons of their clearer bodily emphasis, or in Schilder's phrase, "body image," it was expected that Italian schizophrenics, male or female, would be given to hypochondriacal complaints and to somatic or bodily preoccupations.

As concerns alcoholism in case histories, this was expected to be found more frequently in Irish patients than in Italian. The accompanying table summarizes these seven variables, which must then be considered in their meaningful etiological sense.

With a skeletonized set of differences between the two samples indicated in the table, it remains to account for the development of each kind of pathology. The previous community surveys in New York City contained, for each ethnic group, a whole continuum of persons and families whose behavior ranged from normative or "normal" standards of conduct to those who were aberrant or deviant. When one had studied healthy, or moderately ill, Irish and Italians in their family settings and community groups, one could distinguish the characteristic cultural contributions and backgrounds, and the particular pace of cultural change for each group, with its typical or special patterns of stress in family conflicts. Each ethnic group, Irish, Italian, Puerto Rican, or other, sanctioned or interdicted outlets for emotional expression. In the range of persons and families from the healthy and well-balanced to

SIGNIFICANT VARIABLES IN IRISH AND ITALIAN PATIENTS*

	Irish	Italian	Total
Variable 1: Homosexual types			
Latent	27	7	34
Overt	0	20	20
Total	27	27	54
Variable 2: Sin and guilt preoccupations			
Present	28	9	37
Absent	2	21	23
Total	30	30	60
Variable 3: Behavior disorder			
Present	4	23	27
Absent	26	7	33
Total	30	30	60
Variable 4: Attitude toward authority			
Compliant	24	9	33
Rejecting	6	21	27
Total	30	30	60
Variable 5: Fixity in delusional system			
No	7	20	27
Some	23	10	33
Total	30	30	60
Variable 6: Somatic (Hypochondriacal) complaints			
Present	13	21	34
Absent	17	9	26
Total	30	30	60
Variable 7: Chronic alcoholism			
Present	19	1	20
Absent	11	29	40
Total	30	30	60

* Statistical measures indicated that each of these variables was highly significant in delineating differences between Irish and Italian schizophrenics.

those evidencing pathology, the cultural patterns—even where undergoing change—provided the necessary framework for understanding the meanings of emotional stress and conflict, both in pathogenic families and individuals and in those who seemed to be symptom-free. The crucial point for each cultural group of the eight studied was that it was the normative side of the continuum, the on-going ethnic group, which helped define the kinds of conflict or repression, the types of emotional expression, the system of values, or the functioning of the family for each individual.

While Freud stated long ago that neurosis is the price paid for civilization, the writer found that each culture or subculture contained its designs for living. In each, consequently, there were various stresses and strains, and there were well-functioning families, as well as pathogenic ones. Creative and negative features typified the genius and the pitfalls of each cultural system. Therefore, the writer conducted no such search for a single etiology of a mental illness as characterized inquiry in the nineteenth century. Instead, he insisted upon viewing every family and every patient in their meaningful cultural settings.

Therefore, three variables not included in the table were considered of primary significance. All were earlier-acting in relation to life history than those in the table. The first (Variable A) dealt with the possibilities in each cultural group, by virtue of its family system, for the development of negative and destructive emotions of various sorts. While it is true that, in the schizophrenias, elements of hostility and anxiety may coexist in different degrees, the amount of each emotion in such admixtures, and the means by which it is expressed or controlled, are crucial matters. D. H. Funkenstein's contrast between anxiety states premised on fear and those based upon hate is relevant here. This dichotomy in the schizophrenias (fear versus hate) was taken into account, together with psychoanalytic estimates as to whether these emotions were expressed or denied outlet in typical family structures of a cultural group.

It was noted that in Irish families, particularly in those poorly organized, the central figure is usually the mother. Her authority extends to all matters of household management, including not only child-rearing but the major decisions governing the home. She achieves this status by reasons of her matronage and not infrequently conceives of the distaff as the symbol of authority, of family domain, and of emotional control. Historically, fathers in the southwest Irish counties were frequently in straitened economic circumstances, and were shadowy and ineffectual figures in the home. It was hypothesized, on the basis of this family structure, that anxiety, tinged with fear and hate, would be the resultant emotion in Irish male patients who as sons had been raised to view themselves as "forever boys and burdens." In two-thirds of the Irish cases, this primary anxiety (with some hostility usually compressed by fear) was directed toward all female figures. In only three cases of a total of forty did the father appear more centrally, and in these three the entire pattern of illness shifted to the Italian model in most details. In one of these, as already stated, the mother had died when the patient was three.

In sharp contrast, Italian cultural values set greater store on male parental or eldest-sibling dominance while at the same time reinforcing more direct expressions of the resultant hostile emotions. This acting-out of feelings brought more hostility to the fore in poorly repressed conflicts with fathers or elder male siblings. One Italian patient, for example, entered the acute phase of illness at the time of his older brother's wedding and expressed himself with floridly violent accusations against his father. In practically all cases, there was a strong repulsion from the father, elder brother and even surrogate authority figures. The Italian mothers, in such instances, were often subtly rejecting and preferred the oldest son. In some cases, the mother, playing a subordinate role in the family, had compensated by assuming a mildly seductive and pampering role in relationships with the son. One could trace the effects of a harsh and punitive domineering father. The mother compensated for her own feelings of neglect at the father's hands by building up hostile forms of impulsiveness in these sons, along with features of poor emotional control.

Italian patients, even where labeled like Irish as schizophrenics with paranoid reactions, had more prominent problems of emotional overflow (schizo-affective features) which took the form of elated overtalkativeness, curious mannerisms, grinning and laughing hyperactivity, and even assaultiveness. Even hostility directed toward the self came into evidence when elated excitements gave way to inept suicidal attempts. One-third of the Italian sample showed such periodic excitements, with confusion and emotional lability (catatonic excitements) while the other two-thirds were subject to extreme mood swings in which the depressed and quiescent periods gave way to destructive outbursts, elation, suicidal behavior, or curious mannerisms. In brief, all Italian patients had so much affective coloring, aimed primarily at male figures and images, that the paranoid schizophrenic label seemed to fit them poorly.

A second primary difference in the samples (Variable B) dealt with the central tendencies in each culture for channeling emotional expression. To some extent, this expression of the emotional life in each ethnic group applied also to female patients. Italian culture generally sanctions the freer expression of emotions than does Irish culture, and emotion may be expressed, in lower class groups particularly, in bodily action. The Irish, on the contrary, are famous for a greater constriction of activity; and their most endearing trait, which no doubt compensates for this constriction, is an equally rich fantasy life. In Freudian theory, fantasy may substitute, almost vicariously, for action. The writer has, indeed, already noted the intensity of emotion and its expression in activity in poorly controlled Italian patients. The counterpart in the Irish sample of patients was a fantasy substitute for action. While Italian patients might oscillate between hyperactivity and under-activity, or show an inability to time their activities, thoughts, or emotions effectively, the Irish, with no such difficulties in timing or guarding their emotions, showed an inversely large proportion of rich and extensive fantasy. Their more deeply repressed conflicts consequently took a more delusional and paranoid form. One Irishman, for example, gave for two years a most lurid series of accounts of the death of each family member, blaming his mother for a horrible accident which be-fell the father. (The father had actually died at a ripe old age, in a hospital, of a common ailment.) With each monotonous recital, the father's death in front of the home became more blood-stained and painful. The mother became a cold, emotionless, and witch-like figure described in an affectless tone and cursed as if in ritualistic magic.

Linked with these two primary variables of family authority structure and the channeling of emotional expression were other cultural variables affecting the emotional life. With Italian males, more direct feelings of hostility flooded up from shallowly repressed levels, connected with feelings of being re-pelled by a father, older brother, or surrogate authority figure. As concerns sexual identification (Variable 1 of the table), two-thirds of the Italian sample showed active homosexuality which had at one time or another been overtly practised. This rejection of male identity and strong repulsion from the male role fitted the variables already considered—hatred of the father, lack of stability in the mother, and the cultural sanc-tions for expression of emotion. Impulsiveness, acting out, and emotional overflow might be expected among the ill of this cultural group. This acting-out of impulse was often noted in a background of sociopathic escapades—common in childhood or in youth.

For the same variables, the Irish male patient, beset with anxiety and fear of female figures early in life, likewise lacked possibilities of a firm male identification, but here the fear was centered on the opposite sex; and the sexual repression and the emphases of the culture on sin or guilt made for a repressive, latent form of homosexuality. Instead of the open refusal to be male, or repulsion from the male role as in Italian patients (non-identification in Italians), the Irish had a fearful or anxious lack of positive male identification. Here the latent homosexual tendency was controlled by added distortions and repressions. If repressed sufficiently, the Irish patient was pallidly asexual. Only three, as the table indicates, managed to achieve or maintain the asexual balance in repression. In the 27 who were latent homosexuals, the distortions of body image had already occurred in several who had bizarre delusional misidentifications as to their sexual characteristics. One such delusional form may serve to illustrate: the patient who believed his entire bodily structure in the front was covered by an "apron." This apron had certain feminine characteristics, like periodic bleeding or the capacity to distract the patient's thoughts ("affecting my thoughts"—adversely of course).

Beyond family structure, the problem of sexual identification, and the channels for emotional expression in each culture, lies a further series of the consequences of emotional stress and its pitfalls in poorly organized families. The sexual misidentifications (in Irish males) and non-identifications (or refusals to identify properly in the Italian series) are contrasting types which occur in very different defensive emotional structures. In this sense, Variables 2 and 3 of the table may be considered concomitant variations, or further consequences, of the basic themes of stress problems and affective controls in family structure. Obviously, personality traits exist and function together in the total business of living. Thus the concepts of sin and guilt, particularly in the sexual area, were built up in the Irish patients and were readily accessible in their cultural stock-in-trade. Not only did 28 Irish patients torment and exacerbate themselves with such sin and guilt formulae, but 21 Italians of similar faith did not apply the irritations of sin and guilt to their sexual ideologies. Again, with the Irish, such formulae often become delusional and persecutory. A particular kind of mythology, prominent among nonliterate peoples, and concerning a toothed, castrating vagina occurred in the setting of incestuous guilt about feelings toward sisters and other female relatives in several Irish cases. Contrary to this, 26 Irish patients showed no evidence in the hospital or in life histories of ever having been involved in any sociopathic behavior, whereas 23 Italians showed repeated and marked evidence of behavior disorders. As has been seen, the attitude toward authority (Variable 4 of the table), more consciously expressed in instruments like the Sentence Completion List, or exemplified in life histories and ward behavior, indicated a similar difference in attitude, with 24 compliant Irish patients to almost the same number of more rebellious Italians.

Variable 5 of the table explored the prediction that the Irish patients, with their anxious fantasies, their latent and repressed homosexual trends, and their indoctrinated "sex-is-sin" feelings of guilt, would be forced to build fixed delusional systems. While Irish patients used delusional or fantasy defense against their sexual misidentification problems and shattered self-esteem, the Italians expressed their sense of defeat and hostility mainly in mood swings, excitements and impulsive behavior. Thus delusional fixity occurred in a ratio greater than three to one for the Irish, while exactly two-thirds of the Italian patients had no manifest delusions during the study and half of the remaining ten had changeable and minor delusional episodes. On the other hand, as might be expected, the Italian patients distinctly led in Variable 6 of the table, in the frequency with which hypochondriacal complaints about imagined somatic disorders were mentioned. For Variable 7, only one of the Italian patients had ever been chronically addicted to alcohol although all liked wines, whisky, or beer. In the Irish, on the contrary, almost two-thirds had sought escape from problems in protracted periods of alcohol addiction.

In discussing this relationship between environment and mental illnesses, authors like Stanton and Schwartz in their book, *The Mental Hospital*,[258] or Fromm-Reichmann in her *Principles of Intensive Psychotherapy*,[259] have discussed patients' reactions to ways of handling them, to interaction processes on the ward, or to different psychotherapeutic approaches. These authors concede a general validity to the idea that no patients, not even schizophrenics, live in a cultural vacuum. But the related thought that the course of illness and the very structuring of personality bear a cultural imprint is neglected in the literature. All nine variables discussed so far show inner consistency and integration of defenses which constitute two separate kinds of illness for the two ethnic groups. Psychiatrists, in treating each type, can be more effective if they understand these linkages of culture and personality. What Sullivan called "the schizophrenic way of life" can be related and regeared to more positive cultural determinants only after one understands the differences in family structures, in self-identification problems, and in methods of emotional control which have made up the characteristic blend in any balance of defenses.

A final, or tenth, variable (Variable C) was therefore used in the study to describe this balance of defenses. It was found to favor fantasy and withdrawal patterns for the Irish to the extent of paranoid reactions. The Italian patients suffered from disorders of poor emotional and impulse control. The Irish were most anxious in their relations with persons of the opposite sex and the shaping of the basic personality contained notions of male inadequacy, fear of females, and latent homosexual tendencies, intensified by sin and guilt preoccupation. With the Irish, self-esteem and identification were destroyed at the same time; and weakness, inadequacy feelings, suspiciousness, and paranoid delusions took over. Hence bodily somatizations and hypochondriacal complaints, common in Italians, were rare in the Irish. Delusions became fixed in paranoid channels, and fantasy and distortion were used to preserve the delusional system intact. These were quiet anxious men, fearful of anything which might separate them from the protection of the ward and their well-regulated delusional systems.

Obviously, the Italian patients were different not only on each count, but in the total pattern of symptoms. As different, they represented other problems in management and therapy. A family structure, diametrically different from the Irish, favored overt expression of homosexuality. The different cultural emphasis on emotional expression led to the acting out of impulse. The strength of anger in this emotional liability, the motor excitements or flaring up of affect could throw the patient into confusional affective states, or into the excitements, periodic and sometimes destructive, which characterized an even greater proportion. This balance, or typical resolution of defenses, was most important in the actual handling and maintenance of rapport with each patient.

Cannon, Wolff, Funkenstein and others have each written on the physiological consequences of such long-standing emotional states. Possibly the attack on these problems will benefit from further psychological understanding. Important in the psychotherapy which accompanies and vitalizes such methods will be the joint contribution, no doubt, of psychiatry and anthropology. The former is expert in the guidance of the individual case, and the latter is helpful in indicating the types of family organization and social experience which influence all behavior, normative or pathological. Future research in social psychiatry is now required on various mental disorders, and it is hoped that further explorations of this type will be carried out elsewhere.

CULTURAL DEFINITIONS OF ILLNESS

It is possible to set scenes for this discussion rather quickly. But, to avoid misunderstanding, certain general propositions will have to be set forth first; the examples will follow.

Between anthropology and medicine, a rich field has developed, which, for convenience, we call "social psychiatry." Others have called it "culture and personality," or "medical sociology," and Francis Hsu recently dubbed it "psychological anthropology." Since naming the baby has seemed to me less important than its careful nurturance and orientation, I welcome this babel of terms—all are harmless while the infant is still young.

My former colleague at Cornell Medical College, Dr. Thomas A. C. Rennie, warned his medical contemporaries that social psychiatry was not a new form of psychiatry, but noted that it did contain new challenges, and harbored new areas of interest. Anthropologists will notice that their previous infant care and adult personality studies are now open to the same charges as those with which this observer greeted such early works as E. H. Erikson's *Childhood and Society,* with obvious correctives from his own Ute Indian studies.[260] Sociologists are discovering that quantitative assessment of admission figures, or of people in treatment, are not "prevalence studies," even when labeled "treated prevalence."[261] And Freudians have been overcoming earlier rigidities in favor of ego-adaptation interests. Technically, social psychiatry is included in this list because it is the study of the etiology and dynamics of mental and psychosomatic illnesses, seen in their environmental settings.[262] As such, it must be linked with all the fields just named, and embrace cross-cultural studies and interclass communication problems.

May we add, for the wary, that this field also studies mental health in terms of the prevalence of illness—or its absence and the reasons for that absence. Obviously, it also includes attitudes toward illness, and thus, the cultural assets and liabilities affecting illness.

But somehow, these trends in the modernization of theory and approach to culture and illness phenomena are not enough. We have discussed the matter elsewhere, in two theoretical essays dealing with epidemiological surveys and culture and personality studies.[263] Outstanding in a field including such interdisciplinary efforts as the culture and personality studies of the anthropologist, medical psychiatry, and epidemiology is the need for philosophical clarity. We already know that culture affects normative personality types, as it affects, by the same token, the epidemiology of mental and psychosomatic disorders.[264] With the science of cultural anthropology, and with the potent factor of cultural influences, one introduces a variegated scheme that includes all such differences. However, our new proposals or propositions for discussion are the following: despite this variegated scheme and these differences, *transcultural values may be found, provided we shift attention to process and away from our past preoccupations with the illness entities just mentioned.* Hopefully, the same is true of interclass communication: *values existing across class lines may be perceived, provided one obtains, beforehand, an understanding of the subcultural (barrier) effects of class membership.* Both the Hollingshead-Redlich study in New Haven, and our own Midtown Study with Dr. Thomas A. C. Rennie, in New York City, would seem to point up the necessity for greater interclass communication.[265] Thus, the main burden of this essay becomes clearer if we state, from the outset, that modern man is involved in three processes:

The cultural evolutionists have reminded us, recently, that man is, first of all, involved in a sociocultural process of development. Second, psychiatry would add that he is involved in a maturational process. Third, social psychiatry would add, in relating these two, that modern man, that is, urban man, and his nonliterate cousins, are both involved in an epidemiological process. We should like to discuss the roles of anthropology and psychiatry, or social psychiatry, in these relationships. Our case illustration will be modern Ghana, on which there are abundant data, albeit controversial in part, from the fields of anthropology, psychiatry, and epidemiological survey.[266]

Before dealing with the Ghana data, I should like to indicate how one discussant, Dr. Jerrold E. Levy, and I have benefited by a preliminary correspondence on cultural definitions of illness. Dr. Levy is studying Navaho health concepts and their connection with behavior. My own trips among Navaho around Shiprock, New Mexico, while I was studying the Southern Ute Indians, convince me that Dr. Levy has observed keenly the Navaho. He tells me that among them, individuals who take up antisocial practices like witchcraft are not considered ill. While they are hardly paragons of deportment, they express maladjustments and unhappiness, which we would recognize as such, by accepting the sorcery role. They do not deny that they are witches, and may even try their hand at it now and then. Living lives not in accord with ideal values, they are nonetheless so far from Navaho concepts of illness that I am tempted to say that they fit in well with larger concepts of individualism, and with the need for vigor and mobility, which is a more dominant theme in Navaho-Apache life ways, and one which is found among the neighboring Ute as well.

Dr. Levy's impression of Navaho schizophrenics is that they accentuate less approved withdrawal patterns, and become, in a form different from the Western European, somewhat "catatonic." I am not referring to Donald Jewell's sympathetic account of a Navaho male who was not schizophrenic but, rather, was simply concerned about an unfinished ceremony.[267] The Navaho epidemiological literature has better data on the prevalence of catatonia, as well as clearer cases of depression phenomena, such as George W. Hohmann's case account in the Seward symposium.[268]

The larger concepts of a cultural tradition, which we refer to as *beliefs,* are rooted in the character structure and affective life of a particular people. But, while some have referred to the latter as outgrowth of child-rearing practices, we see them, phenomenologically, as rooted more pervasively, and in an antecedent fashion, in the patterns of thought and patterns of feeling, which, in turn, affect such elements as child-rearing.[269] It is not enough to say that this is a reversal of the classical Freudian conceptions of causation for sociological purposes. In our opinion, it opens the door for the study of Freudian mechanisms—the ego-defense systems—on a cross-cultural basis, despite the fact that Freud was relatively unconcerned with either epidemiology or cultural evolutionary processes. Not only do societies change, but the cultural evolutionary process throws into bolder relief specific cultural societies in which questions of epidemiology, acculturative change and the stresses implicit in a given cultural setting have practical importance. The cross-cultural dimension, and its understanding, are preliminary to an application of social psychiatry.[270] The general evolutionary framework of acculturation studies *is* its setting, if social psychiatry is to be applied.

Thus, Dr. Levy notes that the Navaho who must be brought in for psychiatric help are repressing hostilities, not ventilating them in witchcraft. The real murderer, he says, might often be considered a person temporarily contaminated, rather than chronically sick. Yet, the asocial, rather than the antisocial, persons is the one who is called sick in mind, who must run away "losing his senses," and who is known to be riddled with

conflicting hostilities. Similarly, the Ute recognized the con-
flicted conversion hysteric as standing in need of dream
therapy, since, again, his impulses were poorly controlled, and
protruded, and the currents of wish and resentment were dan-
gerously near the surface. To comment on Navaho, Apache,
and Ute together, they may be called cultures, which, in aboriginal times, valued vigor, mobility, and individualized expression for obvious material reasons. But the antisocial man
receives a rigorously different treatment in the viable horti-
culture of the village Pueblo Indians, for the most part. Here,
the rugged individualist is accused of witchcraft, and the
sanctions, applied sternly, are something quite different from
psychiatric care. The one culture calls the asocial person sick,
and the other reserves this term for the antisocial.

Of course, these are all societies—the more nomadic Atha-
baskans and the Ute on the one hand, and the settled village
peoples on the other—that Radcliffe-Brown, or Herbert
Spencer for that matter, would have designated as societies of
relatively narrow integration. In our own society, there is less
homogeneity, as Robert Redfield noted, and the family forms
are less integrated with a single scheme of values that pervades
the culture as a whole. The heterogeneity exists in subcultural
ethnic and class differences.

We are emphasizing the ethnic and class variables, and for
some time have done so in our own research, for a relatively
simple reason. Not only do such variations or differences characterize modern heterogeneous societies, but they render invalid
the usual Western European psychiatric monoliths erected by
Kraepelin, and others, as universal psychiatric illness nomenclature. This one-system typology for illnesses does not accommodate, as we pointed out in 1956, either the cross-cultural
variations in illness forms, or their historical changes, in the
cultures and subcultures of the world. On a pan-human level,
we are convinced that Freudian defeat is not implied in this
last statement. Freud took the first step with a relatively simple

conception of the defense mechanisms in balance or imbalance, and with a masterly evolutionary scheme for individual maturation, which we designated useful as a general theory—a first step—in a paper in 1942.[271] But the requirement now, in the shrinking world, is to expand this system into its subcultural and cultural variants, and this can only be done by painstaking interdisciplinary research.[272]

A further simple reason for a reorientation in interdisciplinary research should be obvious by referring back to such sequences as Apache-Navaho and Pueblo, or Ute and Aztecan for that matter. The cultural stress system is not an epiphenomenon of child-rearing practices, nor does the definition of illness follow a single pan-human plan. American anthropologists denied the obvious realities of cultural evolution as a realistic, if general, framework for so long during the decades from 1910 to 1950, that, to borrow an analogy from psychiatry, they became rigidly obsessed with the punctilios of particular cultures. This was nowhere more true than at Columbia University, where I studied in the Boas, and subsequent, periods. Of course, it was here that the resurgence of interest in culture and personality studies began. But these studies were developed again on the somewhat anti-evolutionary basis of culture-for-culture analysis, and on child-rearing models.[273] A still later resurgence of interest in evolutionism may be traced, as one could guess, again to Columbia personnel, among others.

When one refers back to the Navaho-Apache and Pueblo, or the Ute-Aztecan sequences, it is obvious that the cultural stress systems not only vary, but they vary according to *the experiential pressures imposed by the culture.* We find Hallowell's work extremely revealing here, although Hallowell seems less willing to consider Ojibwa material as having a more generic significance than we are. I notice that withdrawal and isolation, psychosocially, is also considered asocial here, as with the Navaho, and that the channel for illness behavior is somewhat ordained and stylized. We are impressed by the fact that

typical cultural stresses exist, and that the illness form is chan-
nelized, and certainly related to these stresses. In assessing these
relationships, the cultural stress system may be countered by
elaborate systems for providing cultural safety-valves for typical
stresses. One thinks of endless examples—the *vagina dentata*
myths that are so widespread, cults of sorcery like the *Vada*
cult of the Trobriands, or the *Beloi* cult of Bathonga. Obviously, the cultural stress system, expressing experiential pressures imposed by the culture, may be modified by or mitigated
through a built-in system of safety-valves. Therefore, let us add
to the experiential pressures imposed by a culture its attitudes
toward illness and instrumentalities for channelizing problems.

Let us turn now to a so-called ethnopsychiatric study of rural
Ghana, a book called *The Search for Security,* written by a
psychiatrist and student of anthropology, Dr. M. J. Field.[274]
The book was favorably reviewed by an able Africanist, Dr.
Paul Bohannan, in the pages of *The American Anthropologist.*[275] In our own reviewing of it, we will rely on a wealth of
contrary literature, on studies from the hospital at Accra, on
correspondence and materials provided by the World Health
Organization, Mental Health Section, and on fieldwork discussions with Ghanaians, especially Mr. Frederick Kwadzo
Wurapa, a medical student from Ghana, who has been working with me, on fellowship, on this very problem.

Dr. Field, the author of the full-length study of the visitors
to shrines in a new religious movement of Ghana, has definite
competence in medicine and, besides that, additional training
in clinical psychology and psychiatry. She began her studies in
West Africa in the 1930s, as an ethnologist with the Gold
Coast government. In 1955, she returned to the Ashanti, and,
with support from the British Medical Research Council,
studied shrine cults of the Akan-speaking peoples of Ghana,
utilizing over 2,500 cases. Further, the Northwestern University
series in African Studies is already a distinguished list for
Africanists, so that one expects, and finds in this book, a rich

mine of information for students of human behavior and for those interested in the newly industrialized and rapidly acculturating nations finally coming into their own in Africa.

Dr. Field noted that the shrines of a new religious movement were the places to which pilgrims, some requiring psychiatric care, came for religious psychotherapeutic purposes. After sketching their social, economic, and domestic backgrounds, and their religious ideology, she discusses the concept of *spirit possession,* as this bears on priestly functions and continues this in her chapter 5: "The Troubles and Desires of Ordinary People." Thirteen chapters follow on specific disease entities, with one on mental disturbances of children, and one on stable personalities, for contrast. Obviously, all the cases are not presented in full, or even schematically, but some verbatim excerpts from complaints uttered at shrines give us the flavor of the problem. Special chapters on "Mental Illness Resulting from Physical Illness," and on "Post-Influenzal Psychosis," among this series of 13, remind us that physical ills add a life stress of sizable proportions to these people's problems.

The Achilles' heel of this book is the astounding number of cases (over 2,500) diagnosed by *one* person. In this light, when I read that she located 41 chronic schizophrenics among them, representing a population estimated in 1948 at 4,283 (almost a "0.10 per cent incidence"), and then read: "In Europe and America the expectation of schizophrenia in the general population is usually estimated at about 0.8 per cent,"[276] I, for one, cannot jump on the bandwagon. Granting that the rural Ghana picture is, most certainly, not a functional "primitive paradise," but a rapidly modernizing, acculturated, and stressful scene, this classification in short order of 2,500 cases, including 41 chronic schizophrenics, strikes me as singularly open to error—if accomplished by one English physician in so ridiculously short period of time as that available to her. In charity, I should favor the "stressful acculturation theory," and probable overestimated rates attributable to it. But the unwitting public is bound to go astray on this study in assuming her rates of 0.8 per cent schizophrenics to be accurate. In our New York City study, called the Midtown Study, 81.5 per cent of the total sample were found by staff psychiatrists to manifest significant symptoms, in a range from mild to marked (or greatly impaired) severity. When an attempt was made to locate the numbers of *"probable psychotic type,"* these were found to be 13 per cent in the bottom class stratum (and not 0.8 per cent). Cases labeled severely disturbed were found among 28 per cent of the lower class, and 18 per cent of the middle class. Several years, a large staff, and three psychiatrists' ratings were required. Those rated "well" (or relatively symptom free) were distinctly in a minority (18.5 per cent). Obviously, in New York, by class measures, more serious impairment clusters in the lower classes.

Let us look at a few other background factors in Ghanaian mental health.

Some Possible Sources of Cultural and Mental Conflicts Among Ghanaians

NUTRITION AND MENTAL HEALTH. Although there is a disagreement among psychiatrists as to the significance of malnutrition as a contributing factor to mental illness, the fact that malnutrition is common in the population today leads one to think that undernourishment must be important in the etiology of the various mental illnesses. In a recent report the Minister of Agriculture, Mr. Kodjo Botsio, stated that 10,000 out of 20,000 Ghanaians examined in a project by the National Nutrition Board were found to be victims of malnutrition.[277] Despite the fact that the introduction of antibiotics has cut down the prevalence of diseases like yaws and leprosy, a large section of the total population still suffers from the weakening effects they produce. For, in a country where less than ten years ago most rural people considered diseases like yaws an inevitable part of a child's development, and where malaria is as common as the common cold, one would expect a very febrile population. With such predispositions as these, malnutrition can be a very dangerous precipitating factor of mental disorder.

Another organic disease that can make a malnourished population more vulnerable to mental disorders is trypanosomiasis. Dr. Geoffrey Tooth, as cited by Field, reports: "Eighty per cent of hospital cases of trypanosomiasis have mental symptoms, and Dr. Djoleto, who worked with Dr. Tooth in the Accra Mental Hospital, has noted that trypanosomiasis accounts for the great majority of patients who are brought in 'raving mad,' the parasites being found in cerebrospinal fluid."[278] Neither malnutrition nor the infectious and febrile diseases alone can cause mental illness. However, these two factors are important in the etiology of mental illness because the individual becomes exceedingly predisposed to social factors that produce mental disorders when he already has a poorly nourished body that is also infested by febrile and infectious diseases. Under these conditions, a question one would ask is: How quickly and successfully are the Ghanaians—especially the rural Ghanaians— freeing themselves from disease and malnutrition? Because improvement in a people's diet involves both education toward the change of eating habits, as well as the ability to cope with the economic demands of the new diet, it is only the few well-educated people who can be said to have adequate protection from disease with properly balanced diets.

AGING.   From the description of the Ghanaian family (cited below), it can be concluded that the aged there have traditionally secure positions in the family. A father continues to make decisions, or at least influences them, even when he is so old that the sons and daughters are providing for his welfare. There is very little chance of a feeling of isolation and insecurity in the aged of Ghana. It has to be pointed out, however, that the security of the aged varies among the different regions of the country. In my own opinion, a continuum can be set up, with the most secure aged men being those of the rural areas, and the least secure those of urban areas. In a mental institution, like the one in Accra, in which most of the patients are referred by police magistrates, one might find hardly any mental illness due to the complications of old age. This fact is supported by the study of Dr. Forster, Director of the Accra institution, in which a diagnosis of admissions shows only 14 cases of senile dementia out of a total of 1,010 cases in 1960.[279] In the rural population, where there is even a greater degree of security for the elderly, there are no evidences of high rates of senile disorders. The cases reported by Dr. Field cannot be due to old age, because consultation at the shrines is carried out properly for any ailment, of both young and old alike. Moreover, the cases of the elderly patients are complicated by superstitious beliefs in the influence of the *juju,* the fetish, and witchcraft. In view of the dynamics of the society, it is improbable that the older people at the shrines have any troubles arising from their advanced age.

FAMILY LIFE. The traditional Ghanaian family includes not only a man, his wife and children, but also the next of kin on the father's side (in areas where paternal inheritance is the rule) or on the mother's side (in areas where matrilinear inheritance is practiced). The man and his household are therefore only a part of the whole basic unit—the clan. As a consequence, there are responsibilities that individuals owe to other members of the clan.

There are many examples of customs and traditions that are designed to strengthen the solidarity of the clan, rather than that of the family, in the sense that we recognize it in the Western world. For example, all land is publicly owned, and any member can use any part of it, given the appropriate permission from the eldest or head member of the clan. When one needs help on his farm, his household, as well as members of the clan, can be asked, and assistance is always available. At the time when this kind of social organization was important, most areas of Ghana were almost completely self-sufficient agrarian communities.

It is true that a greater part of Ghana is still agrarian. But there have been some important changes in the economic basis of agriculture that have had far-reaching implications for family life. Introduction of cocoa and coffee, as cash crops, almost overnight revolutionized the system of land ownership. The new motive in farming was no longer production of food for the family, but, besides this, enough cocoa or coffee to sell, in order to fill other economic needs. This new trend necessarily has resulted in much conflict and confusion in the clans. As can be expected, different individuals will adapt to these new ways of self-advancement and individual endeavor at different rates. Thus, in such a transition, one is bound to find many instances of confused people. For example, while previously one could rely on the members of the clan to contribute to the educational cost of an ambitious son or daughter, this became, more recently, the sole responsibility of one person. For a person who does not have enough cash the question then becomes: Shall I resign myself to life as my forefathers knew it, or shall I pursue it the way I see it now? This is a difficult question to answer in view of the many unavoidable social pressures, e.g., the inevitable European modernizing and technological influences that are bound to spread like fire all over Africa. Apart from confusions that can be produced by disease, here is a rather potent source of stress to most people in modern acculturating communities, where class variations arise.

STATUS. Along with the breakdown of the clan as a unit in Akan-speaking society has come change in motivation and status among the people. Although literacy is estimated at only

15 to 20 per cent of the population, no one can deny the fact that since the independence of Ghana, in 1957, the whole country has seen a mass scramble for education, on all levels. A man is no longer satisfied with a family scene (in the Western sense) confined to a village, in which his sons take after him, and make their homes in the same vicinity, while his daughters get married to other country fellows. The new status orientation has become visible in the ability of a person to give the best education to his children. This trend is rather new among most people in southern and central Ghana, and both the boys and girls of school and college age, together with their parents, struggle to acquire it. Whether the quest after this new symbol of prestige is enough to cause any conflict in the minds of the people is not very easy to determine. However, there is one thing that can be said; namely, the personality development under the older system of social organization involved less stress from the side of mixed feelings and aspirations, and therefore less chance for what Horney would have called competitive struggles in the personality structures of large numbers of the people.

JOB OPPORTUNITIES AND MONEY AS A MOTIVATION. As a result of the new push for higher education, monetary rewards have become much of an incentive to the younger generation. This tendency, however, varies from one region to another. Wurapa feels that while the Ashantis, the Fantes, the Akwapims, the Akims, and the Ewes are rather adaptable, and are advanced in this regard (according to Western standards), the Hausas, themselves a conglomeration of many tribes who are mostly Moslems by religion, are more conservative. It is only those Northerners (Hausas) who have lived for a time in the South who have picked up the new motivations.

As Dr. Adeoye Lambo has pointed out, as soon as most Africans become "Westernized," the Western measuring stick can be used to assess them, in the same way that any such

Western society is analyzed. The question then is: How successful have the various tribes in Ghana been in their pursuit of jobs requiring higher education, and, also, the luxury that goes with such jobs, without any unusual stresses on their mental functioning or personalities? Again, it is impossible for me to imagine a high degree of success, in view of the fact that the two types of status referred to make different demands on the individual personality. For example, while success in the achievement of the new status requires a lot of independent or individualized thinking and self-reliance, one could have done quite well under the old system with almost every decision being shared by parents or siblings, or even a member of the clan.

MARRIAGE.   It is only natural that with the trend toward high educational attainment among youth, the customs regarding marriage should also change. Although most people still hold to the formalities connected with marriage, the major change has been greater with the young, and the newly-wedded, who make more individualized decisions in the contraction of their wedlock. While parents used to be charged with the responsibility of choosing partners for their sons and daughters, this is now becoming the sole responsibility of the boy and the girl, with the parents playing a rather subsidiary part. What problems, if any, this change has produced requires further research. But the divorce rate is higher now than ever before, according to statistics available for southern and central Ghana.

RELIGION.   An outstanding characteristic of most tribes in Ghana is their ability to adapt themselves to other ways of life and thought. An evidence of this can be seen in the spread of Christianity and mission education, which missionaries brought to most areas. Christianity is essentially foreign to the people of Ghana. Before they became Christians, most people worshipped various gods, through their ancestors. As already pointed out, the Northern people of Ghana are mostly Mos-

lems, so that Islam is more of an indigenous religion than
Christianity. And the Northern people, being more conservative, are more resistant to conversion to Christianity. The effect
of Christianity on the minds of most Ghanaian Christians can
be aptly described as one of an intrusion leading to a certain
amount of confusion. There can be no case established for the
contention that Ghanaian Christians regard Christianity and
ancestral worship as identical. Most Christians realize the difference between the two, but they are often in a dilemma when
it comes to decisions as to religious behavior. Here, then, is
another source of conflict.

The Cultural Basis of Depression Found Among the Akans

Of the various types and degrees of depression that beset
man, the Akans would seem to have the reactive type of
depression. The external provocation usually is the influence of
one's family and kinsmen. Such things as a person's prosperity
in business, the health of his family members, and the safety of
his *Kra* (soul) are believed to be in some unknown way controlled by the sorcery of friends and relatives. Endogenous depression, i.e., depression without any apparent external cause,
hardly existed, for an Akan would always show a depressive
state as the result of a "damage" to his *Kra* perpetrated by
someone else. An old proverb, present in most of the vernacu-
lars, shows the attitude of these tribes to misfortune and hardships. It states: When one is bitten by a louse, one looks into
one's own clothes if one desires to rid himself of the louse. One's
clothes here refer symbolically to one's closest kinsmen; hence,
the notion that one's relatives and friends can be the cause of a
person's hardships and misfortunes. This does not exclude the
possible interpretation of the individual being the cause of his
own problems. However, any of the above interpretations will
make the theory that these tribes show generalized projections

and paranoid reactions—as Field claimed—rather untenable. Whether these external but close provocations are concrete and real, or even have a basis for popular acceptance, is another matter altogether.

There can be many realistic reasons for the existence of depressive states. Whatever the stated reason may be, depression that has resulted from external cultural stress must be distinguished from similar stresses that are part of a rather stable, less changing culture. There was a discussion of 27 cases of depression in the Field book but, as the author herself pointed out, "the depressed patient is not considered mentally ill, for the patient is correctly oriented, accessible and says nothing which is in ideological setting irrational."[280] At the same time, many cases were recorded as having depressive overtones, and these were used for the establishment of the incidence of such mental illness. Cases with possible depressive backgrounds, according to Field, include 397 cases of complaints of "not prospering," 350 cases of routine "thanks for year's protection," and 151 cases of "complaints of unspecified sickness."[281] Therefore, we cannot equate such reactive forms of depression with mental illness using European nomenclature, when we assess matters for these Akans. Moreover, the swift cultural changes that have been sweeping all of Ghana also make such an equation incorrect. This is because the tribes, during the period of rapid change, have responded to the foreign stresses within the framework of their already existing cultural patterns.

It is important to distinguish the various processes of acculturation, and their effects on these tribes, from the deviations of individuals from normative patterns of behavior that may be part of a changing cultural scene. As Robert A. Lystad, a student of Ghana, has pointed out, acceptance and adaptation of social institutions to changing conditions, whether imposed from outside the culture or emerging from within in response to other changes, is a typical characteristic of Ashanti-Akans.[282] Naturally, the degree of resistance to change, both at the individual and tribal level, varies very widely. This is one of the most cogent reasons why an interpretation of the reaction to change in any of these tribes has to be evaluated with care.

The following is an account of a change that perhaps has been one of the most important for the tribal life of the people of Ghana: the introduction of cocoa-growing as a cash crop. Before the introduction of cocoa, almost every farmer engaged in subsistence farming. Under a subsistence form of agriculture, large kin groups were comfortably accommodated, on small pieces of land, for many generations. The Akans, in particular, had ordinarily a matrilineal type of inheritance; individual ownership of property was not important.

Teteh-Kwashi is believed to have brought the first cocoa pods into Ghana, on his return from Fernando Poo Island, about 1876. This event was synonymous with the beginning of a new era in the tribal life of the people. Cocoa, being a perennial and a cash crop, has brought with it a reorganization of the total agricultural system. Individual ownership of land became necessary. As a matter of fact, the first few farms for cocoa-growing were experimentally cultivated on publicly owned clan property. But, as the economic needs of the people increased, for example, the need for building better homes, sending one's children to school, and so forth, it became necessary for the individual to take care of his own cocoa farms, which then became the main source of his economic power. Older kin relationships gradually broke down. The family (in the Euro-American sense) became the nucleus of the social unit. Even in Ashanti, where matrilineal inheritance had flourished before, the cocoa era saw a man assume responsibility for his children, instead of leaving it to their mother's brother. There was a shift in population, too. Towns located in the cocoa-growing areas of the south and central regions grew from about 500 to about 1,500 in population.

Cultural changes such as those described above undoubtedly

require that the people adjust to the new way of life. In all of the 146 cases of all types, neurotic or otherwise, reported by Field, one can notice the obvious plight of these people in their attempt to adjust to new situations. One realizes that the problem of adjustment involves fundamental conflicts both in social structure and in the individual psyche. Depending on what one believes is more significant in producing psychoneuroses—the social environment or the individual psyche—one has to qualify his deductions accordingly, since the *two* factors are undoubtedly both operative.

One significant fact about the survey of the Akans is that the shrines have grown in number in a manner parallel to their growing cocoa output. The cases of depression recorded at the shrines are examples of the patient's desire to ventilate his conflicts, both in regard to the social structure and his own peace of mind. The fetish priests have also adapted their shrines to meet the needs of their steadily increasing numbers of clients; and, of course, the same prestige is attached to the priesthood now as it was before the cocoa-growing era. According to J. B. Loudon,[283] a Bantu-speaking population would appear to derive most of its psychopathology from social and environmental factors, rather than directly from intrapsychic factors. It appears probable that most of the mental disorders in a society such as the Akan would differ from that of a literate society, whose classification of neurosis is mainly on the basis of a more individualized version of the psyche.

INTERGENERATIONAL CONFLICT. From the foregoing discussion of the changes that are taking place within the various institutions of the society in Ghana, it becomes a matter of course to look for possible conflicts within the society that may be due to intergenerational friction. The ease with which individuals are abandoning older customs in favor of modern trends varies widely in Ghana. In general, it can be stated that the more educated a person becomes, the more willing he is to modify his traditional way of life. Although some individuals are simply conservative, no matter how superficially Westernized they are, it is generally true to say that the nonliterates are more conservative and more opposed to the idea of change than those who are literate.

It has already been mentioned that the Northerners in Ghana are more conservative than the people of the South. But even in the North, the rate of acculturation involving, among other things, more formal education for everyone, has been rapid enough for one to speak of a fair amount of intergeneration conflict, even there. An outstanding example of such a conflict can be seen all over the country in the area of chieftaincy. Chieftaincy has been a long inherited and indigenous institution, by means of which the tribes have been ruled by popularly elected chiefs, through a Council of Elders from a particular royal patrilineal lineage of a clan. Every village has its own chief, and elders, or council of advisers. At the level of the tribe, there is usually an over-all chief, who symbolizes the unity of the various chiefs and their people in the tribe. Thus, the machinery of government of every tribe provides adequate protection for the citizens. Chieftaincy has developed along with the traditional reverence of the elderly, and it is therefore the preferred system among the nonliterate folk.

The advent of Europeans, the British in particular, has certainly produced conflict within the tribes between the adherents of chieftaincy and those who advocate a strong central government, with *little* or *no* authority delegated to the chiefs. The present generation has more adherents of the latter system. This conflict was less noticeable during the days of British colonial administration because the British initiated the central government rather gradually, taking away the power of the chief step-by-step. But the present intergeneration conflict is more serious, as the newly-elected government—since 1957, made up entirely of Ghanaians—has been taking drastic steps to curtail the power of the chiefs. The slogan that has been associated with such measures is.: "United we stand, divided we fall; Freedom for all Ghana as a sovereign state." In the face of these changes, there are those belonging to the more conservative school, who believe in the older system of sovereignty for every group of tribes, with federation only among various regions of the country. The important thing here is that this intergeneration conflict exists on the level of sociopolitical values, at the various levels of organization of government and institutions. Some of these already discussed include family life, village life, marriage, and the life of newly developing urban communities.

A Critique of Field's Epidemiology

In the foregoing, we have indicated that although there is no question as to the existence of forms of mental illness among the rural Akans, the problem of the nature and causes of these mental illnesses is by no means clear cut. One way of establishing the cause of mental illness is to estimate the level and kind of anxiety in a people. Field's analysis of complaints and requests made at routine *Abisa* (shrine supplications) included:

Complaints of not prospering	397
Unspecified sickness	151
Sick children	123
Requests for the birth of a child	112
Requests from pregnant women for safe delivery	110
Thanks for the birth of a child	107
Complaints of long childlessness	100
Complaints by new supplicants for unspecified protection	94
Requests for help in new enterprises	93
Marital problems	59
Thanks for cure of sickness	57

Money urgently needed	55
Protection requested for specified dangers	53
Consultation on behalf of absent sick people	47
Complaint that children born always die	51
Others	555
Total	2,164

Although the area and exact population of the survey was not given, the Ashanti rural population can be estimated at about 1½ million. Assuming that the sampling procedures for the survey were appropriate, this number of reported cases would not be unusual. Moreover, the complaints are mostly those of everyday cares of life, and as such do not signify any unusual anxiety. The patients that have been presented are considered by Field to represent two conditions of mental state. The first group includes the patients with varying degrees of dissociated personalities. The second group consists of so-called chronic schizophrenics.

The first group, and by far the larger section of the patients discussed by Field, certainly contains individuals with unusual anxieties and neurotic conditions. An analysis of the nature and causes of these disturbances cannot be evaluated without a knowledge of the possible organic diseases that most of these patients have learned to take for granted. Without a clear idea as to the impact on such patients of diseases like trypanosomiasis and malaria, it is misleading to interpret any manifested signs of mental illness as belonging to one or another category of psychopathology. Since most of these patients were not medically examined, and much in their case histories was not available, one can say with assurance only that the individual supplicants might be presenting examples of strained affective or emotional constituents of their personalities.

The second group, made up of the so-called chronic schizophrenics, also cannot be said to include only mentally disturbed individuals, for in most of these rural people the term *obodamfo* (mad man) is used indiscriminately as descriptive of mental illness. Most of the people so qualified may actually be victims of epileptic fits or severe delirium following malarial attack.

Although the following example does not serve any purpose of statistical generalization concerning the nature and cause of mental illness in rural Ghana, we have a strong feeling that the common characteristic of poor public health in most rural areas will make such a generalization valid. In the Akan-Krachi district, where my assistant, Mr. Wurapa, lived most of his life, there are seven towns and villages, with about 3,500 population. These people speak Twi, like the Ashantis, and have customs and traditions that are identical. Only three individuals in this area are known who could be classified, according to Field's definition,[284] as chronic schizophrenics, and with them the diagnoses would not be certain. These individuals were unkempt and improperly dressed most of the time. The general opinion among all the inhabitants who live in this area was that they were "mad." One of these men possibly was a schizophrenic, for he was considered a normal individual until his early twenties, and after that was believed to have indulged in bad "medicine" (suman), an antisocial variety of sorcery. He therefore was punished by the gods, according to popular belief, with a confused mental state. The other two, however, both had defective and peculiar gaits and mannerisms of speech. They also appeared much retarded in growth, looking much younger, more ill, and thinner than their own age group. People conjectured that these two men might have some congenital organic defect, which the society and its medical technique were incapable of recognizing. Another possibility suggested was that of acquired defects due to malnutrition.

The above three cases are examples of mental illness caused by sociocultural and organic stresses. According to Field, there is an incidence of 0.95 per cent of chronic schizophrenia. She goes on to note that the expectation of schizophrenia in Europe and America is estimated at 0.8 per cent. There could be an intelligent comparison of the two percentages of incidence if the two populations under question underwent the same epidemiological survey or, indeed, had the same basis for their schizophrenias. At present, there seems to be more mental illness due to organic factors solely, in the rural areas, and it is interesting at this point to speculate as to the changing etiology of mental illness as these rural communities become urbanized. One can conjecture that if the general health of these rural communities is improved along with urbanization, then existing social stresses would become more of a major causative factor of mental illness than is now the case. At any rate, Field's estimates appear to be gross exaggerations.

The problem of what constitutes a "potential schizophrenic" was not discussed by Field. She writes: "In England, Ghana and Nigeria, at the present time, concern is being expressed about the large number of young Africans who go to Britain for study courses and there suffer mental breakdown."[285] She points out that the incidence for young literates of primary school age is, however, even higher in their own homes than in Britain. If one considers the social adjustment that these young students are experiencing, it will be evident that mental breakdown can be fomented, if not produced, in terms of the unusual stress of being away. Even when in Ghana, most of these youngsters used to travel 60 or 70 miles away from home just to attend high school; this entailed considerable problems in social adjustment. But the student who goes to Britain finds himself in an entirely new and unsupporting environment. Most of them remain in England for four or five years, or longer. These students have to grapple with new financial and social problems, especially if they are not sponsored by the government. Under such circumstances, they easily develop excessive anxiety. And that is not all, because even the successful students in Britain have to return later to a less dramatic social adjustment back in their own homes, after several years of life in a different environment.

The Search for Security

The question that M. J. Field has tried to answer; namely, Do primitive people have the same mental illness we do? can therefore be posed in a different form: Do primitive people have the same *basis* for their mental illness as we do? This is a more complete question. For while nonliterate people may have mental illnesses *similar* to those in the Western societies, their cultural environments provide a different basis for their mental problems.

Any ethnopsychiatric study of rural Ghana, and of any group for that matter, must be aimed first at establishing what the normative behavior is in the society. From such a norm, one can set out to describe how its various members succeed, or fail, to adjust to the usual stresses and strains.

In order to determine how many of the supplicants at the various shrines were actually mentally ill, it is necessary to take a look at the customary beliefs concerning fetishes and shrines. The existence of spirits, both good and evil, is universally believed in by most of these tribes. The power of these spirits to bring good fortune, or disaster, in the form of illness, is also accepted as fact. It is regarded a special honor to be called by one of these spirits to serve as a priest, and to interpret the will of the gods to the people. Closely associated with this belief in spirits is the popular idea of life after death, and ancestral worship. The origin of any shrine can be traced to the "call" of an individual to serve the gods. Although these "calls" to serve may in certain cases be influenced by the psychic state of the person being called, it is generally accepted that the spirits call only sincere and devoted persons. In certain cases, however, a priest, after he has been called, can be punished by the gods, and this is usually interpreted by the people as due to a deliberate violation of the supernatural orders.

Once a priest has become established, he becomes the mediator between the people and their past ancestors, who are believed to be living in harmony with the gods. The social role of the priest is therefore a very significant one. The priest is supposed to know the spiritual lot of the individual, and also to have the power of casting out evil spirits and their effects. Since ill health is believed to be caused by the evil spirit, the priest is the man to consult in health and disease. The fact that the shrines are visited by people with reasons ranging from the desire for a cure for a disease to that of asking for the protection of the gods, or giving thanks to the gods for a previous blessing, shows the central importance of the shrines and their priests in their lives. How many of the people visiting the shrines are actually mentally ill, according to the criteria of their tribes? Obviously, the Ashanti do not consider any of the supplicants at the shrines—who, after consultation, return to their communities—as being mentally ill. In my opinion, the socially accepted place of the shrines among these tribes is one of the reasons for the high attendance, which can be wrongly interpreted to mean a high incidence of mental illness.

Rural Ashanti, Akims, and Fantes have many of their traditions and customs rooted in ancient tradition. Adherence to old beliefs and superstitions has been a very strong factor in their attempt to grapple with the superimposed, so-called modern, socioeconomic stresses. Most rural Ghanaians, like any other people in their position in Africa, have been undergoing the fastest change in their lives during the past two or three decades. In many of the cases discussed by Field, it is evident that the individual anxieties are invariably influenced to great extent by the degree to which the patients have accepted the supernatural origin of their troubles. On the whole, ignorance and poverty have resulted in many organic diseases, for which most of these rural peoples have no cures.

Most of the patients classified as literate by the author have at the most completed only the Middle School—equivalent to the American eighth grade. Such individuals can read and write some English, and usually are employed locally as assistant clerks, or as messengers in commercial establishments. As a rule, these so-called literate individuals are not very satisfied, socially and economically. The result is that their educations do not make them any less superstitious than their kin in the villages. One finds in such a group individuals stricken with fear and anxiety. The interesting thing has been that, in their frustration, these people turn to practices and beliefs of their parents as a means of justifying their failures in life. Some writers have referred to such instances as examples of the "scapegoat psychology."

Perhaps the most important factor that has contributed to the seemingly high rate of mental illness Field claims for these tribes has been the dominant sway that witchcraft still holds today on many Akan-speaking people. As B. Malinowski pointed out in his book *Dynamics of Culture Change,* no amount of education has helped to prevent modern forms of witch-hunting in such countries as Germany.[286] It can be expected then that African tribes would have a rather strong belief in the power of sorcery. Cultural contact of many African tribes with the West has not helped decrease this belief in witchcraft. As a matter of fact, indications are that there has been an increase. This paradox has been attributed by some writers to unsuccessful cultural change. Most colonial powers, and even missionaries, have dealt with the problem of witchcraft very ineffectively. The denial of a psychological basis for witchcraft has resulted in a superficial verbal attack on the "evils" of sorcery.

The foregoing paragraphs have not refuted the existence of mental illness among the rural Ashanti, Akims, and Fantes, but they point out the cultural and psychological basis of these continuing customs. When Field says, "the indexes of social breakdown—delinquency, crime, riots, rebellion, mental illness, unemployment, poverty, emigration, diminishing population—do not appear to be appreciably higher than before contact with the White," she could add that it has been only in areas where social institutions change rapidly that these disturbances are felt.

Using a modified form of her approach to the ethnopsychiatric study of these tribes, one would therefore have arrived at a much smaller estimate of prevalence of mental illness. The shrines that she visited represent the sole refuge for the solution of the psychological problems of these people. There is the likelihood that if modern medicine were a popular means for the cure of illnesses of all origins among these tribes, then she would have found fewer patients at the shrines. Also, one is tempted to doubt the statistical validity of the many hearsay reports that Field included in her evaluations. For example, one of her assistants was asked to go and find out how many of his friends were in similar socioeconomic straits as he himself was. It is obvious that the report rendered by such a "sampling device" is bound to be faulty. On many other occasions, Field collected evidence of mental illness about certain patients from their relatives and friends, who might themselves have had undetected biases. These are problems that any investigator of any social problem would have to face.

The most effective way of arriving at moderately valuable conclusions is to attempt to eliminate some of the elements in the investigative procedure that are liable to be undependable. For example, some of the patients could have been followed up beyond a *single, short* interview. Trained native field workers could have helped improve the dependability of the case histories. Above all, one could wait until such carefully collected data had accumulated over a significant period of time before the percentage of incidence or prevalence of mental illness was estimated. The writer could not claim to have studied "incidence," and therefore her "prevalence" is equally open to question. These are some of the problems that all the new states in Africa are facing, and some headway must be made in this direction before a Western type of ethnopsychiatric and epidemiological analysis can be fruitfully applied.

As Lambo has pointed out: "Obsessional neurosis in primitive Africans is usually marked by or mistaken for normal tribal religious rituals. Therefore, the essential prerequisites for a sound diagnosis are a thorough knowledge of the language and the subcultural group to which the patient belongs, for example, his religion."[287]

CULTURE AND CHRONIC ILLNESS:
ON THE EPIDEMIOLOGY OF
DIABETES CROSS-CULTURALLY

In this discussion of chronic illness, we wish to focus on diabetes as an example, specifically on juvenile diabetes. H. R. Leavell and E. G. Clark in their *Preventive Medicine*[288] remind us that diabetes has shown a definite upward trend over the past few years, and they list it among the leading causes of death as our population grows older. While 75 per cent of known diabetics are over fifty, and both morbidity and mortality rates are higher for females, the rapid increase in known cases (50,000 annually being added to a prevalence of one million) suggests that case finding is also on the increase.

If, then, we know about 1¼ million cases in 1963 epidemiologically—the figure given by Hilleboe and Larimore in their *Preventive Medicine*—we know less about an estimated equal number of cases believed to exist in the population. On the other hand, differentiated population studies have for some time alleged that Southern Italian and Eastern European Jewish populations have higher than average rates; and it is interesting to note in passing that these are both cultural groups in which the mother's nurturant and cooking abilities are seen as important functions in maintaining not only health but also quasi-magical dietary excellence. This I have dealt with for the Southern Italian background in an analysis of one female case involving a combination of hypoglycemia and obesity.[289]

Other epidemiological information on diabetes has not been startling.*

While such large-scale epidemiological surveys are certainly social in their implications, they are a far cry from the kind of clinical observations that trace the course of stress in actual lives. For this, we get some glimmers of the process indirectly through animal experimentation. Experiments on rats have shown that those allowed to live together in pairs appeared to resist the development of experimental forms of diabetes (alloxan diabetes) better than those living alone. Similar experiments showed the incidence of spontaneously developing mammary tumors significantly greater in mice caged as isolates than in those allowed to live in groups.

For juvenile diabetes, on the other hand, the peer group of age mates has seemed to be less implicated in clinical studies to date than parents and sibling, though the matter of kinds of social relationships looms large even in the family circle. Indeed, Noyes and Kolb state:

> The illness magnifies the difficulty between the child and the parent. Those parents with perfectionistic, aggressive attitudes may bring their children to good control of the diabetes but with the creation of a behavior difficulty. On the other hand, parents who pity themselves or blame the child and reject it may foster poor control of the diabetes. The need to limit food often becomes a battleground between the child and parents and the child and physician. This is particularly so since the giving of candy or of food is often a token of approval in the family.[290]

The authors go on to indicate the passive weapon of food-

* For comparative materials, see above, p. 268.

refusal the American child frequently wields. Others, starved for affection, express oral aggression and hostility by overeating. They conclude that psychiatrists are required to mediate such parent-child conflicts and can help parents understand such emotional problems in cases of already developed juvenile diabetes. They also conclude that there may be occasions when dietary regimen and insulin requirements must be modified to conform with existing emotional problems. Dr. Frank W. Reynolds, writing in the Hilleboe and Larimore text on screening methods for diabetes, notes that while adult diabetes is often insidious and frequently asymptomatic in onset, juvenile diabetes is usually a severe and symptom-producing disease right from the beginning.

These conclusions lead me to consider the oral and emotional control aspects of the disease in greater detail. We all know that early childhood and infantile patterns are important in psychoneurotic etiology. In the earliest stage of life, the taking of food and sucking is an oral stage optimally connected with tactile stimulation, warmth, and security. Harry Harlow has noted that even with rhesus monkeys, terry cloth mother-surrogates do better than wire-mounted bottles, and of course the rhesus mothers do best of all in providing tactile stimulation, warmth, and security. From the first in his observations, he has stressed the social equivalents of such contact, and perhaps his most crucial experiments have been concerned with the point that peer-group age mates, among the rhesus monkeys, can mitigate the effects of a loss of these mothering functions, likewise producing the tactile stimulation, warmth, security, and we add *social* stimulations needed by the young monkeys in their development. Sherwood L. Washburn, an anthropologist, has similar materials, also in the form of excellent films secured while observing baboon colonies in their natural habitats in Africa. While S. Zuckerman had earlier described *The Social Life of Monkeys and Apes* in the London Zoological Gardens in terms of physical strength and dominance and their continuous patterns of sexual activity, those in natural habitat have a more elaborate system of group behavior, exhibit patterns of cooperation, exploration and even play to a greater extent, and put the negative and quarrelsome behavior of Zuckerman's apes to shame, much as we would expect. Indeed, though they are healthy specimens, they appear to be more "sublimated," to borrow a Freudian term, than the caged baboons of Zuckerman, and more elaborated in behavior patterns, involving groups, than their captive cousins in London, or their phylogenetic ancestors in Harlow's primate laboratory in Wisconsin. The human needs for sensory stimulation, and more than that —for humanly social relationships—hasten the same search for essentially social factors in the studies of psychotic-like effects in sensory deprivation of adults, or of the hygiene-protected but socially deprived children in experiments of René Spitz, John Bowlby, and George Engel.

In his recent book George Engel describes diabetes as a somatic decompensation—a complication of flight-fight patterns—in an already defective system of emotional adaptation. He says:

> In the diabetic, the mobilization of free fatty acids during the flight-fight reaction may elevate the level of blood ketones and thereby increase or provoke acidosis. Hyperglycemia and increased glycosuria may also occur in the diabetic under such conditions.[291]

Of course, it was the classic experiments of Cannon with cats that demonstrated glycosuria when the animals were both overstimulated and enraged. Since then, glycosuria has been noted in football players following a hard game and in students after difficult examinations. Hyperglycemia, similarly, occurred in anxious patients facing an operation, or in soldiers or flyers faced with danger. I. Arthur Mirsky has cast doubt on hyperglycemia as the major factor responsible for the glycosuria accompanying such anxiety states, and he has suggested that the latter occurs mainly because of decreased glucose absorption from the kidney tubules. The present author can offer nothing significant on these refinements in the study of mechanisms in anomalies of sugar metabolism. But it appears that mechanisms described by Engel and by Mirsky, involving larger organ systems, probably do describe the case better for man than Cannon's pioneering experiments with cats. Certainly, the total organism responds in man more elaborately and with more spare adjustive machinery in such complicated end-states as continuous anxiety.

In other words, in alluding to somatic decompensations of one sort or another, we are basically discussing the anxiety theory of Freud[292] as having a dual function in regulatory but pathological behavior. We are suggesting that anomalies of sugar metabolism do become "steady states" and involve larger organ systems as signals of danger mobilizing both the anticipatory and defensive functions of certain kinds of troubled individuals. Freud noted that as a symptom of disordered psychological functioning, anxiety serves as such a signal of danger, and has at first exactly such mobilizing powers. But, unfortunately, when the stress continues to be too intense or protracted, and the simple striving mechanisms are inadequate to the problem, greater anxiety may appear in the setting of disintegrative states in which such defensive maneuvers are frantically overused and may themselves wear thin. It is for this reason, we think, that Noyes and Kolb have noticed that overcontrolled juvenile diabetes may come into good control of the diabetes, but erupt on the psychological side with more serious behavior problems. Again, this implies a total human being responding to his meaningful environment and treatment as a whole person. If this is true, it would mean parenthetically that there is probably not a single, or simple, personality type with a few well-defined traits of character that inclines toward diabetes; but instead there may be more generic types. Doctor T. A. C. Rennie wrote persuasively many years ago of hypoglycemic states accompanying anxiety; and it seemed to me then as now that in some bipolar system these were the persons who exemplified more of a neurasthenic withdrawal, or "flight reaction," or who, in other words, had "lost fight." Getting back to the type we are describing at this contrast point of hyperglycemic reaction forms, most authors have described a passive form of aggression, with hostility just below the surface and fluctuating with the organic signs, for the diabetic syndrome. The oral-aggressive patterns of obesity have also been noted. And brittle diabetes, of course, may connote more complex problems and reaction forms.

From the anthropological standpoint, one thing seems clear and it is that nonliterate peoples utilize conversion hysterias where we "moderns" show rising rates of psychosomatic disorders. The chief reason seems to be that we largely lack the social supports for expressing emotional entanglements in emotional language; whereas nonliterate peoples need not convert these voltages into body language. Instead of using the giving of food, or its withholding, as a token of love and affection, most nonliterate peoples recognize fixed social obligations, equally reciprocal in character, in gift exchanges involving edibles. One cannot read Malinowski's prolific writing on the Trobriand Islanders, a gardening people, without recognizing the tremendous importance in inland to seacoast trade, or even in inter-island trade, of both feasting and the almost ritual gifts of yams. But my point is that such exchanges are regularized and not at all the passing whim of an affectionate impulse. Even among the Siriono of Eastern Bolivia, a hunting and gathering people whose marginal economy, in Allan R. Holmberg's description, unleashes tremendous publicly expressed anxieties about food, the point is that these *are* publicly expressed, and not, again, the result of personal whim or fancy. We can contrast these conditions in primitive agriculture and gathering with our own tokens of approval or affection to children or to assorted females of candy and other comestibles, or of dinner "dates" for that matter, recently extended to business or professional acquaintances in the ritual "love magic" of our commercial and professional establishments.

Perhaps we can make the point of contrast clearer by selecting from the anthropological and medical literature an example where food and comestibles strongly connote love and affection, or its withdrawal, and where rates of diabetes are alleged to be exceedingly high. In India, where obesity is not in the least implicated in relation to diabetes, cultural patterns emphasize the giving of food as a major expression of regard and approval. We are not implying that these patterns are structured as ours are, in terms of the basic confusions unleashed in children by such standardized exhortations as, "Eat it for mother's sake," "Eat it because it's 'good' for you," etcetera. We probably derive much of our slang jargon from the common currency of such memory traces, and here I think of the meanings of "being fed up" for *angry*, "filled to the gills" for *overeating* and *overdrinking*, and countless other terms for annoyance or discomfort. Nor do we feel that all such patterns are to the same end, as with the Southern Italians' concern for healthful nurturance and girth, believed to be symbolized in red vegetables "making good blood" or *pasta* producing "more strength, larger girth and vigor." Similarly, an Eastern European Jewish mother's "making of the Sabbath" is, in the Zborowski and Herzog book, *Life is With People*,[293] primarily centered in the maternal nurturant and protective rituals, like the Italian mothers,' quasi-magical in character. Moreover, nonliterate cultures and these later examples too allowed no option or choice between nursing infants and bottle feeding them.

On the other hand, the Asiatic Indian culture, where food is not only surrounded by ritual but connotes also the individualized bestowal of love and affection, is a prime example of high rates of diabetes. A. K. Raychaudhury, in commenting on these high rates in contrast to other rice-eating peoples, attributes the

Hindu example to the role of suffering in their society and their allegedly "masochistically inclined" tendencies. The present author cannot frankly find real evidence for masochism in Hindu society, but he does find fascinating Raychaudhury and others typical noting of the high Hindu rates for diabetes, and in particular the still greater susceptibility of women to the disease.[294] For not only is food of ritual concern among Hindus, but its bestowal is also a personal act of love and affection. Further, the Hindu woman is notable not only for the higher rates of diabetes, but in regard to purely functional emotional disorders, the hysterias are most common in India and women again are the prime victims with the highest rates. Of course, social factors are crucial since the Hindu women, involved in family arranged marriages, must live in the husband's village, subject at many points to the authority of his kin. The rest of Raychaudhury's description—far from masochism—now falls into place. He mentions the vacillating nature of the diabetic, his dependent leaning, the concomitant annoyance, the repression of hostility, the resulting excess of glucose in the blood, the "extra work" required metabolically.

While Southern Italian, East European Jewish, and Hindu examples are instructive, the variations in prevalence of diabetes among American populations are no less important for epidemiological insight into possible etiology. "We moderns," so to speak, do not suffer from diabetes on the same scale or in uniform rates throughout a population.*

This intergenerational conflict between parents on the one side and age-mates on the other, which we claimed in the Midtown Study, was a kind of cultural marginality—a push toward one cultural set, and a simultaneous pull toward another—also has been credited by Thorsten Sellin as a factor explaining low rates of crime in first generations, followed by higher delinquency rates in the second generation. In the setting of psychosomatic studies, more specific psychodynamics must be dis-

* For comparative materials, see above, p. 270.

cerned, but for diabetes they may well be found in the area of overdetermined and emotional reactions to food. Here we are reminded that the "oral component" in medical practice, and use of the physician in a threatening or rewarding sense by parents who relate badly to their own children, can involve the doctor in repetitions of parental conflicts of juvenile diabetics. No doubt, medical practice has always been so involved, ever since the classic cults of Hygeia in ancient Greece proposed that sanatoria always conduct therapy to include regulation of food (dietetics). In the same sense today, surgeons frequently encounter the diabetic with peripheral complications in which diet, insulin, and foot care were neglected in a fairly hostile fashion. By this we mean that what looks, at first blush, like masochistic neglect may represent a seething transference of basic hostilities from the patient, and unless the physician can modulate the countertransference properly, he will be caught unwarily in the same pattern of intergeneration conflicts. This is why clinicians commenting specifically on the control of juvenile diabetes refer to the oral component chiefly in two forms. Flanders Dunbar,[295] Hilda Bruch,[296] or D. P. Barr[297] all suggest such poorly controlled kinds of hostility, and all assure us that nine out of ten diabetics in our society have some previous history of obesity.

Besides the factors traceable to culture, ethnic group, and intergenerational conflict, and the predisposing factor of weight gain as a precipitant of diabetes, its growing proportion in the American population generally is a matter for further concern. In American culture and ethos, in the broadest sense, we live amid values that stress immediate gratification, and children today hear less of delayed gratification than its opposite. Perhaps for commercial as well as technological reasons, "quick service," "instant foods," and overeating, particularly of sweets, is a part of a complex of bestowing quick gratifications or denying them. Thirty years ago W. F. Osborn noted that goods and services were being supplied increasingly from without the household confines, as the American family changed from a multigeneration, rural family in the main to an urban or suburban status. While the family was losing economic functions of food production and household maintenance, the affectional factor, he said, grew proportionally in significance among its functions as a whole.[298] Where functions of the family become thus limited, and the family form itself shrinks to the nuclear one of parents and children, overeating, sweets included, easily becomes a regressive substitute for dependency and love, especially where sweets become the symbol for either. For these reasons, we feel, the orality and passive or childlike seeking for affection have been stressed by clinicians. This basic pattern is elaborated by Rosen and Lidz stating that diabetics react to sibling rivalry by regressive means of requiring maternal attention, in other words, by "becoming helpless, demanding or negativistic rather than through more active measures."[299] Mirsky wrote about the same time of basic conflicts involving the "frustration of infantile wishes for care."[300]

The studies by Hinkle and Wolf have traced related emotional factors in management of the disease. For example, the glucose-tolerance curve becomes more abnormal when the patient is hostile and depressed, and is nearer normal when he feels cared for and accepted.[301] Implying some sort of balance wheel to the chronic abnormalities, significant alterations in ketonemia were present, though inconsistently, with similar emotional states. In patients who are mere children, feeding problems are frequently added to problems of insulin regimen, whereas adolescents in our society are prone to become over-concerned about their "difference" from age mates. Both the Rosen and Lidz and the Hinkle and Wolf studies show that deviations from diet occur as protests against such added frustrations. Recently, among Africans who are newly adapted to the frustrations, racial discrimination, and confusions of urbanism in Johannesburg, diabetes has been reported to have reached striking proportions.[302] One can predict that as nonliterate peoples are swept into colonial, urban, and nuclear family conditions, psychosomatic conditions will become more prevalent.[303]

SENRYU POETRY AS FOLK AND COMMUNITY EXPRESSION

The following account deals with a type of poetry produced in a wartime community under federal jurisdiction. The locale is the Tule Lake Center for Japanese-Americans in northern California. The federal agency is the War Relocation Authority of the United States Department of the Interior. The authors are, respectively, the Community Analyst assigned to this Project since May 1943, and one of his Assistants in the Community Analysis Section.

Tule Lake is one of several centers originally established to house Japanese-American citizens and aliens evacuated from the west coast under military order. For more than a year it had been a Relocation Center, like the rest, with a portion of the population found ineligible for "leave" into the outer communities. However, in the summer of 1943, the Center was designated for the purpose of segregating evacuees who, for one reason or another, failed to qualify for relocation back into the normal stream of American life. Immediately, Tule Lake witnessed a vast reshuffling of population. Those ineligible for residence in Relocation Centers arrived in Army-commandeered trains and those ineligible for residence in the Segregation Center were sent to other Centers. Before the trainloads had arrived, a tall manproof fence enclosed the Project area. Back behind the fence, people looked warily at their new neighbors; families from all parts of the west coast and some from Hawaii were now thrown together. In the older generation, uprooted from American soil, were represented many provinces, or kens, of Japan of fifty years ago.

The poetry discussed below is an expression of the community during this turbulent period. Yet the individuals and families who came to Tule Lake and those who remained behind represented many different points of view and types of background. There were farmers and merchants, artists and laborers, professionals and illiterates. There were a few rich and many poor. There were women and children born here, and aged immigrants who after a half-century of toil in America without benefit of citizenship wished to end their lives in the land of their birth. There were youthful citizens who came simply out of a desire to accompany their parents as so-called voluntary segregants. There were families with emotional ties to close relatives abroad and families who believed that the future was destroyed for them here. There was the farmer, the businessman who saw his community stakes uprooted, the foreign-educated with his language handicap. There were the impecunious large families who saw no hope of re-establishing in communities farther east. To understand the poetry, one must understand the people. In general, they were all, except the very young, embittered and disaffected by the journey inland.

The poetry bears this out. In the new community, a tall manproof fence with barbed wire slanting inward surrounded the blocks of tarpaper shacks. Here lived families who once resided in the cities and rural districts of Washington, Oregon, and California. Guarding installations, watchtowers manned by sentries, and floodlights commanded the village of the minority which, "on the outside" at least, was once famous for low crime and delinquency rates, for generous support of Community Chest and Red Cross, and for frugal and industrious habits which brought families into middle-class brackets and sent children through college. All individuals in Tule Lake were fingerprinted and processed, screened and catalogued as to loyalty or disloyalty—all except children. Soon roughly half the adult community found jobs on project maintenance, and families earned stipends of $12, $16, and $19 per month, depending on the kind of work. Mass feeding was accomplished as before through huge mess-halls in all the blocks. Evacuee wardens patrolled the camp grounds under the surveillance of a Caucasian police department which grew notably in size and equipment. Before long, jeeps and peeps backed up the Army sentries at the gates. Life within the narrow Center confines became dull and prosaic, if not sternly regimented. Senryu poetry records much of this story. It is one way in which people in an abnormal community find an outlet—in painting and music and Hollywood movies for the sophisticates, in baseball, basketball, and jitterbug for the Americanized youth, in poker and sake for the man of the world, in Japanese checkers and chess and theatricals for the gentlemen of Japan, and in Senryu poetry and Utai singing clubs for the older esthete.

Three Forms of Japanese Poetry

In Japanese poetry there are three principal forms of metric composition. They are:

1. Chyo-ka (Long Song) composed of any number of stanzas. Each stanza usually consists of four or eight lines. Each line has two phrases, a first of five syllables and a second of seven. This form is as old as the Kojiki, the earliest systematic recording of Japanese history. It probably emerged as one of the results of the influence of Chinese poetry, the Kojiki being written about 1,200 years ago when Chinese culture was assiduously introduced to the Japanese court. Yet Chyo-ka never occupied an important position in Japanese literature until Japan came in contact with Occidental culture. Then, the

Chyo-ka form began to be used frequently in translations of American and European poems.

2. Tan-ka (Short Song), or Wa-ka (Japanese-style Song). Tan-ka and Wa-ka are two names for one and the same form with only slight variations. The former is the more common variant. In it, the number of syllables is limited to thirty-one. On occasion, an extra syllable is allowed if it is a single vowel or "*n*." These thirty-one syllables are divided into five phrases or "meters," each phrase containing a fixed number of syllables in the order 5-7-5-7-7. This particular form of Tan-ka is said to have originated in the mythological period of Japan's history. Since it came down to the present, it obviously suited Japanese poetic taste. Depending on the historic period, various themes —deep national spirit, or samurai loyalty, or appreciation of nature, flowers, or a moonlit night—all find emotional expression in the Tan-ka form. A felicity in composing Tan-ka is considered one of the finest accomplishments in Japanese literature.

3. Senryu and Hai-ku are, in contrast to the above, more recent forms. About two hundred years ago, when the Tokugawa Era was at the height of peace and prosperity, there arose in Osaka and in Yedo (Tokio) a school of poetry which created a form still shorter than the Tan-ka. This school was composed of prosperous merchants, doctors, and in general a rising middle class with an interest in literature and leisure enough to appreciate it. In structure, the new form was merely the first three phrases of the Tan-ka, omitting the last two. The arrangement of syllables in phrases therefore was 5-7-5. The new form was called Hai-ku, and its topics or themes principally concerned the seasons and nature and such items as autumn moon, blossoms, or the old pond. Generally, there was more freedom in choice of subject matter and more versatility in treatment. Occasionally the Hai-ku composer dwelt on human affairs and emotions, looking for the common and universal aspects of the mundane world as it affected man, but

handling these matters in the light of discriminating literary taste. Either to compose Hai-ku or appreciate it in its full emotional impact and economy of line required the cultivation of esthetic taste to a high degree. Hai-ku tended toward the universal emotion and the mundane world, but remained, in the last analysis, a delicate and cultivated form nurtured under glass. It grew in the guest rooms of sophisticates and never became a folk, or mass, art.

It is difficult to ascertain the chronological relationship of Hai-ku and Senryu. But it may reasonably be assumed that Senryu branched out of Hai-ku shortly after the latter came into existence. At any rate, the name, Senryu, which means "River Willow," was simply the nom de plume of one who proposed to his poetry circle to compose Tan-ka by means of two persons, the first poet writing the initial three phrases of 5, 7, and 5 syllables, and the second adding the last two phrases of 7 syllables each. Apparently, the artistry depended on final unity and consistency in both the meaning and phraseology of the finished product. It was like certain forms of folk art in which more than one person participates in the development of a theme, a story, or a coherent idea. It appears that the people who flocked around Senryu, unlike the poets of the Hai-ku School, displayed greater interest in human affairs than in the well-worn objects of nature. What Senryu lost in delicate and effete refinement, it gained in popularity, vigor, and hearty good humor. The Senryu cultists were commoners, men of the street, rather than esthetes. Naturally their products were in a lighter vein for the most part, although full of penetrating insight, sarcastic comment, and tender emotion.

Soon, however, a movement began in Senryu circles to differentiate the form further from the Hai-ku. The opposition won out by proposing that the last two phrases of 7 syllables each be discarded, thus making Senryu exactly the same as Hai-ku as to form. Yet in its contents, Senryu retained the more common and popular values and became firmly established as folk art. Thus, Senryu required no "high brow" culture, no fixed mannerisms. But to its neophyte there still remained the danger of falling into vulgarisms.

Today, among literary hobbyists, Senryu and Hai-ku are almost equally appreciated, and much ink has been spilt concerning the difference between the two. The most feasible conclusion is that in Hai-ku one perceives nature in terms highly colored with human emotion, whereas in Senryu one touches upon human affairs even through the medium of natural objects. Thus a "blossom" might be a fittting topic in Hai-ku poetry. But when "blossom" becomes a metaphor for a lovely girl, one is in the realm of Senryu.

The Tule Lake Senryu Circle

It is not surprising that a folk art, popular in the Japan of fifty years ago, found fertile soil in the Tule Lake community. The practice of composing Senryu here, as at other Centers, did not await the establishment of Tule Lake as the Segregation Center. The formation of a Senryu circle marked no sudden trend toward Japanization. Rather, this element of Japanese culture which had lived among the first generation, or Issei, as a part of their cultural heritage, was revived when west coast communities were uprooted, careers interrupted, and the long, uncomfortable trek inland begun on the shortest notice. Senryu poetry, then, is one aspect of the cultural revivalism which occurred within the first-generation age group when they realized that their futures might be uncertain in this nation. As we shall see below, this cultural activity provides escape from the drab realities of Center existence. It also recaptures Japanese cultural values of an apolitical sort. Here the farmhand and housewife, working within a cultural form, can retain a kind of folk expression which has, at times, an artistic quality. Working within the same form, they are able, on occasion, to comment satirically upon the monotonous existence they seek to escape. This "backward glance" at the conditions of Center life has been successful in catching the emotionalism of the residents, so that once again the folk art is expressive of the folk society.

THE TULE LAKE SENRYU KAI. Literally, the name of this group means "Senryu Association." In actuality, it was a more or less informal club, organized at Tule Lake in September 1942, when the evacuees felt reasonably settled and adjusted in the then-Relocation Center.* The club closed up shop in November 1943 because of the much-publicized "Tule Lake Incident." It began again in February 1944. Later, it was holding regular weekly meetings every Tuesday night in the Ironing and Utility Room of Block 14.

MEMBERSHIP. Up to November 1943 the Tule Lake Senryu Association had over thirty persons on its membership roll. Six were women—housewives and widows. All of these women were Issei or first-generation. One elderly widow had a fine educational background in Japan and also spoke English fluently. The men ranged in age from thirty to sixty years, about ten of the younger probably being Kibei (a United States citizen who has lived, and possibly been educated in whole or in part, in Japan; literally "returned to this country"). In education, about one-third of the men had higher than grade-school instruction in Japan. As employed on the Project, they were farmhands, block janitors, truck drivers, officers of the Tule Lake Cooperative, and a social worker. According to their pre-evacuation experience, they were farmhands, sawmill workers, businessmen (and some business women), housewives, restaurant operators, hotel proprietors, and so forth. Anyone could become a member by leaving his

* Mr. F. Obayashi, who compiled these data, was a member of the group from May to November 1943. Without him, this article could not have been written.

or her name and Center address. Of course, there were occasional visitors.

REGULAR MEETING. The chairman of the Tule Lake Senryu Association from May to November 1943 was foreman of the block janitors. In education, he presumably had nothing better than the grade school in Japan, but he had composed Senryu for more than twenty years. He presided over regular meetings as follows.

A box was prepared containing many topics for composition, each written on a small, folded slip of paper. The topics, furnished by the members, were replenished from time to time. By order of the chairman, a member picked out one of these slips, unfolded it, and announced the topic. The members were then required to compose Senryu on the theme mentioned. Each person wrote one to three Senryu on each topic, recording these on pieces of scratch paper, but leaving them unsigned. When the topic was announced, the chair appointed a critic, or grader, of all the Senryu written on that subject.

When the chair felt that enough time had been spent on a given theme, he announced that "the time is up." The compositions were then collected and submitted to the critic. Usually a member takes about forty-five minutes on a given subject, and then another topic is chosen, the same procedure repeated, while the critic is grading those composed on the previous theme. A meeting ordinarily covers three topics.

At the end of the last period of composition, the chair requested the critic of the first set of Senryu to announce the "grades." The critic, to do this, read aloud one Senryu after another beginning with the lowest grade. After each Senryu was read, its author answered by calling out his or her name. Then, and then only, the critic learned who had composed each poem. When there are some Senryu graded below par—and in each meeting there are a few—the critic spares the composer the embarrassment of reading them aloud. Occasionally, however, the critic states why some were rejected. The commonest defect is "too flat," possessing neither originality nor freshness. Those ambiguous in meaning are also left ungraded. Although relations between male and female, or husband and wife, are allowed as subject matter, frank indecency or vulgarity is never tolerated. For example, under the topic, "Shoes," the following Senryu was rejected on grounds of indecency:

> Ara fushigi (Oh, incomprehensible!)
> Yamome no heyani (In a bachelor's room)
> Onna gutsu (Woman's shoes)

THE CHOICE OF TOPIC.   In collections of Tan-ka verse, classical and modern, a frequent topic is war. As a matter of fact, a number of poems are found which actually were composed on the battleground. In Hai-ku or Senryu verse, on the other hand, we find very few which have a warlike theme, probably because both forms were products of peaceful times, express emotions in "a lighter vein," and the classical authors of these forms were mainly civilians from various walks of life. However this may be, the Tule Lake Senryu Kai unconsciously turned its back on the topic of war. Though the poems were hardly "products of peaceful times," members never discussed the war at the meetings, and even afterwards, when they fell to gossip, made no mention of it in their conversation. It was as if there were an unwritten code among them. The war was something to forget, and the meeting accomplished this if only for a few hours. While, in general, escape was an unconscious motive, life in the Tule Lake Center could not go unnoticed. On this, we shall comment later.

THE TOPICS CLASSIFIED.   The following topics were found in a collection of Senryu made into a volume by the members of the Tule Lake Senryu Kai. The collection covers an eight-month period from January 4, 1943 to August 31, 1943. They have been grouped into three classes.

1. *Topics Expressed by Verb, Adverb, Adjective, and Preposition:* Too, or Again; Probably, or Seemingly; Then; Against, or Opposing; Spring Comes; Above All, or Further; Until Arriving; Given Up; Doubled; Worrying; While Awaiting the Downpour; Being Obedient; Peeping; Giving Up; Home Coming; Getting Ready, Careless; Worthless; and so forth.

2. *Topics Expressed by a Common Noun:* Wall, or Partition; Records; Ice; Road; Mouth; Fagot; Lamplight; Tea; Horizontal Stripes; Socks; A Hurry-Scurry Fellow; Father; Companion; Children; Idiot; Screen; Finger; Evening; Razor; Skeleton or Spine; Wheels; Baseball; Vinegar; Eye; Diary; Bag; Next Door; Tobacco; Shoes; Thread; Sake (rice-wine); Landscape; and so forth.

3. *Topics Expressed by an Abstract Noun:* Daytime; Making Money; The Unexpected; Convenience; Connection; Yawning; An Addition; Action, or Moving; Soliloquy; Working Steady; Orientation, or The Objective; Red; Consolation; Grumbling; Trouble; Dreams, or Castles in the Air; Rest; Pleasing, or Charming; Green; Hara (literal translation is "belly," but here the connotation is "Being Phlegmatic"); The Act of Thanking; On Being Emotionally Stirred; Alone; Scent; Argument, or Discussion; One; Nearsighted; Relying, or Trusting; Games (including Gambling Games); Peace of Mind; A Refined or Polished Person; The Broad-minded; Carrying More Than One Responsibility; Sun-burnt; Something Coarse; A Period; Self-conceit; Complexity; Front; Inner Circle; Impromptu Performance; Appearances; Dreams; The Pretext; New Styles; A Letter, or Calligraphy; Disturbances; and so forth.

The above linguistic classification, based on a sampling of the topics recorded, shows that the abstract idea predominates as subject matter in the Tule Lake Senryu Kai. More precisely, those topics which in Japanese are expressed by abstract nouns represent nearly 48 per cent of the entire collection. Mr. Obayashi, who analyzed the collection and translated from the Japanese, stated that if one added to this figure those topics in the first group which can, in translation, be considered as abstract nouns, then a total of 68 per cent of all topics may be said to be rather abstract in type.

Center Life as Subject Matter

One purpose of this analysis was to discover the extent to which Senryu poetry furnished escape from the inadequacies of Center life, and conversely how much it expressed reactions to that life. Again, taking the period from January 4, 1943 to August 31, 1943, two topics were selected from an average of twelve for each month to illustrate the degree to which Senryu topics in general became vehicles of escape or instruments of social comment. To prevent exaggeration of the escape motif, Mr. Obayashi selected as his two topics of the month those subjects which had under them the greatest number of recorded Senryu concerning Center life. He then constructed the table on the following page.

From the table, it is obvious that Senryu concerning Center life at best do not exceed 17 per cent of the entire number of 558 Senryu. It may therefore be concluded that the members preferred as subject matter topics unrelated to life at Tule Lake. It may further be assumed that they desired to forget the drab existence in the Center, and as a matter of fact sought in Senryu a method of escape from it. Cultural revivalism and folk expression are, then, the prime purposes of Senryu poetry. The cultural form itself provides the refuge, the recreation, and the escape.

While Senryu is, in the main, a vehicle of folk expression which provides escape, it is also, though in a lesser degree, an instrument of community expression. The following examples

1943	Topics	Senryu under the topic	Senryu concerning Center Life
January	"Daytime"	24	14
	"Wall"	30	8
February	"Being Happy"	36	2
	"And Then"	45	5
March	"Doubled"	31	3
	"Consolation"	28	4
April	"Waiting"	36	6
	"Green"	21	4
May	"Seemingly"	38	4
	"Finger"	30	2
June	Miscellaneous	50	8
	"Games"	25	3
July	"Being Obedient"	40	4
	"Farewell"	25	12
August	"Bag"	44	9
	"Next Door"	55	9
Total		558	97

have been selected from the collection of 558 Senryu to indicate the nature of such social comment. It may be said, parenthetically, that these social poems catch the emotionalism of the residents toward Center life in its characteristic intensity and bitterness. That there are not more of them is probably best explained by the fact that conversational comment of this type is daily and uninterrupted, the satire stale by repetition, and Senryu after all too dignified a form of folk expression, too convenient an escape, to dwell on the humdrum level of life as it is lived. When the Senryu group remembers Center life, however, the comment is pungent and the dislike studied. They then again become the "exiles," on "budgets" of $16 a month, who pass the day with "frequent yawns."

The Style and Appreciation of Senryu

This selection of twenty Senryu illustrates the restraint, suggestiveness, and studied understatement characteristic of the form as a whole. In old Japanese prints of, say, Kunihiro or Hiroshiga, the space left empty bears an important relationship to the entire composition. So, in Senryu and Hai-ku, what is left unsaid but suggested in the economy of line etched in with only seventeen syllables has an emotional impact on the hearer. In the above examples, therefore, we have included in parentheses the reader's imagined comment. If, by chance, the social comment appears at points to be an overly satiric or witty reflection on Center life, the reader unaccustomed to the social psychology of Relocation Centers must realize that the actual feelings are still more bitter and the urge to satire keener. He must take our word for it that Japanese circumlocution, restraint and understatement are still here.

Both to illustrate the style and feeling of Senryu poetry and to measure the emotional intensities of the above examples, Mr. F. Obayashi has selected from among classical Senryu an example which shows how much meaning Senryu conveys without "saying." The poem tells also how closely the form is interwoven with Japanese social life, customs, and values:

> Hosu sode ni (Sleeves which must be dried, and also)
> Nururu sode ari (There are wet sleeves)
> Doyo-boshi (In midsummer sunning)

(Free translation)

> With kimono sleeves drying,
> Sleeves are slightly moistened,
> In midsummer's sunning.

	Original	Literal Translation	Free Translation
	Shyu-yo-sho	The Center,	In the Center,
	Akubi majiri no	Of yawning, mixed,	With frequent yawns
	Hi o okuri	A day is spent.	A day is passed.
	Sore kara no	Since then,	Since that time,
	Yosan jyu roku doru de	The budget, by sixteen dollars,	A budget is limited to sixteen dollars.
	Sumi	Is done.	(One manages on $12, $16, or $19 a month—if employed.)
	Mata shimon ka to	Again, the fingerprints,	"So, finger-printing again!"
	Oyaji no	The old man's	See the old man's bitter face.
	Nigai koa	Bitter face.	(We are not criminals.)
	Ryo donari	Two neighbors,	Neighbors on either side:
	Batten ben ni	Batten (colloquial) and	One from Batten-ken, the other from Gansu.
	Gansu chyo	Gansu (inflection).	(Batten is colloquial for people from Kumamoto province; Gansu, for those from Hiroshima. People are thrown together.)
	Yume dakega	Dreams only,	Only in dreams,
	Jiyu no ten chi	Of freedom and earth and sky,	In a world of freedom,
	Kake meguri	Running about.	Earth-bounded, we walk.
			(And here, the fence.)

Shyu-yo-sho Fuyu no hiashi mo Oshiku nashi	The Center, The steps of a winter day, Not minded.	In the Center, The shortness of a winter's day, Is not repined. (As there is so little to do.)
Sake no aji Hai sho e mademo Tsuki matoi	The taste of rice-wine, Even there, to the place of exile Clinging around.	The craving for rice-wine, Even in the Center exile, Clings tenaciously. (Rice-wine has its uses.)
Koko mo mata Sumeba miyako no Suna ni nare	Here, too, A metropolis, when residing, Accustomed to the sand.	Here stands our metropolis, Once we dwell long and feel At home in sand and dust.
Tsuma mo mata Teishyu no namini Gekkyu toru	Wife, too, Same as husband, Works and earns a salary.	Wives also, Now earn the same amount As husbands. (Why not *more*, my dear husband!)
Sakuno uchi Mata kaki hitoye Mawari michi	Within the fence, One more fence, A round about way.	Within the Project fence, All other barriers Make a circuitous road. (With apologies to Frost, manproof fences make poor neighbors.)

Original	Literal Translation	Free Translation
Kibana naki Haru o zoka ni Miru haisho	With few natural flowers, Spring is seen in the artificial flowers, In the Center.	Here, where natural flowers are rare, Spring is seen In artificial ones.
Dehairi ye Kiroku towareru Shyu-yo-sho	On coming in, on going out, The record is requested, In Relocation Centers.	On arrival and departure From the Center, One's past record is exhibited. (To keep in mind past mischief.)
Ashi-ato ga Tsuiteru kabe mo Shyu-yo-sho	Footprints, here, On the wall remain, In the Center.	Here, upon the wall again, Footprints stamp the nicety of Center life. (When were the barracks last painted?)
Kanshito Nogare rarenai Tokoroni ari	The watchtower Where no one can escape, Is standing guard.	Where escape is never dreamt of, There the watchtower Stands guard.
Ho-o-shin no Oyako de kawaru Sakumo uchi	On future plans, Differences between parent and child, Within the fence.	Discrepancy as to future plan, Often divides parent and child In Center life.

Here in the exile's
Monotonous life,
Only the seasons change.

Be self conceited as you will
But know that here you are
Another exile.

Here, reminiscence comes,
When looking at
The endless rows of barracks' roofs.

"Loyalty," "disloyalty,"
Such words to plague us yesterday, today,
In eyes made red with weeping.

Disturbed though men's minds
Are behind the fence,
Someone still prepares for marriage.
(Life marches on.)

Changeless
In the place of exile,
Is the temperature.

Self-conceited,
Yet here it is merely
A place of exile.

The uniform roofs,
Looking at, lost in reminiscence
In the Center.

Loyalty, disloyalty,
The words make eyes sore,
Yesterday, today.

Man's mind imprisoned and
Disturbed behind the fence,
Prepares for marriage.

Henka naki
Haisho ni henka
Aru kion

Unuborete
Mitaga haisho no
Nakano koto

Onaji yane
Nagamete shinobu
Shyu-yo-sho

Chyu, fuchyu
Mojiga men-shimu
Kino-o, kyo

Jin shin no
Midaru saku nimo
Yomejitaku

The explanation of this delicate etching is that, in Japan, the rainy season of about a month precedes midsummer, when clothes and other objects which absorb moisture (and are in danger of getting moldy in the storeroom) must be dried. It was customary, in old Japan, to dry these articles under the blazing midsummer sun. In the above Senryu, a person, presumably a woman, while sunning the stored clothes, comes upon the clothes worn by a beloved one who passed away. The tears well up and kimono sleeves are moistened. There were sleeves drying and sleeves moistened under the hot, drying sun of midsummer.

Conclusions

Today, almost two hundred years after its birth, Senryu, unlike Hai-ku, is still accepted as a folk art and folk expression.[*] It is a means of developing pungent humor, a form of mental recreation and, no less, an esthetic instrument of personal refinement.[†] As folk art, it is socially organized, and in

[*] J. F. Embree, *Japanese Peasant Songs* (Memoirs of the American Folklore Society, 38, 1944) 5–8. This volume, published in 1944, was available for reference after the Senryu analysis was completed. It was reassuring for the authors to learn that Embree's discussion of the formal and literary aspects of the Tan-ka and Hai-ku is strictly comparable. In his discussion of rural folksong, Embree differentiates a number of folksong forms from "the much studied literary tanka and haiku."

[†] The difference between Embree's collection of Kumamoto peasant songs and Tule Lake Senryu in regard to obscenity may be explained as follows: the former involves a peasant situation in which expression is ordinarily freer with sexual reference, while the latter is consistent with a somewhat urbanized, popular form of poetizing which did not grow directly out of the songs of the peasantry, but was rather a city folk derivation of Hai-ku as explained above. Some of the Kumamoto peasant songs, moreover, are widely known in both city and countryside. The functions of vulgar ditties are therefore well served, and Senryu, like Hai-ku, is free to preserve its own code of "outlawing obscenity." Senryu is more of a cultivated art, in contrast to peasant songs, even though it remains a popular commoners' art. Obscenity is common currency; Senryu, on the other hand, are collected and published.

Japan three or four monthly periodicals carry on the popular tradition which stemmed, as a commoner's art, from the romantic movement of Hai-ku poetry. At Tule Lake, also, the Senryu Association carries on, holding its regular weekly meeting in the Ironing Room of Block 14. Here, in addition to the esthetic and formal values mentioned above, Senryu keeps green the memory of folk culture and poetry. As such, it provides a point of pride and refuge for the exile who seems himself dispossessed and tossed aside. It leaves open an avenue of escape from the drab realities of Center life. And finally, when Center life rears its "ugly head" in Senryu poetry, it receives a rebuke which is sharp and incisive, restrained and dignified, witty and pungent.*

* It would be false to confuse this emotional reaction with politcalized thinking. The evacuation period and all the subsequent events which have caught up and embittered the residents of Centers, particularly at Tule Lake, led to two culturalized types of reaction. The first was the escape and refuge found in cultural revivalism. Assembly Centers and Relocation Centers witnessed the efflorescence of flower arrangement, utai singing, Senryu poetizing, and the like. Shut off from the mainstream of American life, surrounded by fences, forms, and investigations, familiar objects of culture offered solace and restored courage. The second culturalized reaction was the necessary response to the new conditions of existence, and for a proud people satire and bitterness served best. The welding together of these two reactions is frequently through art forms. For example, the analyst has noted that the traditional songs sung at wedding banquets are often in the same satiric vein. One priceless example heard recently, which brought down the house, concerned the seagulls who fly into Tule Lake in summer. The translation obtained for the chorus went as follows:

The sea-birds fly inland to the dry and waterless desert.
They stop here, but will not stay. Too dry, too dreary here.
They fly away. Even the sea-birds find no reason to remain.

The satire of "social pride," group pride, at the same gathering took the form of a lampoon on sentimental English songs when one man, in mock sadness, sang a soulful version of: "It's a Long, Long Way to Tipperary."

CULTURAL DILEMMA OF A KIBEI YOUTH

The patient, Jiro, was a Kibei male youth detained at one of the War Relocation Centers, California.* In keeping with Japanese attitudes toward mental illness, he was brought after dark to the hospital by his father. For some time, Jiro had avoided his family and lived in another barracks apartment with Kibei boys who reported that his conduct had become strange. He was mute and withdrawn. While under observation in a bare hospital room, containing only a cot and chair, Jiro had attempted suicide by hanging. When helped to the cot, he rose and sat stiffly on the straight-backed chair. He remained there, with an alert and frightened look, eyes staring intently at any intruder. He refused most nourishment and ate only if left alone.

The last interview with Jiro before commitment showed him to be catatonic and rigidly controlled, but not entirely out of contact. Initial attempts at the usual handshake or bow elicited no response. When patted on the shoulder, the immobile facial muscles relaxed for a fleeting instant into the merest smile of recognition. He began to mouth the word, "Sensei," and succeeded only after difficulty to manage the first syllable.† Minutes passed during which Jiro shifted uncomfortably and stiffly in his chair. Slowly and quietly the examiner addressed him as follows: "Jiro, you don't have to

* For detailed information concerning the project from which this case was taken, see E. H. Spicer, M. K. Opler, et al., Impounded People (Washington, D.C.: U.S. Government Printing Office, 1946).

† "Sensei" for professor, any teacher or physician, in Japanese, was his common term of address for the author.

speak now if you don't want to. What is bothering you will pass away soon, I hope. Better feelings will take their place. I will shake your hand, and either write or come to see you." His face changed almost imperceptibly to the former look of alertness and fright and there were no further signs of recognition. When he shook hands, his arm seemed weak and his hands were cold and clammy. But years later he repeated these four sentences perfectly and added, with enthusiasm, that they had helped.

Cultural Background

THE "NOTHINGEST." Jiro was twenty years old at the time of acute onset. He had been living in a center barracks-apartment with four Kibei boys for about a year. As the center enlarged, following government policies of segregation affecting Kibei as a class, his group moved to the newly built ward or district known as "Manzanar." At the time, Jiro, who seemed to evidence prodromal symptoms, explained, though not too convincingly, that he was glad to move because he disliked being near his family in the old ward.

In appearance, Jiro was smaller than most California Nisei age mates. He seemed, at twenty, younger than his years. Shy and withdrawn, he was also more self-deprecating than is demanded by good Japanese etiquette. He had no outlets or interests and, in comparison to his four roommates, he described himself as the *nothingest*.

Jiro had returned to the United States in 1940 at the age of fifteen, having gone through Japanese middle school. The year following, as an adolescent still trying to get his bearings in a strange new world, he was perplexed by the prejudices unleashed in wartime and the social rejection implied by forced relocation to the centers. Living in centers from age sixteen to twenty, he confided that his horizons had shrunk to the one square mile of barracks and that his various interests had gradually diminshed accordingly. His favorite phrase, complementing his own feeling of nothingness, was that here, or in the future, there was nothing. Since his feelings of hopelessness were not duplicated in hundreds of other Kibei in similar circumstances, it seemed important to pursue Jiro's story further.

FAMILY SETUP IN AMERICA.　His family was not atypical in composition. It consisted of an elderly Issei father of sixty-one years, bent on retiring as his sons came of age. His mother was a conservative Nisei woman of forty-five, obedient and compliant. Much rivalry was felt toward a brother, two years his junior, who towered more than a head above him in height. In view of Jiro's conflict with and distaste for his family, there was allusion to this brother's becoming the future family head. A sister, three years younger than Jiro, had nothing in common with him. At the point of commitment, all family members were concerned about the blot on the family reputation since mental disturbance, like venereal disease, tuberculosis, or outcaste status, could prevent good marriages. Both Jiro's trip to the hospital at night and the general family embarrassment could be interpreted partly in this light.

At Jiro's birth, his father was forty, but his paternal grandfather had reached the official Japanese age of retirement, sixty-one. Birth was attended by the customary registry of his name in family records abroad, along with solemn agreement, after the letter of announcement, to send him abroad for education to the grandparental home following his weaning. This custom was viewed as an act of filial duty of sons who could not themselves return to lighten parental burdens or hasten their actual retirement. Accordingly, two years later in the company of a paternal aunt, Jiro traveled abroad. His mother, to impress her father-in-law's ménage, saw to it that he was toilet trained after a fashion and weaned by the end of the first year. She reported that he walked before a year and a half. As

to her own feelings in the matter, they were expressed as follows: "After marriage, a wife no longer belongs to any family
but her husband's; when I was married, the white wedding
dress was our color of mourning—of leaving our family behind."

Jiro's father had come to Sacramento Valley at thirty years
of age. His pioneering history was a typical one. He hired out
as a farm laborer after failing to get steady work in San Fran-
cisco. Farming was his métier, but he found the methods quite
unlike those of the family farm outside of Hiroshima. In both
instances the land seemed poor, but the rocky, tree-stump hill-
sides of the valley were more untamed. A first assignment—to
plow a contoured hillside—found him coaching the horse the
night before to familiarize both man and beast with the task.
The story of the tired horse, sweaty and spuming foam, was
exchanged good-humoredly with other exiled farm hands, but
his father was dedicated to sobriety and hard work. Lacking a
citizen's right to own land, he had worked his way tirelessly as
tenant, removing the stumps and boulders in the pioneer days
of this fruit orchard country. He married soberly at forty, after
nine years of sweat and toil, picking a daughter of the small
Japanese-American community duly selected by the *baishakunin*, or go-betweens, of his own and a neighboring family.

The couple, quite disparate in age, hardly knew each other.
Jiro's mother was a hard-working and dutiful daughter whose
elder sister had yielded a son to her parents by *yoshi-marriage**
two years before. This son-in-law's adoption led to his taking
the in-laws' surname, and made this second nubile daughter
somewhat superfluous. She had done a man's work on the
farm, consistently being eclipsed by her sister. Gaunt and appearing older than her age, anyone would have taken her to
be the Issei wife of an Issei husband. In the center, freed for

---

* Yoshi-marriages among Japanese occur where a couple without male
offspring adopt a husband for their daughter, calling him "son," bestowing
their family name on him, and making him legal inheritor.

once of her daily labors, she spoke Japanese almost exclusively, visited her available relatives, and attended classes in flower arrangement, tea ceremony, dressmaking, and the functions of the Buddhist Church. Her Nisei children, quite the opposite, were versed in California slang and before segregation wore the saddle shoes, bobby socks, *yogore* (slang for *pachuco* or zoot-suit) costumes of typical West Coast Nisei. Somewhere in this intergeneration conflict and in the confusion of relocation and its aftermath, Jiro's homecoming was lost.

Both parents agreed that the artificialties of center life estranged the generations. Their conservatism, however, increased as their former tenancy holdings were wiped out, along with other tangible property, by relocation and enforced segregation from the mainstream of American life. They learned the small farm had gone to other tenants and deteriorated beyond repair. As economic, political, and social securities slipped away, they clung to their last vestige of respect—a cultural identity. An enlargement of the father's photograph had gone into one of the five suitcases brought to the center. This was bowed to before and after school and, now, upon leaving the barracks or on return. The mother referred to her husband as *anata,* spouse or lord, and never by name. The father's generally sober nature turned dour and tyrannical with his fears of the future. In the rifts between Issei and Kibei occurring generally in the center, his anger exploded on Jiro. Despite a life of unremitting labor, he had now reached the age of retirement only to see his efforts brought to nothing. The *nothing* was repeated, even if the thin barracks' walls and limited privacy allowed little else to be said. With Jiro he would insist on the ultimate respect demanded by filial piety, even as he had insisted before in sending the boy to his own father in Japan.

For this family, there was no way out of the segregation center. Although Jiro had, in fact, returned to this country at age fifteen because dual citizenship made him eligible for future Japanese military draft, American policy labeled him

Kibei and, hence, suspect. Were he older at the time of relocation, better versed in American ways and language, or eligible for service, he might have found his way out. In his own conception, the decade and a half from 1925 to 1940 had made Japan itself brutally harsh and military, but here in the United States he was just as much a citizen without a country. To political insecurities were added pervasive psychological insecurities.

FAMILY SETUP IN JAPAN. Jiro's Hiroshima-ken grandparents were delighted, in principle, to receive a two-year-old grandson, but the grandfather was by this time sixty-three and had suffered financial reverses. The grandmother was sickly. To add to the inauspiciousness of the moment, anti-American feeling ran high, particularly in Hiroshima, due to our Japanese Exclusion Laws. To cap it all, Jiro himself was violently ill on the voyage and remained so for two months afterwards. The family reports "stomach trouble" with violent retching and vomiting. According to the aunt's account, her trip also was made difficult and it was not easy to welcome Jiro to his new home.

EARLY EVENTS IN JAPAN. Both Jiro and the family were able to piece together subsequent events. The grandmother's illness went from bad to worse, and she died when Jiro was in his fourth year. Hushed rumors in the household mentioned tuberculosis. In Japan, venereal, tubercular, or mental illnesses are, like former outcaste or *eta* family origins, topics not to be discussed in polite society. Any one of these dread diseases is enough to prevent a good marriage and is searched for by the diligent *baishakunin*. Jiro long remembered the rumors and the threat they aroused. He recalled the lowered voices and polite circumlocutions used. Years later, when his grandfather spoke bitterly of Jiro's adding more than the grandmother could bear, he felt the whole weight of impossible obligations heaped upon himself and merged with terrifying scenes of his grandmother's coughing and grasping her sides. The sense of feeling worthless and lonely, of having done wrong, again took root, and he experienced a helpless sense of embarrassment and the wish to be sent away. He reported memories from before school age of a widowed aunt helping with his care and of his being carried astride her back to and from work. In the early school period, the austere image of the grandfather again intervenes, along with the harsh stiffness of the teachers. There were shameful episodes of enuresis, rare in Japanese schools. Three years before Jiro's return to the United States the grandfather died, and he recalls his sense of relief as he went to live with the widowed aunt while completing his education.

Early Symptoms

SEXUAL FEARS.   Sexual interest was recalled as beginning and ending abruptly during this period of flight from patriarchal authority. Masturbation was denied throughout. Intersex bathing in the large wooden tubs of hot water, used for soaking in the evening, is described for more than one farmhouse. At one, contiguous to his aunt's, there were fantasies and daydreams concerning a female cousin. Besides the semipublic bathing, household nudity was common. Much of this evolved into private sexual guilt if not shame. Because of the circumlocutions in his grandfather's household concerning tuberculosis, venereal disease, and kindred matters, he was fearful of prostitutes.

At one gathering, the more elderly ladies became drunk and ribald. One of them, the most boisterous, spirited Jiro outside. She weighed more than he and, in her state of agility, she threw him on the ground calling him little boy, a term reminiscent of his grandmother's call. She attempted to have intercourse, but he was overwhelmed with shame and disgust.

Having visited dubious restaurants in Hiroshima City with his grandfather, he recalled the raw, direct, and gaudy pornography at which he had stolen furtive glances, the scenes on cups and dishes and wall drawings. The net result was to increase his revulsion and distaste, whereupon the last raucous laugh of the elderly lady was left ringing in his ears. Comparing notes with others of his age, he imagined he had become impotent. Refusal to visit the city for the purpose of going to a house of prostitution lost him his best friend soon after.

INFERIORITY FEELING. Accounts of early memories concerning symptomatic items are sketchy in the extreme. Much of this Jiro later helped to assemble. He recalled a stomach disorder, with violent retching, for several days following the incident with the elderly lady. Earlier fantasies and daydreams concerning the female cousin do not appear to be significant symptomatological clues. Throughout his most commonplace accounts of events, however, his sense of inferiority, in households, sports, or school, is a consistent thread. He felt weak and insecure, small and insignificant or, at times, helpless and afraid. In school, the parading of the amazing deeds of patriots and historical figures convinced him, "I shall never be a man like these." Revenge stories of the Forty-Seven *Ronin* or Masterless Retainers, who after years of waiting conspired to wipe out shame visited upon their Lord, inspired him with terror. Japanese movies with the same themes of vendetta or revenge, which form an equivalent of American westerns, upset him. The more fantastic ones of marvelous magicians and transformers left him soothed and satisfied.

Return to the United States

FACT AND FANCY ABOUT HOMECOMING. Strangely enough, Jiro's social and personal history took a turn for the worse as he re-entered the land of his birth. On the surface, home-coming should be auspicious for the eldest son of an Issei father and a conservative Nisei mother, particularly where he is conversant and moderately well educated in things Japanese. But just as Jiro had been *persona non grata* in the decade of the Twenties in Japan, following our Exclusion Laws, so in the wartime Forties in America he found himself an unwelcome citizen. While he arrived on these shores in a time of uneasy peace, his family, especially his siblings, had changed during the dozen years of his absence to the point where they no longer resembled the Japan that he knew.

From the viewpoint of his own insecurities, Jiro could hardly make the accommodation quickly. He had always been jealous of friends abroad who enjoyed the pleasant pampering of their own families, and he had been almost distrustful of their tolerance for his awkward, shy manners. Homecoming had long been viewed with intangible yearnings, with fancies that Japanese education would count for much among the Japanese-Americans of the United States, both young and old. He hoped that his status as first-born son would insure him immediate prestige in his own home. A sister of the same age as the erstwhile female cousin would have her circle of schoolgirl friends. And in this Japanese-American oasis, far from the "White" gangster males and loosely disciplined, immodest females who peopled the America of prewar Japanese propaganda, Jiro felt he could regain his human dignity.

The *dramatis personae* of these homecoming fantasies had been built up for some time in the haze of social distance. His father was well along in years and, like his dead grandfather, figured vaguely. His mother, much younger, was cast in the role of the vivacious paternal aunt. Instead, he was greeted by a sombre and exacting father, by a mother who seemed as worn and exhausted as his grandmother had been, and by other relatives who seemed distant and meant nothing. A brother of thirteen and his highly Americanized friends towered above Jiro. His sister's clique of sophisticated schoolgirls, obviously critical of his speech and manners, unnerved him. In general, the Nisei, with their smattering of Japanese and their even more incomprehensible Japanese-American slang, were different from all expectations. Both his English and his parents' Japanese, with archaic terms and curious additions, seemed untranslatable.

HOSTILITY TOWARD FATHER AND BROTHER. At first, the Nisei, within and outside his family, were the target of his well-controlled hostility. Their preferences in clothes and food were different. They danced, the sexes together, in athletic gyrations which seemed to him undignified or immodest. While his mother adopted the shuffling female gait of Issei women (toes inward and hunched-over shoulders), he himself seemed to walk more stiffly, in his rapid, mincing step, than either brother or father. Already shy and self-conscious, all speech, gait, and gesture seemed awkward or inappropriate. In Japan, fixity of etiquette and polite consideration for the feelings of others constantly sanctioned even the most commonplace behavior; in the U. S. such sanctions were strangely wanting. So fully occupied were his own siblings in their adolescent groups, that the first day home he walked three miles to speak with another Kibei and, as he put it, felt all alone.

In time, however, his father proved the greatest disappointment. Reared to respect age and paternity, it was hard to discover in himself the true nature of these feelings. Many Issei who came to this country in the early waves of immigration, before Exclusion, were disgruntled second sons who could never inherit in impoverished Japanese families. So it was with Jiro's father. Arriving in this country long past youth, penniless, unmarried, and with no trade but farming, he had toiled and sacrificed to attain marital status and patriarchal dignity. Jiro regarded his mother's lack of information about modern Japan as pitiable, but his gruff father also struck him as being hopelessly behind the times. He felt that his own status as first-born son was not honored by a father who had himself been "a second son." He resented his brother, Ichiro, for his very name since that name meant *eldest son*. It was as if he, Jiro, was written off as dead and sent to Japan at his brother's birth. In Japan, there is a phrase, "A brother is a beginning of a stranger." Jiro felt this rivalry in every way possible, and it was linked with even greater dislike for a remote and distant father who, in poor times, had hoped his eldest son would somehow make his way in Japan. That it was not customary to name a second son "Ichiro" was part and parcel of the many barbarisms of the household, for which he secretly blamed his father. He felt that his father had awakened too late to the thought that the future of his united family lay in America. Now this father, like the grandfather before, viewed him as a burden.

Since the age of fifteen is less confused and more focused than four, all hostilities toward the irritable grandfather that had been dissipated in infantile helplessness were mobilized in new form. He was estranged from brother and father. Later, in the center, as the Issei-Kibei rifts widened, the father was blamed in a variety of ways. When the family future in remote Northern California seemed a thing of the past, Jiro would ask, "Why did you bring me back? To rot in a concentration camp?" Or taunt, "Now I suppose your Ichiro will grow up to hold land in America!" The theme was disillusionment, insecurity, and hopelessness.

Because Ichiro knew American ways, because he could hold land when of age or help in dealings with the surrounding community, the father looked to him as a mainstay. On countless occasions, Jiro would be called almost absent-mindedly to do some task and then dismissed with reminders that he could not accomplish that particular job. In the primogeniture system, sibling rivalries are bound to ensue; but where every family decision and most tasks hinge upon the abandonment of this rule, the normal tensions are exacerbated. A father of retirement age increases this potential. Where he is indecisive or confused about his own family's future, there is no mitigating set of sanctions anywhere in Japanese culture. Here, indeed, the father insisted on sole and continuing authority with sons who had not yet come of age. But in this family, uprooted and at bay in wartime relocation, the father clung to authority at the risk of reducing Jiro to helpless ineffectuality. And so the clock was turned back to the same helpless fears that marked childhood in Japan. Jiro described this quite well. Before the center period, there were recurrences of childish nightmares, night sweats, sleeplessness, and terrified awakenings.

ESTRANGEMENT FROM SISTER AND PEERS. During the same period, "A brother is the beginning of a stranger" applied to his relations with his sister. In Japanese custom, an elder brother, of age, may regulate a sister's conduct to unusual lengths. He may sanction or prevent her marriage, and, until she moves to her husband's household, he is, like his father before him, the custodian of her morals and protector of a family's good name. With his sister of the soda-drinking, bobby-sox set, Jiro was at once the stranger in quite another sense. Ichiro's friends were greatly preferred. In the sister's presence or with such groups, Jiro found himself more than usually inarticulate. Between being tongue-tied in public, and issuing peremptory commands to her in the household, Jiro felt more and more that their relationship was untenable. The sister, in turn, like others of her group, was either amused or frightened by the gruff manners and curt address of the Kibei. He avoided the school or country church dances in part because dancing was strange to him, but even more so because Nisei added to his feelings of fright and estrangement.

Some of these feelings, in the peer group, were not due to empty fear and embarrassment. Like other Kibei, Jiro overheard discussions of himself and others of the Kibei class. He was doubly resentful that these young people, so sure of themselves, did not even know the many rules for preventing face-to-face embarrassment, minimizing shame in others. These girls, who knew other rules, who rose as if at a signal to dance with boys, and whose sense of propriety was fixed less by family than by gossip and rumor, succeeded in adding to his anger and resentment. In the same context, he disliked the lordly Issei all the more for prattling about old-fashioned ways while they controlled none of these changes. It seemed that the upstart Nisei escaped family surveillance even more than his kind who were expected, in passive solidarity, to differ from the majority of the younger generation.

These girls and women of his mother's generation, Issei picture brides or Nisei, were separated by a deep gulf. The older generation was passively the property of their husbands. Dressed in shapeless calico, dutiful daughter types were not like the younger generation. He missed the type, well-known in Japan, who through intelligence or connivance almost ran the home from behind the scenes. Or else the family solidarity, down through generations, seemed lacking. Whatever it was, few older women seemed capable of the dignity or even of the ribaldry and abandon he remembered from earlier years. His mother, sickly and worn, he saw only as a pale and helpless reflection of paternal authority. She appeared colorless, imitative, and, like himself, passively dutiful. He even felt that, in these qualities, he took after her. At any rate, going full circle in his family group, Jiro found no solid attachment. He was thrown back upon his own sense of loneliness and ineffectuality.

During the year before relocation, these attitudes crystallized rapidly. Morose at home, he found companionship only with a few scattered Kibei acquaintances. He avoided sports, like the ubiquitous baseball (*basu-boru*). Intersexual contacts were absent. Speech and manner became, if anything, more awkward and constricted. Energy went into suppressing anger and controlling the tongue. Private rages found him tearing away handfuls of leaves and grass or biting his fingers. He became restless and, he thought, quite different from other Japanese, always trained for poise and patience. The Nisei California slang contained a characteristic phrase, "waste-time," for anything useless. He thought of the phrase constantly as he deliberately wasted time on lonely, aimless walks. Angrily he thought, "Where are the Nisei, with their bad manners, hurrying to? Where are *they* going?"

The Uprooting of Relocation

MOUNTING TENSION.   The answer came abruptly after Pearl Harbor. With the first events, he was momentarily glad of American citizenship, of avoidance of further training abroad. For once he understood briefly the Americanized Nisei who were flocking toward enlistment. However, they were rejected on obvious grounds of prejudice. As this happened repeatedly, his sarcasm grew, along with a sardonic sense of their being, after all, somewhat like himself—with no roots anywhere.

Soon, however, he realized what was really happening. Families, by Western Defense Command dogma and decree, were uprooted and herded en masse into such Assembly Centers as the converted stables at Santa Anita and Tanforan race tracks. From there, the trek to hastily constructed and half-finished centers seemed like a bad dream. Faced with bare barracks and a few army cots and potbellied stoves, with pine knotholes gaping into neighbors' rooms, anger and helplessness became endemic and diffused. In some families, fathers were interned elsewhere. In any case, families were literally thrown together. Privacy was minimal. Mass feeding at twenty cents a day per capita began. The Nisei took over center work at $12, $16, and $19 per month, the last restricted to technical or professional services. At first, there was not enough resurgence of things Japanese for most Kibei to function. As a group, their common resentments grew. Many insisted, as Jiro also felt, that Issei blind compliance and the Nisei knuckling-under were the wrong way, and that, first and foremost, citizenship rights should be restored.

MOTHER'S ILLNESS.   In the general and hasty exodus from the valley the mother became ill, and only months later, in the center, did she recover. Jiro felt in his mother's illness and long convalescence the same pangs of shame and undercurrents of rejection and helplessness that attended his grandmother's death earlier. From the coughing, he was afraid that tuberculosis was involved, and here in center conditions, this was not something which would remain a private family affair. Even without a hospital diagnosis of tuberculosis in the family, the fear continued. With no privacy, the merest dispute with his father now declined into a silently endured paternal lecture in a barracks room apartment where the neighbors on each side could hear all. The custom grew in the center, particularly during loyalty registration, for Kibei boys to room together for self-protection. At first, he and the four Kibei friends took up their separate living quarters in the same ward as his parents— known as "Sacramento" district. It was later, during the transformation of the center into a segregation camp, that the group moved to the "Manzanar" ward of the project.

BREAK WITH FAMILY.   Many center events are interwoven with Jiro's final break with his father and family. Loyalty registration was incorrectly presented to the center residents as an army draft of the loyal. With some families still disunited, and all resentful of the sudden forced relocation of all men, women, and children, rumor and confusion beset the center. An Issei committee, sensing this, requested time for the program to be presented accurately in both Japanese and English to all the population. They even offered to conduct the governmental education plan. This suggestion the project director refused. Kibei were categorically blamed for the confusions which further ensued, since some Kibei had requested careful elucidation of the program. Their bachelor quarters were searched in the center. Not until Issei and Nisei leaders were browbeaten and beaten literally did the program of a few days get under way. Even then, it dragged on amid confusions for several months. A modicum of real peace was never fully restored at the center.

Community analysis was instituted shortly after the height of difficulties, and it was then that we met Jiro and his roommates. If not Jiro himself, then his circle, had made attempts to control hotheads in the center. His family felt hopeless about the center as well as the future; and they were in that part of resident population which had adopted a *shikatiganai* (a hopeless and fateful "it-can't-be-helped") attitude. They had, at first, recoiled from the center turbulence, hoping to register loyalty when the confusion died down. It never did, whereupon they hoped to hold together as a family—the last remaining security. In this interim, not only were Japanese-American Citizens League leaders beaten, but Kibei bachelor quarters became storm centers of the general turbulence.

One event stands out in Jiro's mind as a measure of his inadequacy during this period. His small group, like many of the "Sacramento" ward, was rumored to have registered loyalty already. Another Kibei group of *judo* and *sumo* (wrestling) experts decided to pay a serious call. Jiro's judoist friend was absent at the time or matters might have gone differently. Instead, Jiro was alone when he saw the visitors approach, and he quickly hid himself under a cot and barricaded himself with blankets. He was, of course, found and, being unable to talk from fright, he was beaten for no good reason at all. The quarters were ransacked. Since word passes quickly in a center, his friends soon reappeared and saw the chaos. In subsequent weeks, his group circulated throughout the ward, explaining intricacies of registration to confused rural people. Jiro did not. By the time the center had cooled down, the joking sobriquet his friends had given him was widespread. The words implied "at home, but at the same time not there." When able, he registered affirmatively to loyalty, but with the popular Kibei qualification, "if my citizenship rights are restored." His brother, Ichiro, registered a simple "Yes." In the further confusions of segregation time, his brother and sister were eligible to move to another center. But Jiro and his friends were blocked by Kibei status, and his own case was doubly confused by the qualified answer.

SEGREGATION AND EMOTIONAL ISOLATION. Before segregation and the second family separation, Jiro and his friends moved to the "Manzanar" ward of the project. His resentment of his father's inability to carry him through relocation outside center confines grew apace. Segregation which brought endless factions of Kibei from all the centers estranged him even from this category of persons. By now, he was by no means the most popular member of his small group of five. Their various sustaining interests in art, literature, or Japanese sports had left him far behind. At this point, without family and with only attenuated friendships left, we note a rapid crystallization of symptoms. He became lazy and slovenly in habits. His restlessness at night was noted, and he would fall asleep over a Japanese book in the daytime. His literary choices became more and more juvenile, with badly written collections of fairy tales and myths prominent. In comparison with his earlier tastes, there was greater tolerance of stories about vendetta and revenge.

The altercations with his father, on brief visits before their departure from the center, gradually died down. The family noted that he was becoming morose and distant. As the time for departure approached, they appealed for the right to take Jiro with them. His status was clouded as a Kibei as well as by the first qualified answer on citizenship rights. No Kibei in such status could go elsewhere. In Jiro's description, the fences closed in on him and fear took over.

Before departure, his father arranged to bring him to the hospital for observation, as his friends had obligingly and politely suggested. The father did so with a finally hopeless, passive, and mutely compliant Jiro in his wake. Lacking center facilities in this barracks town of almost twenty thousand people, even rudimentary therapeutic approaches to mental illness were reduced to the phrase, "for observation purposes." The choice of site for this purpose could only be in a private ward of a distinctly overcrowded community hospital on center grounds. There was enacted the scene with which this chapter opened.

The Outcome

BREAK WITH REALITY. Psychiatric examination disclosed that Jiro was confused, depressed, frightened, and inwardly hostile. When not mute, he referred to officialdom in uncomplimentary terms. He refused to answer personal questions. He was frightened enough to appear entirely tongue-tied, but a few phrases and syllables could be uttered here and there. Following family departure, he became completely mute. With the targets of primary hostility now hundreds of miles away, an awkward suicidal attempt quietly transpired.

There were no hallucinations reportable then or in later hospitalization. In the hospital, after two months of practically no speech—a few phrases in a week's period—Jiro could become voluble when he chose. His own account indicates that he was affectively confused, but at times afraid of being laughed at: "my words would not have made much sense anyway." A lack of confidence, a certainty of being confused and ineffective, and feelings of strangeness and isolation mark his accounts for this period.

Concerning periods when communication was better established, Jiro recalls suddenly occurring needs to talk with someone or to hear from someone. There was, at such times of breaking through, the feeling that if contact did not occur, everything would become worse and again be unbearable. Generally stiff and awkward, even by Kibei standards, there was evidence of greater rigidity and inability to relax in the period of illness. Besides shyness and lack of spontaneity, a major ingredient of the rigidity was an attempt to control a flood of hostile impulses, along with a fear that they were becoming, in fact, uncontrollable.

In one discussion, Jiro remembered the helpless rage that boiled up to the surface. It was at this point that he recalled the tearing at grass and leaves, the jealousy of siblings, and the anger at father and grandfather "for trying to get rid of me." The rages were everywhere aimed at events as well as attributed to feelings about people. "I was angry that my grandmother died, or that my mother was sick when I needed help." In the center one could add the massive angers attached to whole categories of persons. There were the Issei, even beyond the father image, lacking in wise and omnipotent guidance. There were the Nisei pre-empting the attractive roles of center life. There were the adolescents and post-adolescents with their studied rejection. Or, finally, there were the family members as a group, seen in vivid terms of separation, lack of real welcome, and final departure. Certainly, the years abroad had robbed him of more than citizenship. Together with the jarring experiences of relocation and the political embroilments of the center, he had become, like many Kibei, the doubly rejected.

CULTURE CONFLICT AND PERSONAL STRESS. It is interesting to speculate as to whether balances in this family, the actual roles influenced by culture conflict, would have reached some equilibrium had not relocation and the swift march of wartime events intervened. Ultimately, under center conditions, this situation was not merely the introducing of new strains into family structure, but the literal tearing apart of a cohesive pattern. As the center continued, and as segregation was heaped upon the inequities of relocation, more people became mentally ill, and a disproportionate number of these were Kibei. Moreover, Jiro's case does not stand alone. Others like him had periods of acute onset at times when center stresses were at their height and equally dramatic recoveries in hospitals outside center confines. Under hospitalization, Jiro himself indicated that the stresses which had magnified family conflicts into large-scale cultural conflicts disappeared in his attitudes and feelings in but a few months. A therapist could become like a different species of "father," serene, untroubled, and supportive. Staff were, in certain persons, likened to "the family I never had." For a time, other patients were frightening, but later, as in Buddhist tenets, one learns "to help one another."

RELIEF AND RESTITUTION. A final visit to Jiro following remission, and in connection with later field work, disclosed that other Kibei and relocation center acquaintances were friendly to him despite his hospitalization. The old communities were re-establishing in California. Several had revived in the valley, and now, for once, there was a sense of common experiences, ineradicable, of former center life. Center Kibei who were younger, like his former roommate, were again selected as friends, no doubt because one could compete somewhat more successfully with them or at least tolerate comparisons. With time, it was recognized that not all Kibei are fallen stars and not all of life an endless series of disappointments.

Remission had come rapidly in Jiro's case. The six months of hospitalization were calmer than the four years of relocation history. The great wave of Kibei immigration before the war had contained few with as much repetitive and traumatic experiences as Jiro. He was now ready to call it bad luck, rather than helpless and hopeless fears. Since the family, in turn, can now plan without being held in official duress, they are fully aware of pitfalls in his fears of rejection, his awkward shyness, and his rigid controls of impulse. They have responded to his quest for equal rights, not only in citizenship, but in achievement and recognition. A whole second generation is now coming into its own, and the first generation, while nostalgic, is today more gracefully accepting the shift in authority and responsibility.

Projective data by test instruments were unavailable at the time of Jiro's acute illness, and his remission was almost too rapid to come within hospital testing programs. As one would guess, he showed a rather weak ego integration with a good deal of compensatory fantasy and concern about impulse control. Those traits have vastly diminished, and Jiro lives today in his family setting in which all members have learned much about their cultural identities, their changing pattern, and their need for cohesiveness. While no symptomatology is markedly in evidence in Jiro or in others of the family, the father's authoritarian attitudes, buttressed by older Japanese standards, were hard to soften in his own deprived existence. In this cultural group, the second generation, youthful at the time of World War II, has now taken firm root. With the passage of years, the mother's hypochondriacal defenses and "crisis illnesses" are gone. In this family, as in any other, we see how the illness of one affects the health of each member. In the group, uprooted by relocation, we discern the marks of overwhelming stress. But the Japanese family is ideally built for unified solidity over generations. A second generation, unmolested and given time, can put down roots deep in American soil.

DILEMMAS OF TWO PUERTO RICAN MEN

Spanish Family Values and Acculturation Problems

Most Puerto Rican migrants come to New York to avoid the poverty and population pressure of the Island. They may carry with them the burdens of an original cultural heritage Spanish-American in spirit and tradition and quite different from the variegated pattern of beliefs in the metropolis. This cultural orientation will have stemmed from Spain and been modified in the rural districts of the Island or in the slums of San Juan. But if it is Puerto Rican at all, it will stress the dominance of males in most social activity, in paternal authority, and in patriarchal responsibilities, according to specific ideas of honor, respect, and shame. Families should be large as indicators of male potency. Providing adequately for them is a routine matter of honor and prestige. The lines of authority in the family go lineally from father to son, brooking no interference from subordinated female roles. The latter are to be protected within the family setting, with collateral male kin performing this function. Beyond this magic circle, all unprotected adult females are fair sexual game, and the young girls chafe at the perennial roles of baby-tender and sheltered homemaker.

This is the common warp of Latin cultures in the Island or south of the Rio Grande. But everywhere, in cities and industrialized plantations, the weft of urban processes challenges such values. To the extent that women work for wages in some parts of Puerto Rico, man's role is less crucial. Besides this, countless women become dissatisfied with the role indoctrination of childhood and adolescence. They may become, in subtle ways, destructive in the intersexual and familial relationships that come within their control. The weakening of male role has meant higher rates of desertion in the lower class and of separation in middle-class population. Marriages are brittle, adding to the childhood deprivation and internal strains within the family. These strains, greater in lower classes, may be found either in San Juan or in New York City.

But besides these social and economic strains on family life, cultural conflict also takes its toll. There is the great gulf between ideal or original cultural expectations, already mentioned, and what the migrants find existing on the mainland. Their values—what they deem desirable, proper, or good—are rarely found. Male job downgrading and unemployment are more drastic here for males than for females. One street song begins, "I would not trade Puerto Rico for a hundred New Yorks!"

With such dislocations and the rapid pace of acculturation, the number of adjustment problems of Puerto Rican youth grows also. Here we describe two Puerto Rican young men caught in such culture conflicts. They are both second sons, in their early twenties, and both, not uncharacteristically, have fathers absent from the home scene.

The first was studied in a public hospital facility following hospitalization for a few months in the navy. His naval tour of duty had been short and his diagnosis was schizophrenic reaction, paranoid type. He was white and from the lower-middle-class stratum of San Juan. In the latter respect he contrasted with the second case, a colored ambulatory schizophrenic with paranoid traits who was from the lower class of San Juan's worst slum.

A Lower-Middle-Class Veteran

Let us call the lower-middle-class veteran Alberto. He is twenty-one years of age. Both parents came from the lower-middle-class stratum of the city of San Juan. The father was twenty-three and the mother eighteen at the time of marriage, whereupon the father, after several lesser jobs and minor clerkships, secured the enviable post of policeman.

ALBERTO'S FATHER: GUAPO OR POLICEMAN? Alberto's father, from all accounts, was a much-spoiled eldest son of indulgent parents. The neighbors knew him by the Puerto Rican term, *guapo,* a lad who takes liberties—a headstrong adventurer. Alberto's uncle in New York described his elder sibling as having a swashbuckling exterior, but being really attached to an ambitious and manipulative mother. Alberto's paternal grandmother had prevailed upon her husband to sell his interest in the small family farm and join the general exodus of rural families from the district to the city. There her ambitions for an easier life ran counter to her husband's distaste for the new surroundings. The paternal grandfather felt his social and economic independence dwindle as his new responsibilities grew. With Alberto's father, he encouraged the *guapo* tendencies, vented sudden fits of anger and alternately allowed him every breach of discipline. Alberto's father, first as *guapo,* and later even as policeman, found it hard "to settle down." He was impulsive and volatile in temperament, the darling of his mother, and always in some scrape with authorities.

EARLY LIFE IN SAN JUAN. In San Juan, where Alberto's mother and the maternal grandparents lived, the household had consisted of the paternal grandparents, Alberto's parents, and the four children whom we shall call Roberto, Alberto, Melinda, and Elena. Alberto's mother had been subjected to the usual strict upbringing of Puerto Rican girls. She and her parents had lived in the rural countryside before they, too, settled in San Juan. Alberto's mother had viewed the marriage, arranged by her own father, as an escape from pressures of being an only daughter. She was married off at age eighteen.

Roberto, the elder son, was born in the second year of marriage, and Alberto, a year later. Neither pregnancy nor birth was unusual. The mother hoped to nurse both boys for well over a year, but in her rigid concern for this self-imposed schedule of nursing, she complained that Alberto's arrival had interrupted the suckling of the elder son. To compensate for this, "a better job" was done "for Alberto," who was nursed for two years. Both boys walked at about a year and a half, and were toilet trained, under constant urging, before two.

Both mother and paternal grandmother laid great stress upon learning language through constant repetition of words. In this, as in every aspect of child care, the manipulative older woman and rigidly strict mother vied and quarreled with each other. Disassociating himself from these female battles, Alberto's father would assume his most manly, decisive (and *guapo*) manner on the rare occasions when he was at home. Issuing orders in a deep, guttural voice, his decisions were peremptory and arbitrary. Often, he would side with his mother for no apparent reason or indulge in frequent fits of anger. In time, the sinecure on the police force led to illegal scrapes and shady deals, salted with a series of the extramarital liaisons sanctioned in this culture for males. The number of alcoholic sprees with boon companions increased. Alberto's mother salvaged her all-important marital status by rigid adherence to the routines of a meticulous housewife, becoming overly clean, orderly, and compulsive.

CLEANLINESS RITUALS. The boy's toilet training was one such instance. The mother exulted in claims that Alberto *wanted* to use a receptacle because Roberto used it. She argued with the grandmother that she was not forcing him—and the issue was drawn. Both boys were pitted against each other in the contest of cleanliness. Alberto, perhaps less accomplished than his older sibling in toilet training, had the advantage of occupying a hammock adjacent to his parents' bed.

Besides the possible confusions of genital and anal functioning, he early began to cater to his mother's phobic fear of "city dirt and disease." In the daytime, he never liked to sit on the floor as did most children; he wished to be bathed by his mother frequently; and he delighted her by constantly washing his hands.

ANAL FEATURES: PSYCHOPHYSIOLOGIC REACTIONS.   As the boy grew, these themes took other forms. The mother commented that Puerto Ricans often went barefoot whenever the occasion afforded itself, but Alberto preferred to wear shoes to be clean. With the central controversies over toilet training ringing in the household, he buttressed his claims to exemplary cleanliness by periodically developing severe constipation. As early as two and three years and on through latency, the mother gave a weekly, almost ceremonial dosage of castor oil or milk of magnesia. This was accompanied by considerable discussion of bowel movements. As the triumvirate of mother, boy, and grandmother dwelled on the bodily function, the father, in his sudden, brief appearances in the household, shouted his beliefs and decisions about these same matters. Alberto's confusion and desire to please everyone at all costs crystallized in the organ language of colitis, whereby constipation alternated with diarrhea throughout his life.

The matter did not even rest there. He and his siblings also had their share of worms, the childhood plague of Puerto Rico. In addition, two siblings, both girls, were born when the patient was, respectively, five and six years old. With all siblings, the castor oil was administered to counteract *Worms* and *Constipation,* the twin evils, but since Alberto's bowel involvement was the greater, he drew the greater attention on both scores. By age seven, when his female siblings required infancy care, his mother began to give him hot water enemas at least once a month. Later, at eighteen, during the acute onset of his schizophrenic illness, he tried to self-administer such an enema, but failed because he feared too much hot water, and complained, for the first time in his life, that his mother had given the children laxatives and enemas "when we didn't need them." To this was added, "it was done when father was away and he didn't care about the house anyway."

During the childhood diseases of whooping cough, measles, and chicken pox, further efforts were made to monopolize his mother's attention. Each siege was followed by a month-long period of being run down, requiring the mother's continuous care. By sixteen, a continual nasal discharge began. While his physical condition was excellent in all reports, the rhinitis and alternating bowel patterns were part of a larger series of vaguely shifting hypochondriacal complaints including claims of stomach trouble, dizziness, and poor sleep.

ANAL FEATURES AGAIN: SEXUAL BEHAVIOR. Sexual life is described as beginning in adolescence, coincidental with the father's separation and shortly after arrival in New York. Masturbation occurred frequently in showers and toilets, either before or after bowel movements. Heterosexual excitements are claimed in New York's crowded apartments, but despite more talk of divorce and desertion than in San Juan, he himself had neither dates not girl friends and denies any homosexual experience. In late adolescence, masturbation began to evoke guilt. "It makes you dumb or dull and pimply." One should also know where to go for sex with women. His own busy life began to require his attendance at college in evening classes while working overtime as clerk. The patient added that there was too much preoccupation with homosexuality in Puerto Rican neighborhoods, but he was, at first, unaware of his selective attention to this matter.

Perhaps the most striking symptom on this score was the patient's compulsive need for having bowel movements in public toilets. At first, he was unaware of the homosexual motivations for this, but explained that he stopped several times at subway stations for this purpose. This pattern occurred about three times a week, with anxiety about going to work, and masturbation occasionally to lessen this anxiety. His notion of the homosexual had no shadings and was limited to one type not infrequent in Puerto Rican culture. In his definition, this was a man "who cannot make the grade, and doesn't want to be a man—instead he wants to think and be like a woman." Having studied biology in college evening session, he had come away with the notion that the adrenals stimulate either sex to its characteristic types of activity. To this he added that homosexuals are all passively oriented, masturbating and paying each other like prostitutes. Later, in the hospital, the projection of passive attitudes was indicated in his asking the psychiatrist, "Am I getting paid while I am kept here?"

FAMILY BURDENS. The patient entered public school at the usual age, skipped grades, and completed high school in less than the four years, at almost sixteen. He was graduated with honors and college was envisaged for the future. Since this was not economically feasible, he entered trade school and, at the same time, became a clerk. He contributed two-thirds of his small salary to his mother's household expenses. It was at this time that the rhinitis began and the fear and resentment toward his father turned to open hostility. The father, in turn, had succeeded in going from bad to worse, had lost his sinecure through shady deals and had moved the family to the mainland city of New York for economic reasons. A year later, the parents separated and Alberto's father deserted the family.

Alberto described how his father went from storekeeper to factory worker, how in New York he constantly used the phrase, "In Puerto Rico, even a dog can bark," alluding to thin walls in crowded New York apartments; and how he finally returned to the Island. Roberto, the older brother, regarded the father as "just no good." He himself entered the navy and completed a successful tour of duty. When Alberto's

normally placid, cooperative, or suggestible. Although ideas of persecution continued ("people" talking about him), he began to discuss with insight his hostilities aimed at father, mother, and brother. His restlessness persisted only in a desire to travel and join the merchant marine after full recovery.

DREAM ANALYSIS.   Dream material was recounted. *Dream 1:* He dreamed he owned a horse; and stated, "You wake up and find it's no horse." *Dream 2* reflected similar doubts of male potency, and concerned driving a car which magically transformed into a broom or stick incapable of motion. This dream was quickly associated, in frank Puerto Rican terms, with others about sexual intercourse. Alberto stated: "I think I need sex with a woman—dreaming of intercourse and waking up with night losses or wet dreams; the body must get rid of sperms because they accumulate." *Dream 3* concerned travel on a ship to Spain where he saw the Pyrenees covered with snow; it all changed to clouds as he awoke. In *Dream 4* an older nightmare was evoked; he was dying, and all the persons around him were busy nailing him into his coffin; he wished to tell them he was really alive, but could not speak. In *Dream 5,* he was breaking windows and doing this fearfully, but he could not run away like the friends with him. "I felt like I was nailed down to the floor." *Dream 6* had him married and settled down with a girl he knew back in New York; she was described as being brunette and small, and was a person occasionally seen in real life.

Still greater content was developed in a later series of dreams, with undistorted and insightful interpretations. In *Dream 1* a boat moving slowly out of harbor finds him staring down at the eddying, green water which seems to bubble with slimy dirt stirred up by the ship's wake; with nausea, he wishes to vomit at its stench. His commentary reminded him of his mother, and the bowel movements with enemas. *Dream 2* concerned a tall priest and nun to whom he explains his wish to marry; there is a figure of a girl, covered with rags, but looking like Melinda in age. The nun in white disappears while he is explaining, and the priestly figure becomes a voice shouting farther away. The associations indicated that the adult figures may have been parents, and his father disappeared when most needed. He liked his sister nearest in age, and felt sorry for her, "although sometimes I think my sisters have fewer troubles and worries growing up." *Dream 3* finds him in possession of a small, pearl-handled knife which becomes a large switch-blade; he attempts to cut down clowns painted white on a platform, but as he tries, the knife becomes "runt-sized" again with blood on it. His father shouts that Puerto Ricans do not use knives, "People just say that," and he takes it away. No free associations of this seemingly obvious dream were elicited. In *Dream 4,* he is a child dirtied by other children who try to burn him with a stick-and-paper torch; he is afraid his family will catch him in this state, but can neither move nor talk. Comments included that the fire warmed him through the mud, and he really liked the way it felt. In *Dream 5* he wants to drink at a public fountain, but the dirt and gum in the bowl make him sick; when he drinks, it tastes like hard liquor and turns his stomach. Here associations were made to negative training of the mother and feelings of revulsion toward the father.

MOTHER'S LACK OF INSIGHT INTO PATIENT'S PROBLEMS.   The mother, when visiting the patient in the hospital, proved to be an extremely attractive, carefully groomed woman of forty-one, with surface warmth and affability, who at the same time gave the impression of underlying coldness. Her icy manner developed in discussions of the family, particularly the father's role in family separation. There was distinct defensiveness about the patient's illness, of which she had no real understanding. Her English was halting at times only because of concern about the effect of her statements. What emerged most clearly was the strong-willed and rigid drive to be accepted and admired.

While the patient was aware of the seriousness of his illness, the mother denied any understanding of what had happened to him, being more concerned with her expectations for him. In her eyes, the outlook was good if only one realized he had been a good boy, clean in childhood, and abstemious with women and alcohol in youth—in contrast to the uncontrolled behavior of his father. She paraded his successful school career and willingness to help her financially while working his way through college as almost official reasons why nothing serious could be wrong. True, the patient had complained of being tired from the combination of overtime work and college attendance, but he slept well and possessed a good appetite. Finally, to clinch it all, there was no history of mental illness in the family and she was overly vehement in denials of nervousness or tension in the patient's entering service. Like most Puerto Ricans, she preferred to describe mental illness as a simple matter of bodily malfunction (nerves), possibly brought on by overwork.

PATIENT'S GOOD INSIGHT AND PROGNOSIS. In Alberto's accounts of his two sisters, it is clear that they had become, for him, somewhat seductive figures representing, as did the mother, both a sexual threat and an unwelcome burden. The Melinda of the dream recounted above was ready for marriage. In one dream, he associated that he had seen his sisters naked and was obviously embarrassed. While the mother denied sibling rivalries and negative emotions in the home climate, Alberto's accounts indicate the daughters' resentment of their mother's authority, the sons' open rivalry, and the mother's nagging and planful means of getting her own way. Alberto never felt that happiness or accomplishment was for himself. His seemingly useless gifts to his mother, his castration fears and self-punishment patterns, his anal and homosexual preoccupations, and his passivity were not in accord with the appropriate pattern of masculinity in this culture. But neither was his home headed by an adequate father. It was fatherless and controlled by a manipulative, rigid, and demanding mother. As Alberto grew up, these reversals of role in his Puerto Rican family became increasingly untenable.

The patient's future, however, is not bleak. Disappearance of acute symptoms occurred rapidly with insight. The family has learned that he cannot continue to develop insight and alone carry the burdens of a problematic family in a setting far different from that of San Juan. His plans to travel are undoubtedly a means of removing himself further from the strong maternal control. Hostile and inwardly suspicious, he nevertheless is able to perceive the blocks to further self-realization. Alberto has learned to read the mapping of his own symptoms —the passivity in hypochondriacal complaints, the earlier lack of firm identification, and the long-buried resentments and hostilities. With good intelligence, verbal facility, and growing insight into a traumatic past, Alberto is catching up with the half-lost years.

Lower-Class Colored Puerto Rican Man

BRUTAL BACKGROUND. The next case, an ambulatory male schizoid, we shall call Ramon. Like Alberto, he was in his early twenties when interviewed and also the second son in a family of four siblings. In contrast, however, Ramon was partly colored. His father, also partly colored, had abandoned the family. The mother and four children promptly moved to the worst slum of San Juan, and on the few occasions when the father visited the city, the parents fought violently. Ramon remembers his father beating the mother brutally and once trying to kill her with a gun. As a child, both parents punished him mercilessly, the father using his belt and the mother her broomstick. Ramon, whose lot fell with the mother ultimately, felt that she showed him no vestige of real affection. The slum was recalled as a place where "we were brought up among savages." Killings and beatings forced the young men to join gangs of hoodlums for survival. When baseball or swimming seemed boring, sadistic sports were substituted. One game involved being thumped on the back with a stick as long as one could bear the pain. Today, Ramon's brother is hospitalized and under treatment for mental disorder, following several aggressive and assaultative episodes.

BEHAVIORAL CONSEQUENCES. Ramon's aggressive and excited behavior is indicated in an account of his trip to the hospital with an interviewer. With mirthless excitement, Ramon appeared on the street to walk to his medical appointment. To any young woman whom he met on the way, he yelled, "Hello, Beauty!" At every corner, he hesitated to cross, explaining that in New York City drivers run you over like dogs. Since he was going to the clinic for a knee injury, he complained of this, calling it arthritis. To the list was added neuralgia and other worries about his health. His account of endless physical disabilities was interlarded with his exploits with prostitutes. Ramon seemed to be saying, "I am ill and worried about my health, but on the other hand I am also a pre-eminent male."

In subsequent discussions, it appeared that his hypochondriacal complaints included ailments which caused him almost constant pain and discomfort. His joints were arthritic. He had a rhinitis reaching asthmatic proportions. A stomach "upset" was almost continual. Where organic ailments stopped, he complained of trouble with sleep, dizziness, tension, and frequent colds. Like Alberto, he smoked continually and stated he had succeeded in getting some maternal attention, if not affection, by protracting childhood health problems. He had also never dated, had girl friends, or married. Ramon impressed one immediately as a tense, overactive individual, looking younger than his given age and overly concerned about his health and sexual identity. Ramon's fears and emotional constriction were early developed. Hostility toward frankly rejecting parents could not be expressed. Far from becoming merely callous, Ramon was afraid to be alone and terrified of being ridiculed. He learned to avoid punishments, tried to escape parental tongue-lashings, but developed a lengthy covert set of fears including high places, strange people, drunkards, food poisons, and being cut. The stern expectations of his mother bred in him a feeling that things should be done perfectly, that one should not show emotions to others, and that one should always be guarded with people. The introjection of these rules, based on suspicion and hostility, he recognized as being far from Puerto Rican values. Yet Ramon preferred to keep such opinions to himself and to trust no one.

HEALTH PREOCCUPATIONS. For as long as Ramon can remember, his chief concerns were about his health and unnamed or unspecified enemies. Discussions of his loneliness, though persistent, had a curious quality of being diffuse and disjointed. It was as if Ramon, like Alberto, hardly understood himself, while at the same time he described frankly his hostilities, his sense of inadequacy, and his emotional isolation. While appearing cooperative on the surface, he seemed blocked, disorderly in appearance, and constantly nervous and agitated. His ailments and imagined sexual exploits, such as nights spent with half a dozen prostitutes, seemed hollow and unconvincing. His suspiciousness and rigid compulsions were as frankly expressed in the same contexts and even more deeply rooted.

For example, Ramon's health rules were thought of as the only road to precarious survival. Though restless and energetic, he complained of being exhausted. This necessitated going to bed early, often in the evening, and above all, making sure of getting proper food. There was no use of drugs or alcohol. As with Alberto, Ramon disdained his father's heavy drinking and became totally abstinent. While his fantasy accounts of sexual exploits were many, he thought of sexual activity as being debilitating or dangerous to health.

ORAL FEATURES: SOMATIC AND MASOCHISTIC REACTIONS. While not stereotyped into a system of defensive controls, Ramon's behavior was at times most bizarre. Like Alberto's enema to rid him of mounting dangers, Ramon too had regulations centered less in the bowel than in the stomach. The upset stomach required certain foods at certain times and enough rest to digest that food properly. The arthritic pains, in his private folklore, were connected with unmet needs for just the right nourishment. While Alberto had centered his concerns on anal levels, Ramon's aggressive orality emphasized his nutritive needs. The arthritis he attempted to cure by eating certain foods and avoiding certain food poisons. When this failed him, he poured boiling water on his leg to ease the pain. The burns were extensive enough to require hospitalization. A comment on the entire masochistic episode was Ramon's cryptic remark, "A person with an incurable disease should stick a bullet through his head and that's all."

Apparently, this sense of hopelessness was early in development. His mother described him as having no real friends as a child and reacting to problems by going off by himself. She described the time that he took iron rods and, in a fit of pique, went out in a violent thunderstorm to see if the lightning would strike him. Despite some contrasts in type of aggression, from Alberto's passivity and dependence to Ramon's oral aggressiveness, both men had lengthy histories of masochistic and self-destructive tendencies. Ramon's nervous stomach, lightning test, and burnt knee episode were not all. He would taunt his elder brother until he was cruelly beaten. While fearing pain, he was often hurt.

FATHER AS A NEGATIVE MODEL. Ramon's father deserted the family, as in Alberto's case, during the boy's adolescence. The father complained that family burdens were heavier than he could bear. The extramarital exploits, the periods of unemployment, and his drunken appearances made the decision a welcome one for his wife. But before this frankly pronounced desertion, Ramon's difficulty in identification with his father is well described. The father, a peddler, was a person only to be avoided. As for the mother—nagging, demanding, and punitive in his absence—Ramon resented her even more. Since the father was colored, and the mother lower-class white, Ramon was mulatto and open to her further rejection, especially after they had moved to New York. On the mainland, the ethnic discriminations led Ramon to feel doubly stigmatized, both as lower-class Puerto Rican and as mulatto. The mother reinforced the social rejection, taunting him with the knowledge that in their tenement he was at first not allowed into the building, ostensibly for racial reasons.

While many Puerto Rican males would not work in the women's garment industry, Ramon does. Excluded from certain aspects of community life, he visits no neighbors and has no friends. His entertainment is exclusively through mass media. On these grounds, too, the battles with the mother are constant and openly antagonistic. In sentence-completion tests, the father is described as "anyone who wants to beat you." The definition of a mother is grounded in mutual exploitation. Ramon has firmly decided never to marry.

MOTHER AS SOURCE OF ORAL DEPRIVATION. The mother's pathology is more overt than in the case of Alberto's family. Generally, in this group, the acting out of lower-class persons is franker or more overt than in the class above. Here the mother, obese and overeating, ostensibly because of Island food deprivations, states that she is "rotten inside" because of constant suffering. For the most part, she and her children had always been hungry and deprived. Her son reported hunger in Puerto Rico that had even robbed him of sleep, and he recalled feeling at such times the most unhappy person in the world. The boys begged food from neighbors and learned to steal. In this period of the lean years, Ramon's oral concerns and resentments grew. "My stomach was ruined then and it was there that I developed a big appetite." In field work, he asked a Puerto Rican interviewer for money repeatedly or begged him to buy coffee and snacks for him. The impression was that Ramon wished to use the interviewer as a "good provider" who bestowed gifts and thus compensated for the rejecting and punitive father.

RESISTANCE TO SCHOOL. Schooling was likewise resented. One story concerned a teacher on the Island who, according to Ramon, pushed him and pinched him. He responded by running away. Ramon never liked school and had, at times, to be absent for want of clothes suitable for the classroom. The mother disagreed with the boy's attitude, stating, "Educate a person and you make him a man of worth rather than a *bandito*. Besides, here the only friend one has is the dollar in his pocket." At sixteen, completing third grade with the teacher incident recounted above, Ramon had obtained a bush knife from his father's cart and threatened to kill him with it.

IDEAS ABOUT SEX AND MARRIAGE. Ramon's persistent childhood fears included the danger of being cut. On receiving a small scalp wound from a falling tree branch in a storm, the sight of blood had terrified him. Ever after, he was afraid of being cut. Possibly related psychodynamically was fear that he might "injure" a girl. An attempt at intercourse on the Island is described with tremendous anxiety. Because the girl cried, he felt he had injured her fatally, and he regrets the incident to this day. His rules for marriage include a drastic improvement in health, a steady job, and plenty of money. Yet he discounts the possibility of his health's ever improving. As for the wife, the criteria are equally rigid. She must be white, second-generation American, wealthy, fluent in English, and a hard worker. He despairs of ever finding such a person among the Puerto Ricans, and until there is, he must find solace in fantasies of prostitutes. His habit of complimenting all passing girls whom he does not know is, for Ramon, a persistent daily habit.

DREAMS AND FANTASIES.   Ramon's dreams include several in which he plays a passive homosexual role. In one, he is slashed by a man with a knife, but emerges unscathed. Psychological tests* such as the Rorschach indicate that he maintains the tenuous balance of a bizarre schizophrenic. Paranoid ideation was consistently shown on all instruments, including TAT and Sentence Completion. There was confusion in distinguishing between genital behavior on the one hand, and oral or anal behavior on the other. On the Rorschach, for example, one of the cards is seen as an old man with a cat-face in which the "cat" is distinctly used as a feminine symbol. The story continues with the young man "somehow having intercourse," whereupon the old man of the story becomes angry because the younger has eaten everything. On Card III, following incoherent rambling about ostriches and a bow tie, the subject jumped up "to have coffee." After nervously gulping water, he complained that he saw eyes staring from the cards, and continued only with animal responses and poorly delineated entrails.

Interviews also evoked the same oral-sexual confusion. During them he begged for food, coffee, money, cigarettes, a particular pencil which caught his fancy, and a hot dog. Most symbolisms of this type were frankly phallic, and many of the supposed sexual exploits with prostitutes of his fancy were described seductively in terms of orgasm without intromission.

DIAGNOSTIC IMPRESSION.   The leading diagnostic impression from the tests was that of a schizophrenic reaction, paranoid type, with sharp mood swings as well. Having heard from his

---

* Unfortunately the original protocols are not available.

mother throughout life constant devaluation of both femininity and of male potency, Ramon apparently adopted a pattern in his own symptomatology of his mother's hypochondriacal complaints, her concern for survival and her displacements to oral emphasis. He is certain that he once irreparably harmed a girl. His male identifications are largely guilty ones, and his rules against female companionship or seeking a marital partner are insurmountable except in fantasy. His personality integration and emotional balance have not progressed far beyond that of his starved childhood—of being the "unhappiest person in the world."

Alberto and Ramon Compared

CHANGING FAMILY ROLES. In any culture, the intrapsychic status depends, in part, on family stability, on continuous structural settings for that stability, and upon cultural values capable of supporting, in realistic fashion, both family and structural setting. The family thus becomes an interdependent small group organization. It functions, for better or worse, as the major recognizable unit of a larger social system. It transmits, in more or less coherent patterns, those meanings and values of a culture which find support or meet rebuffs in the realities of a social world. In the family of Puerto Rican and Spanish-oriented cultures generally, extramarital and premarital liaisons for males in lower strata are sanctioned as part of a pattern of total masculine control or dominance. But these patterns are open to change and have changed with the movements of rural population to industrialized centers like San Juan and New York City.

While larger role expectations may consistently demand a father's economic contributions to enhance his total cultural prestige and honor, the challenge of this general pattern is hollow and meaningless if the economic position of the male changes to the extent it has in Puerto Rican families. Instead, the father, ideally representing the weight of authority within the home, sees his economic role diminish, and with it his importance and real authority. Thus, the economic pressures at the bottom of the social scale in contemporary Puerto Rico are much like those intensified in the New York scene itself. Males undergo a general downgrading in jobs available and the marriages become as evanescent as their dominance role. There is no barrier in a weakened Catholic religious system to formal separation or simple desertion. Both occur increasingly. As families bear the ultimate of poverty, migration, and cultural dislocation, so their component members may break under the strain of rapidly changing or burdensome family organization.

FATHER.   Alberto's and Ramon's fathers, reflecting separation and desertion norms of their respective classes, emerge from two backgrounds. The middle-class father stems from a background of maternal overprotection, and Ramon's still weaker and less effectual father, from his own background of neglect. Both are weak paternal figures. Caught in the transition to urbanism, which, for Puerto Rican culture means increased status for women, the masculine roles of each are further challenged and undermined.

MOTHER.   Alberto's mother, beyond the uniqueness of her particular struggle for independence, represents a psychological compromise between the cultural ideals and the expanded role of the Puerto Rican woman. By sustaining the family through a compulsively organized manipulation of her egocentrically conceived status of matron, she exploitatively uses what the culture designates as her best weapons in life—her sons. Through techniques of seductiveness, increasing narcissism, and competitions between siblings, she produces a passively oriented, masochistic, compulsive, and ultimately confused second male child. Ramon's mother, fighting a more stark battle of survival with fewer means, develops in her child the aggressive forms of hostility which are closer to the surface, out of a welter of neglect. Both children fail to make a masculine identification and both avoid any real interests in female companionship.

EFFECTS ON BOYS. In each case, the cultural expectations for male role performance are channeled for a time into male sibling rivalry which serves to reinforce hostility toward the fathers. Alberto experienced his repulsion from any actual role a few days after enlistment, and thereupon played his grotesque satire of the male world as he knew it. Ramon built his rules against marriage and the female world slowly and carefully over the years. Outside of parental and sexual relations, Alberto felt a hopeless lack of confidence and self-esteem, social and sexual inadequacy, and a poverty of positive emotions. Ramon's concerns about each of these areas was long in developing, but the combination of Puerto Rican and colored status finally crystallized his negative self feelings. Perhaps because of stricter lower-middle-class standards, Alberto's insecurities received less ventilation, leaving him for long behind a façade of successful accomplishment in school and work. His passive dependent and anal orientations were slowly and relentlessly imposed from without, held in rigid control, and finally transmuted into manneristic and carefully fashioned symbols. With Ramon, the acting out of aggressive and sexual impulse was more constant and gradual, consistent with his cruder slum background. The oral deprivations and affect hunger are mirrored in symptoms which center around eating.

Alberto's formalized and rigid defenses have as frantic a quality as Ramon's fantasies and rules. For both young men, the lack of a positive father figure finds no compensation in the culture beyond what a male "should be." Social norms do not exist as personally experienced reality, and acculturation has robbed each, through social and economic processes, of any stable context for behavior. To father desertion, more violent in Ramon's case, and male job downgrading, more obvious in Alberto's one may add the brittle marriages and parental instabilities on the distaff side as centrifugal forces disruptive of binding home influences.

For Alberto the imagined solution was to flee from the family scene, while for Ramon, always more lonely, it was to lose himself in urban anonymity. Therefore, despite his colored status, Ramon was unwilling to leave New York while Alberto pinned his hopes on extensive travel. In both men pent-up affect was siphoned into somatic symptoms in accord with their psychodynamic needs. In their psychoses they show much sudden discharge of affect. Alberto, with better education and advantages, has settled down into the passive role of patient and must measure, with his own insight, the steps to maturity. Ramon, with fewer such assets, vacillates between a long-ingrained will to survive and his depressive reactions and suicidal trends.

CULTURAL FACTORS IN TREATMENT.   Treatment in each case requires not only seeing defenses in balance but noting the cultural conflicts, the social experiences, and the role expectations of both men. Lacking the devious disguises of presumably more sophisticated people, such patients describe or act out their real problems with less evasion. Where they block, as in Alberto's occasional repetitions and symbolizations, or Ramon's interruptions of Rorschach, the signs are usually frank and direct as to what the individual can, and cannot, bear in amnestic material. Ramon remembers his childhood hungers with severe intensity, but his emotional hunger, like Alberto's, must be measured before one can proceed. Beyond the class-differentiations, seen largely in the greater tendency to act out in the lower and to control in the middle classes, these cases appear to be "typical" among Puerto Ricans.

Bibliography and References

1. HALLOWELL, A. I.: The self and its behavioral environment. *Explorations: Studies in Culture and Communication, 2;* 106-165, 1954.
2. OPLER, M. K.: Psychoanalytic techniques in social analysis. *J. of Social Psychol. 15;*91-127, 1942 (*Vide*, p. 115).
3. SULLIVAN, HARRY STACK: *The Interpersonal Theory of Psychiatry.* New York, Norton, 1953 (*Vide*, pp. xi, 365, 371, 376).
4. HALLOWELL, A. I.: *Popular Responses and Cultural Differences*, Rorschach Research Exchange, Vol. IX, 1945.
   HALLOWELL, A. I.: The Rorschach technique in the study of personality and culture, *Am. Anthropologist, 47:*No. 2, 1945.
5. THOMPSON, LAURA: *Culture in Crisis: A Study of the Hopi Indians: or,* Attitudes and acculturation. *Am. Anthropologist, 50:*No. 2, 1950.
6. HALLOWELL, A. I.: *Acculturation Processes and Personality Changes as Indicated by the Rorschach Technique.* Rorschach Research Exchange, Vol. VI, 1942.
7. DuBois, CORA,: *The People of Alor.* Minneapolis, Univ. Minnesota Press, 1944.
   GLADWIN, THOMAS, AND SARASON, S. B.: *Truk: Man in Paradise.* New York, Wenner-Gren Foundation Publications in Anthropology, No. 20, 1953.
8. HALLIDAY, J. L., *Psychosocial Medicine: A Study of the Sick Society.* New York, Norton, 1948.
9. KROEBER, A. L., AND KLUCKHOHN, C.: *Culture.* Papers of the Peabody Museum, Vol. 47, 1952 (*Vide*, p. 118).
10. CANNON, W. B.: *Bodily Changes in Pain, Hunger, Fear and Rage.* New York, Appleton, 1929.
    WOLFF, HAROLD G., Protective reaction patterns and disease. *Ann. Int. Med., 27:* 1947.
    GRACE, WILLIAM: Relationship of specific attitudes and emotions to certain bodily diseases. *Psychosom. Med. 14:*No. 4, 1952.
11. LIDDELL, HOWARD S.: Conditioning and emotions. *Scient. Am. 190:* No. 1, 1954. (Reference is also made to current work of Horsley Gantt.)
12. BLEULER, EUGEN: *Dementia Praecox or The Group of Schizophrenias.* New York, Internat. Univ. Press, 1950 (*Vide*, pp. 336, 463). See also: ZILBOORG, G. AND HENRY G. W.: *A History of Medical Psychiatry.* New York, Norton, 1941.
13. YAP, P. M.: The Latah reaction, *J. Men. Sc., 98;* 515-564, 1952.
14. HARE, E. H.: The ecology of mental disease, *J. Men. Sc. 98:*579-594, 1952.

15. FELIX, R. H., AND BOWERS, R. V.: Mental hygiene and socio-environmental factors. *Milbank Mem. Fund Quart. 26:*125-147, 1948.
16. BENEDICT, RUTH: Anthropology and the abnormal. *J. Genet. Psychol. 10:*59-82, 1934. Cf., HORNEY, KAREN: *New Ways in Psychoanalysis.* New York, Norton, 1939. Also, REDLICH, F.: The concept of normality. *Am. J. Psychotherapy,* 6:551-576, 1952.
17. PARSONS, TALCOTT: *The Social System.* Glencoe, Illinois, Free Press, 1951.
18. FELIX, R. H., AND BOWERS, R. V.: *op.cit.,* p. 125.
19. DIETHELM, OSKAR: The Psychopathologic basis of psychotherapy of schizophrenia. Symposium, *Am. J. Psychiat., 111:*422-425, 1954.
20. DIETHELM, OSKAR: *Report of the Payne Whitney Psychiatric Clinic, New York Hospital,* 1953 (*Vide,* pp. 11-12).
21. GERARD, D. L., AND HUSTON, L.: Family setting and the social ecology of schizophrenia. *Psychiat. Quart.,* 27, 1-12, 1953.
    GERARD, D. L., AND SIEGEL, JOSEPH; The family background of schizophrenia, *Psychiat. Quart., 24:*47-73, 1950.
22. HYDE, ROBERT, *et. al.* Studies in medical sociology. *New England J. Medicine, 231:*543-548, 571-577, 612-618, 1944.
    STOTT, L. S.: Environmental factors in relation to personality adjustments. *Rural Sociology, 10:* 1945.
    COUNTS, R. M., AND REGAN, PETER F.: Chronic schizophrenic reactions. *Monatsschr. f. Psychiatrie & Neurologie, 127:*47-60, 1954.
23. EATON, J. W., AND WEIL, R. J.: The mental health of the Hutterites. *Scient. Am. 189:* No. 1, 1953
    EATON, J. W., AND WEIL. R. J.: The Hutterite mental health study. *Mennonite Quar. Rev.,* January, 1951.
24. HOLLINGSHEAD, A. B., AND REDLICH, F. C.: Social stratification and psychiatric disorders. *Am. Sociological Rev. 18:*No. 2, 1953.
25. DIETHELM, OSKAR: The alcohol problem. *Bull. New York Acad. Med. 29* (2nd Series): No.12, 1953.
26. FELIX, R. H., AND BOWERS, R. V.: *op.cit.*
27. RENNIE, T. A. C.: Prognosis in the psychoneuroses: benign and malignant developments, in HOCH, P. H., AND ZUBIN, J.: *Current Problems in Psychiatric Diagnosis.* New York, Grune & Stratton, 1953.
28. POWDERMAKER, HORTENSE: *Mass Communications Seminar.* New York, Wenner-Gren Foundation for Anthropological Research, 1953 (*Vide* especially, LASSWELL, HAROLD, Characteristics of media, pp. 82 ff.).
29. JONES, MAXWELL: *Social Psychiatry.* London, Tavistock Publications, 1952. See also: HEALY, WILLIAM, on the Borstal System.
30. RENNIE, T. A. C.: Psychiatry. *Ann. Rev. Med.,* pp. 253-260, 1953.
31. LING, THOMAS M.,: *Mental Health and Human Relations.* London, Lewis, 1954.
32. COTTRELL, LEONARD S., AND GALLAGHER, RUTH: *Developments in Social Psychology: 1930-1940.* New York, Beacon House, 1941.

33. LEMERT, E. M.: Exploratory study of mental disorders in a rural problem area. *Rural Sociology*, 13, 1948. See also: LEMERT, E. M.: *Social Pathology*. New York, McGraw-Hill, 1951.

34. COMPARE, LEMKAU, PAUL, TIETZE, CHRISTOPHER, AND COOPER, MARCIA: A survey of statistical studies on the prevalence and incidence of mental disorders in sample populations. *Pub. Health Rep. 58:* (December 31, 1943) (with methods and findings of the Roth-Luton Survey).

35. MANGUS, A.R.: *Mental Health of Rural Children in Ohio*. Ohio Agricultural Experiment Station, Research Bulletin, 682, 1949.

36. STOTT, L. S.: Environmental factors in relation to personality adjustments. *Rural Sociology, 10:* 1945.

37. EATON, J. W.: In defense of culture-personality studies. *Am. Sociological Rev. 16:*No. 1, 1951.

38. WOODARD, J. W.: The relation of personality structure to the structure of culture. *Am. Sociological Rev. 3:*No. 4, 1938.

39. BRILL, A. A.: *Lectures in Psychoanalytic Psychiatry*. New York, Knopf, 1949 (Lectures first given in 1924).

40. SELIGMAN, C. G.: Temperament, conflict and psychosis in a stone age population. *Brit. J. Med. Psychol. 9:*187-202, 1929.

41. DHUNJIBHOY, J.: Brief resume of the types of insanity commonly met with in India, *J. Ment. Sc., 16:*254-264, 1930.

42. STAINBROOK, E.: Some characteristics of the psychopathology of schizophrenic behavior in Bahian society. *Am. J. Psychiat. 109:*330-335, 1952.

43. VAN LOON, H. G., Protopathic instinctive phenomena in normal and pathologic Malay life. *Brit. J. M. Psychol. 8:*264-276, 1928.

44. DEVEREUX, G.: *Reality and Dream: Psychotherapy of a Plains Indian*. New York, Internat. Univ. Press, 1951.

45. SACHS, W.: *Black Hamlet*. Boston, Little, Brown, 1947.

46. MENNINGER, KARL: The contribution of psychoanalysis to American psychiatry. *Bull. Menninger Clin. 18:*85-96, 1954.

47. STAINBROOK, E.: *op.cit.*

48. STAINBROOK, E.: *op.cit.* Compare, for a general account of interior Brazil and coastal regions: LOPEZ, C., Ethnographische Betrachtungen über Schizophrenie. *Ztschr.: Ges. Neurol. u Psychiat., 142:*706-711, 1932.

49. CANNON, W. B.: Voodoo death. *Am. Anthropologist, 44:*No. 2, 1942.

50. GILLIN, JOHN: *The Culture of Security in San Carlos*. New Orleans, Middle American Research Institute, Series No. 16, 1951 (*Vide* pp. 112 ff.). See also:
GILLIN, JOHN: Magical fright. *Psychiatry, 11:*387-400, 1948.

51. HENRY, JULES: Anthropology and psychosomatics. *Psychom. Med. 11:* 216-222, 1949.

52. EBAUGH, FRANKLIN G., Psychosomatic medicine, *International Forum*, Vol. 2, No. 3, 1954.

53. WINSTON, E.: The alleged lack of mental disease among primitive groups. *Am. Anthropologist. 36*, No. 2, 1934.
MEAD, MARGARET: *Coming of Age in Samoa.* New York, William Morrow, 1928.

54. JOSEPH, ALICE, AND MURRAY, V. F.: *Chamorros and Carolinians of Saipan: Personality Studies.* Cambridge, Harvard, 1951.

55. RÓHEIM, GÉZA: Racial differences in the neuroses and psychoses. *Psychiatry, 2-3;* 375-390, 1939.
YAP, P. M.: Mental diseases peculiar to certain cultures: a survey of comparative psychiatry. *J. Ment. Sc. 97:*313-327, 1951.

56. CARPENTER, E. S.: Witch fear among the Aivilik Eskimos. *Am. J. Psychiatry, 110:*No. 3, 1953.

57. BERNDT, R. M., AND BERNDT, C.: The concept of abnormality in an Australian aboriginal society, in: WILBUR, G. B. AND MUENSTERBERGER, W.: *Psychoanalysis and Culture.* New York, Internat. Univ. Press, 1951.

58. JACOBSON, A., AND BERENBERG, A. N.: Japanese psychiatry and psychotherapy. *Am. J. Psychiatry, 109:*No. 5, 1952.

59. MITTELMAN, B., WOLFF, HAROLD G. AND SHARF, MARGARET: *Emotions and gastroduodenal functions. Psychoso. Med. 4:*51-61, 1942.

60. STOUFFER, SAMUEL, et. al.: *The American Soldier:* Vol. IV, *Measurement and Prediction.* Princeton, Princeton Univ. Press, 1950.

61. ACKERKNECHT, E. H.: Psychopathology, Primitive medicine and primitive culture. *Bull. Hist. Med. 14:*30-67, 1943.

62. PARSONS, TALCOTT: Some comments on the general theory of action. *Am. Sociological Rev. 18:*618-631, 1953.

63. FELIX, R. H. AND BOWERS, R. V.: *op.cit.,* pp. 131 ff.

64. HENRY, JULES: Family Structure and the transmission of neurotic behavior. *Am. J. Orthopsychiat. 21,*800-818, 1951.

65. GORDON, J. E., O'ROURKE, E., RICHARDSON, F. L. W., AND LINDEMANN, ERICH: Preventive medicine and epidemiology. *Am. J. Med. Sc. 223:* 316-343, 1952.

66. GRUENBERG, E. M.: Community conditions and psychoses of the elderly. *Am. J. Psychiatry, 110:*No. 12, 1954. (The psychoses dealt with are cerebral arteriosclerosis and senile psychosis.)

67. HOLLINGSHEAD, A. B., AND REDLICH, F. C.: Social stratification and psychiatric disorders. *Am. Sociological Rev. 18:* No. 2, 1953.

68. FARIS, R. E. L., AND DUNHAM, H. W.: *Mental Disorders in Urban Areas: An Ecological Study of Schizophrenia and Other Psychoses.* Chicago Univ. Chicago Press, 1939, p. 53.

69. SCHWARTZ, MORRIS S.: The economic and spatial mobility of paranoid schizophrenics and manic depressives. Master's Thesis, University of Chicago, 1946 (unpublished).

70. ROBINSON, W. S.: Ecological correlations and the behavior of individuals. *Am. Sociological Rev. 15:*351-357, 1950.

71. JONES, MAXWELL, *op.cit.*

72. LEWIS, AUBREY: Social aspects of psychiatry. *Edinburgh M. J., 58:* 214, 1951.

73. SPITZ, RENE A.: *The Psychogenic Diseases in Infancy: The Psychoanalytic Study of the Child.* New York, Internat. Univ. Press, 1951.

74. BOWLBY, JOHN: *Maternal Care and Mental Health.* Geneva, World Health Organization, Monograph Series No. 2, 1951.

75. BALES, R. F.: Cultural differences in rates of alcoholism. *Quar. J. Stud. Alcohol. 6:*480-493, 1946.

76. HYDE, ROBERT, *et. al.: op. cit. New England J. Medicine, 231:*Part III, Table III, 1944.

77. STRAUSS, J. H. AND STRAUSS, M. A.: Suicide, homicide, and social structure in Ceylon. *Am. J. Sociology, 58:*No. 5, 1953 (*Vide,* Table I, p. 462, and commentary).

78. CHESS, STELLA, CLARK, KENNETH B., AND THOMAS, ALEXANDER: The importance of cultural evaluation in psychiatric diagnosis and treatment. *Psychiatric Quart. 27:*102-114, 1953

79. LEWIS, AUBREY: Points of research into the interaction between the individual and the culture, in: TANNER, J. M.: *Prospects in Psychiatric Research.* Oxford, The Proceedings of the Oxford Conference of the Mental Health Research Fund, 1953.

80. LEMERT, E. M., *Social Pathology, op. cit.*

81. STANTON, A. H., AND SCHWARTZ, M. S.: Observations on dissociation as social participation. *Psychiatry, 12:*339-354, 1949.

82. REDLICH, F. C. AND BINGHAM, JUNE: *The Inside Story: Psychiatry and Everyday Life.* New York, KNOPF, 1953, pp. 192-3.

83. DIETHELM, OSKAR,: *Annual Report of the Payne Whitney Psychiatric Clinic,* 1953, *op. cit.,* pp. 9-12.

84. SAPIR, EDWARD: The unconscious patterning of behavior in society, in: DUMMER, E. S., *The Unconscious.* New York, Knopf, 1929, pp. 114-142..

85. KLUCKHOHN, FLORENCE R.: Dominant and substitute profiles of cultural orientation. *Social Forces, 28:*No. 4, 1950.

86. DUNHAM, H. W.: The social personality of the catatonic-schizophrene. *Am. J. Sociology, 49:*508-518, 1944.

87. CLAUSEN, JOHN A., AND KOHN, M. L., The use of the ecological method in social psychiatry. (Mss. from the Laboratory of Socio-Environmental Studies.) Bethesda, Maryland, National Institute of Mental Health, U. S. Public Health Service, 1954.

88. SCHAFFER, LESLIE, AND MYERS, J. K.: Psychotherapy and social stratification. *Psychiatry, 17:*83-93, 1954.

89. ALEXANDER, FRANZ, AND SZASZ, THOMAS S.: The psychosomatic approach in medicine, in: ALEXANDER, FRANZ, AND ROSS, HELEN, *Dynamic Psychiatry.* Chicago, Univ. Chicago Press, 1952 (pp. 369-400).

90. ALEXANDER, FRANZ: *Psychosomatic Medicine.* New York, Norton, 1950.

91. RUESCH, JURGEN, *et. al.*,: *Chronic Disease and Psychological Invalidism.* Berkeley, Univ. California Press, 1946.

92. CAUDILL, WILLIAM, REDLICH, F. C., GILMORE, H. R., AND BRODY, W.: Social structure and interaction processes on a psychiatric ward. *Am. J. Orthopsychiat. 22:*314-334, 1952.

93. DEVEREUX, GEORGE: Psychiatry and anthropology. *Bull. Menninger Clinic. 16:*167-177, 1952.

94. MACKAY, D.: A background for African psychiatry. *East African M. J., 25:*1-10, 1948.

95. CAROTHERS, J. C.: *The African Mind in Health and Disease.* Geneva, World Health Organization, Monograph Series No. 17, 1953. (This study is a careful collation of data from almost two hundred references and direct studies of African psychiatry from various parts of the continent. For accurate summarization and intelligent sifting of data, it is recommended; for inept statements of "the African mind" in general, as reflected in the title, it is not recommended.)

96. LAUBSCHER, B. : *Sex, Custom, and Psychopathology.* London, Routledge, 1937.

97. CAROTHERS, J. C.: A study of mental derangement in Africans and an attempt to explain its peculiarities, more especially in relation to the African attitude to life. *Psychiatry, 11:*47-85, 1948. (Here the above comment on Carothers' recent work applies with greater force. His other work on "frontal lobe functioning" in the African, questionable from the point of view of physical anthropology, may be found in: CAROTHERS, J. C.: Frontal lobe function and the African. *J. Med. Sc. 97:*12-47, 1951; Also, *J. Ment. Sc. 93:*548,1948).

98. TOOTH, G.: *Studies in Mental Illness in the Gold Coast* (Colonial Research Publications No. 6) London, His Majesty's Stat. Offi. 1950.

99. BROCK, J. F., AND AUTRET, M.: *Kwashiorkor in Africa.* Geneva, World Health Organization, Monograph Series No. 8, 1952.

100. CAROTHERS, J. C.: *op. cit.*, 1953, p. 140. (Cf., Carothers, J. C.: *J. Ment. Sc. 97:*12, 1951.)

101. CAROTHERS, J. C.: *op.cit.*, 1953, p. 159.

102. MALZBERG, BENJAMIN A., *Social and Biological Aspects of Mental Disease.* Utica, New York, State Hospitals Press, 1940. (Comprises journal articles published elsewhere.) See also: MALZBERG, BENJAMIN A., Rates of mental disease among certain population groups in New York State. *J. Am. Statistical Asso. 31:*1936; and article by MALZBERG, in KLINEBERG, OTTO: *Characteristics of the American Negro.* New York, publ. Negro in American Life Series, 1944.

103. CAROTHERS, J. C.: *op.cit.*, 1953, p. 163.

104. AUBIN, H.: *L'homme et la Magie.* Paris, 1952.

105. CAROTHERS, J. C.: *op cit.*, 1953, p. 142.

106. CAROTHERS, J. C.: *op. cit.*, 1953, p. 148.

107. CAROTHERS, J. C.: *op. cit.*, 1953, p. 161.

108. BEAGLEHOLE, ERNEST: Culture and psychosis in New Zealand, *J. Polynesian Society,* 48:144, 1939.

109. BEAGLEHOLE, ERNEST: *Some Modern Hawaiians: Culture and Psychosis in Hawaii.* Honolulu, T. H., Univ. Hawaii Research Publications, No. 19, 1939.

110. HALLOWELL, A. I.: *Acculturation Processes and Personality Change as Indicated by Rorschach Technique.* Rorschach Research Exchange, Vol. VI, 1942, pp. 42-50.
HALLOWELL, A. I.: Culture and mental disorder, *J. Abnor. & Social Psychol. 29:*1-9, 1934.

111. LANDES, RUTH: The abnormal among the Ojibwa Indians. *J. Abnor. & Social Psychol. 33:*14-33, 1938.

112. COOPER, J. M.: Mental disease situations in certain cultures. *J. Abnor. & Social Psychol. 29:*10-17, 1934.

113. HALLOWELL, A. I.: Cultural factors in the structuralization of perception, in ROHRER, J. H. AND SHERIF, M.: *Social Psychology at the Crossroads.* New York, Harper, 1951.

114. HALLOWELL, A. I.: Some psychological aspects of measurement among the Salteaux. *Am. Anthropologist. 44:*No. 1, 1942.

115. JOSEPH, ALICE, AND MURRAY, V. F.: *Chamorros and Carolinians of Saipan: Personality Studies.* Cambridge, Harvard, 1951, p. 199.

116. ABERLE, D. F.: 'Arctic Hysteria' and Latah in Mongolia. *Tr. New York Acad. Sc. 14:*291-297, 1952.

117. ACKERKNECHT, E. H.: Psychopathology, primitive medicine, and primitive culture. *op. cit.,* 1943.

118. VAN LOON, H. G.: *op. cit.,* 1928.

119. DEVEREUX, G.: A sociological theory of schizophrenia. *Psychoanalyt. Rev. 26:*315-342, 1934.

120. DEWEY, JOHN: *Human Nature and Conduct.* New York, Henry Holt, 1922, (part II, section 5, p. 131).

121. BAILEY, FLORA L.: Navajo motor habits, *Am. Anthropologist, 44:*No. 2, 1942.

122. ASTROV, MARGOT: The concept of motion as the psychological leitmotif of Navajo life and literature. *J. Am. Folklore, 63:*45-56, 1950.

123. BELO, JANE: The Balinese temper. *Character and Personality, 4,* 120-146, 1935.

124. DEVEREUX, G.: Mohave Indian verbal and motor profanity, in ROHEIM, GÉZA, *Psychoanalysis and the Social Sciences.* New York, Internat. Univ. Press, 1951.

125. BARNOUW, VICTOR: The fantasy world of a Chippewa woman. *Psychiatry 12:*67-76, 1949.

126. HALLOWELL, A. I.: Shabwan: a dissocial Indian girl. *Am. J. Orthopsychiat. 8:*329-340, 1938.
SPENCER, KATHERINE: Mythology and values: an analysis of Navajo Chantway myths. Doctoral thesis, submitted for publication in Papers of the Peabody Museum, Harvard, 1952.

127. LINCOLN, J. S.: *The Dream in Primitive Cultures.* Baltimore, Williams & Wilkins, 1935.

412

128. SPENCER, D. M.: Fijian dreams and visions, in DAVIDSON, D. S.: *Twenty-Fifth Anniversary Studies.* Publications of the Philadelphia Anthropological Society, 1, 199-209, 1937.
129. EGGAN, DOROTHY: The manifest content of dreams. *Am. Anthropologist, 54:*No. 4, 1952.
130. EFRON, DAVID: *Gesture and Environment.* New York, King's Crown Press (Columbia University), 1941.
131. LOWIE, R. H.: *Social Organization.* New York, Rinehart, 1948. (For the points made, *vide,* pp. 15, 281, 318, ff., 322, 387).
132. LEMKAU, PAUL, AND DESANCTIS, CARLO: A survey of Italian psychiatry. *Am. J. Psychiat. 107:* 401-408, 1950.
133. BERNE, ERIC: Some Oriental mental hospitals. *Am. J. Psychiat. 106:* 376-383, 1950.
134. WHITEHEAD, ALFRED NORTH: *Introduction to Mathematics.* New York, Henry Holt, 1911, p. 223.
135. OPLER, M. K.: *op. cit.,* 1942.
136. FROMM, ERICH: Sex and character, in GEDDES, DONALD P., AND CURIE, ENID; *About the Kinsey Report.* New York, New American Library, 1948, pp. 56-7.
137. LEMKAU, PAUL, PASAMANIK, BENJAMIN, AND COOPER, MARCIA: The implications of the psychogenetic hypothesis for mental hygiene. *Am. J. Psychiat. 110:*436-442, 1953.
138. HENRY, G. W., *Sex Variants: A Study of Homosexual Patterns.* New York, Hoeber, 1941 (2 Vols., pp. 1179; *vide,* summaries of male cases: pp. 3-14; and of female cases, pp. 549-556).
139. ROBB, J. H.: Clinical studies of marriage and the family: a symposium, on methods. *Brit. J. M. Psychol. 26,* 215-221, and parts 3, 4, 1953.
     NAEGELE, KASPAR D.,: Hostility and aggression in middle-class American families. Doctoral thesis (Unpublished), Harvard, 1951.
140. SULLIVAN, HARRY STACK: *The Psychiatric Interview.* (Edited by Helen S. Perry and Mary L. Gawel.) New York, Norton, 1954, pp. 28-32, 37-38.
141. ROBERTS, BERTRAM H., AND MYERS, J. K.: Religion, national origin, immigration, and mental disorders. *Am. J. Psychiat. 110:*759-764, 1954.
142. OPLER, M. K.: Cu'tural perspectives in mental health research. *Am. J. Orthopsychiat. 25:*51-59, 1955.
143. FREUD, S.: *Die Traumdeutung,* 3rd Ed. Leipzig and Vienna, Transl. by A. A. Brill, *Interpretation of Dreams.* London, George Allen, 1911.
144. OPLER, M. K.: *op cit.,* 1942 (*Vide,* pp. 118-127). See also:
     OPLER, M. K.: The Southern Ute of Colorado, in Linton, Ralph (Ed.) *Acculturation in Seven American Indian Tribes.* New York, Appleton, 1940.
145. STUNKARD, ALBERT: Some interpersonal aspects of an oriental religion. *Psychiatry, 14-4:*419-431, 1951.
146. OPLER, M. K. (with SPICER, E. H., AND LUOMALA, K): *Impounded People.* Washington, U.S. Department of Interior, 1946.

147. OPLER, M. K.: Anthropology, in HARRIMAN, P. L. (Ed.): *Contemporary Social Science.* Harrisburg, Pennsylvania, Stackpole, 1953. (*Vide*, section, Culture-Personality Theory: A Methodological Review of a Current in American Anthropology, pp. 328-344).

148. SAPIR, EDWARD: The contribution of psychiatry to an understanding of behavior in society. *Am. J. Sociology. 42:*862-870, 1937.

149. KLUCKHOHN, CLYDE: The influence of psychiatry on anthropology in America during the past one hundred years, in HALL, J. K., ZILBOORG, G., AND BUNKER, H. A.: *One Hundred Years of American Psychiatry.* New York, Columbia Univ. Press, 1944.

150. KLEIN, G. S., HOLTZMAN, P. S., AND LASKIN, D.: The perception project: progress report for 1953-54. *Bull. Menninger Clinic, 18:*260-266, 1954.

151. HARTMANN, HEINZ: Ego psychology and the problem of adaptation, in RAPAPORT, DAVID: *Organization and Pathology of Thought.* New York, Columbia Univ. Press, 1951.

152. KRIS, ERNST: On preconscious mental processes, in RAPAPORT, DAVID: *op. cit.*

153. RAPAPORT, DAVID: The autonomy of the ego. *Bull. Menninger Clin.* 15:113-123, 1951.

154. HSU, FRANCIS L. K.: Suppression versus repression. *Psychiatry, 12-3:* 223-242, 1949.

155. WEGROCKI, H. J.: A critique of cultural and statistical concepts of abnormality, in KLUCKHOHN, CLYDE, AND MURRAY, H. A.: *Personality in Nature, Society, and Culture.* New York, KNOPF, 1948.

156. LaBARRE, WESTON: *The Human Animal.* Chicago, Univ. Chicago Press, 1954.

157. FEIBLEMAN, JAMES K.: Towards an analysis of the basic value system. *Am. Anthropologist 56:*421-432, 1954.

158. KLUCKHOHN, CLYDE: Values and value orientations, in PARSONS, TALCOTT, AND SHILS, E. A.: *Toward a General Theory of Action.* Cambridge, Harvard, 1951 (*Vide*, p. 411).

159. CASSIRER, ERNST: *An Essay on Man.* Garden City, New York, Doubleday, 1953 (*Vide*, p. 62).

160. STANTON, A. H., AND SCHWARTZ, M. S.: *The Mental Hospital.* New York, Basic Books, Inc., 1954.

161. FROMM-REICHMAN, FRIEDA: *Principles of Intensive Psychotherapy.* Chicago, Univ. Chicago Press, 1950 (*Vide*, pp. 82-84).

162. FROMM- REICHMAN, FRIEDA: *op. cit.*, pp. 32-33.

163. SIMMONS, LEO, AND WOLFF, HAROLD G.: *Social Science in Medicine.* New York, Russell Sage Foundation, 1954 (*Vide*, pp. 196-197).

164. REDLICH, F. C.: The concept of normality. *Am. J. Psychotherapy, 6-3:* 551-576, 1952 (*Vide*, p. 558).

165. EDEL, ABRAHAM: The concept of values in contemporary philosophical value theory. *Philosophy of Science, 20-3:*198-207, 1954 (*Vide*, p. 204).

414

166. WHITE, LESLIE A.: *The Science of Culture*. New York, Farrar, Straus, 1949, pp. 55–117.
167. *Ibid.*, p. 145.
168. BENEDICT, RUTH: *Patterns of Culture*. Boston, Houghton Mifflin, 1934, pp. 24, 46–48, 237.
169. LINTON, RALPH: *The Cultural Background of Personality*. New York, Appleton-Century, 1945; *The Tree of Culture*. New York, Alfred A. Knopf, 1955.
170. LINTON, RALPH: *The Study of Man*. New York, Appleton-Century, 1936.
171. LINTON, R.: *op. cit.*, 1955.
172. SOROKIN, PITIRIM A.: *Social and Cultural Dynamics*. 4 vols. New York, American Book Co., 1937–1941.
173. BENEDICT, RUTH: Psychological types in the culture of the southwest. *Proceedings of the Twenty-Third International Congress of Americanists* (New York, 1928), 1930, pp. 572–581; Configurations of culture in North America. *American Anthropologist*, 34:1–27, 1932.
174. GOLDENWEISER, ALEXANDER A.: Four phases of anthropological thought. *Publications of the American Sociological Society*, 16 (*Papers and Proceedings of the Sixteenth Annual Meeting, American Sociological Society, 1921*): 50–69, 1922; Diffusionism and the American school of historical ethnology. *American Journal of Sociology*, 31:19–38, 1925.
175. BENEDICT, R.: *op. cit.*, 1932, 1934.
176. BENEDICT, R.: *op. cit.*, 1930.
177. SAPIR, EDWARD: *op. cit.*, 1929.
178. SAPIR, EDWARD: Do we need a superorganic? *American Anthropologist*, 19:441–447, 1917.
179. SAPIR, EDWARD: *op. cit.*, 1929; The emergence of the concept of personality in a study of culture. *Journal of Social Psychology*, 5: 408–415, 1934.
180. SAPIR, EDWARD: *op. cit.*, 1934; The contribution of psychiatry to an understanding of behavior in society. *American Journal of Sociology*, 42:862–870, 1937.
181. SAPIR, EDWARD: *op. cit.*, 1929.
182. MALINOWSKI, BRONISLAW: *Sex and Repression in Savage Society*. New York, Harcourt, Brace and Company, 1927; Culture. *Encyclopedia of the Social Sciences*, 4:621–646, 1931; *Coral Gardens and Their Magic*. 2 vols. London, George Allen and Unwin, Ltd., 1935.
183. Cf. ALEXANDER, FRANZ: *Our Age of Unreason*, rev. ed. Philadelphia, Lippincott, 1951.
184. OPLER, MARVIN K.: *op. cit.*, 1942; *Culture, Psychiatry, and Human Values*. Springfield, Illinois, Charles C Thomas, Publisher, 1956a.

185. BENEDICT, RUTH: Continuities and discontinuities in cultural conditioning. *Psychiatry,* 1:161–167, 1938.

186. SAPIR, EDWARD: *Selected Writings in Language, Culture and Personality,* ed. by David G. Mandelbaum. Berkeley, University of California Press, 1948.

187. LINTON, R.: *op. cit.,* 1945.

188. KARDINER, ABRAM, with RALPH LINTON, CORA DuBOIS, and JAMES WEST: *The Psychological Frontiers of Society.* New York, Columbia University Press, 1945.

189. OPLER, M. K.: *op. cit.,* 1956a.

190. RÓHEIM, GÉZA: Psychoanalysis and anthropology. In *Psychoanalysis and the Social Sciences,* ed. by Géza Róheim, vol. 1, pp. 9–33. New York, International Universities Press, 1947.

191. Cf. NADEL, S. F.: *The Foundations of Social Anthropology.* Glencoe, The Free Press, 1951.

192. BOAS, FRANZ: The limitations of the comparative method of anthropology. *Science,* 40:901–908, 1896.

193. BOAS, FRANZ: The aims of anthropological research. *Science,* 76:605–613, 1932.

194. JENKS, ALBERT ERNEST: Report on the science of anthropology in the Western Hemisphere and the Pacific Islands. In *Reports on the Present Condition and Future Needs of the Science of Anthropology,* by W. H. R. Rivers, A. E. Jenks, and S. G. Morley, pp. 29–59. *Publication of The Carnegie Institution of Washington,* 200, 1913.

195. ALLIER, RAOUL: *The Mind of the Savage.* New York, Harcourt, Brace and Company, n.d.

196. WAITZ, THEODORE: *Anthropologie der Naturvölker.* 6 vols. Leipzig, Friedrich Fleischer, 1859–1872.

197. KROEBER, A. L.: History and science in anthropology. *American Anthropologist,* 37:539–569, 1935.

198. BOAS, F.: *op. cit.,* 1932.

199. *Ibid.,* pp. 608–9.

200. *Ibid.,* pp. 612–13.

201. GOLDENWEISER, ALEXANDER A.: The principle of limited possibilities in the development of culture. *Journal of American Folklore,* 26:259–290, 1913.

202. OPLER, M. K.: *op. cit.,* 1942; *op. cit.,* 1956a; Entities and organization in individual and group behavior: A conceptual framework. *Group Psychotherapy,* 9:290–300, 1956b.

203. OPLER, MARVIN K.: Cultural perspectives in research on schizophrenics. *Psychiatric Quarterly,* 33:506–524, 1959a.

204. FREUD, S.: Psychoanalytic notes upon an autobiographical account of a case of paranoia. *J. Brit. Psychoanal. Psychopath.,* 3:9–68, 1911.

205. BRENNER, CHARLES: *An Elementary Textbook of Psychoanalysis.* New York, International Universities Press, 1955.

206. FREUD, S.: *The Ego and the Id.* London, Hogarth Press and Institute of Psychoanalysis, 1927.

207. FREUD, S.: *Totem and Taboo* (1913). London, Routledge & Kegan Paul, 1950.

208. OPLER, MORRIS E.: *An Apache Life-Way.* Chicago, University of Chicago Press, 1941.

209. OPLER, M. K.: *op. cit.,* 1940; The influence of ethnic and class subcultures on child care. *Social Problems, 3*:12–21, 1955a.

210. Driver, H. E.: *Indians of North America.* Chicago, University of Chicago Press, 1961.

211. Steward, J. H., and Faron, L.: *Native Peoples of South America.* New York, McGraw-Hill, 1959.

212. Mead, Margaret: *Male and Female.* New York, Morrow, 1949.

213. FORD, C. S., and BEACH, F. A.: *Patterns of Sexual Behavior.* New York, Harper & Row, 1951.

214. RADO, S.: *Psychoanalysis of Behavior.* New York, Grune & Stratton, 1956.

215. OPLER, M. K.: *op. cit.,* 1959b.

216. BOGORAS, W.: *The Chukchee. Jesup Exped. Rep.* (New York, American Museum of Natural History, 1904–1909), 7 (Memoir 11).

217. HARLOW, H. F.: Love in infant monkeys. *Scient. Am.,* 200 (68), 40, 63–74, 1959.

218. CALHOUN, J. B.: A behavioral sink. In E. L. Bliss (Ed.), *Roots of Behavior.* New York, Harper & Row, 1962.

219. RADCLIFFE-BROWN, A. R.: *The Andaman Islanders.* New York, Free Press, 1948.

220. GOLDMAN, I.: *The Cubeo, Indians of the northwest Amazon.* Urbana, "Ill. Stud. Anthrop. No. 2," University of Illinois Press, 1963.

221. BENEDICT, R.: *op. cit.,* 1934.

222. *Ibid.,* chapter 6.

223. ERIKSON, E. H.: *Childhood and Society.* New York, Norton, 1950. Cf. also his later position: ERIKSON, E. H.: The problem of ego identity. *J. Amer. Psychoanal. Assn.,* 1956, 4, 56–121.

224. OPLER, M. K.: *op. cit.,* 1955a.

225. LOWIE, R. H.: *Social Organization.* New York, Holt, Rinehart & Winston, 1948.

226. HOLMBERG, A. R.: *Nomads of the long bow.* Washington, D.C. "Smithsonian Inst. Soc. Anthrop. Publ. No. 10," 1950.

227. PIAGET, J.: *The Origins of Intelligence in Children.* New York, International Universities Press, 1952.

228. SULLIVAN, H. S.: *op. cit.,* 1953.

229. FROMM, E.: *The Sane Society*. New York: Holt, Rinehart & Winston, 1955.

230. SROLE, L., LANGNER, T., MICHAEL S., OPLER, M. K., and RENNIE, T. A. C.: *Mental Health in the Metropolis: The Midtown Manhattan Study*. New York, McGraw-Hill, 1962.

231. OPLER, M. K.: Epidemiological studies of mental illness: methods and scope of the Midtown Study in New York. In *Symposium on Preventive and Social Psychiatry*. Washington, D.C., Walter Reed Army Institute of Research, 1958a.

232. FREEMAN, H. E., LEVINE, S., and REEDER, L. G. (Eds.): *Handbook of Medical Sociology*. New York, Prentice-Hall, 1963.

233. GRAHAM, SAXON: Ethnic background and illness in a Pennsylvania county. *Soc. Problems*, 4:76–82 (July) 1956.

234. OPLER, M. K.: *op. cit.*, 1956a.

235. OPLER, M. K. (Ed.): *Culture and Mental Health: Cross-Cultural Studies*. New York, Macmillan, 1959b.

236. SZASZ, T. S.: *The Myth of Mental Illness*. New York, Hoeber-Harper, 1961.

237. SPIRO, M. E.: Cultural heritage, personal tensions, and mental illness in a South Sea culture, in Opler, M. K., *op. cit.*, 1959b.

238. OPLER, M. K.: *op. cit.*, 1956a.

239. OPLER, M. K.: *op. cit.*, 1959b.

240. OPLER, M. K.: Probleme der sozialpsychiatrie. *Schweizer Monatshefte*, Heft 8:691–702, November, 1958b.

241. BINSWANGER, L.: The case of Ellen West, an anthropological-clinical study, in R. May, E. Angel, and H. F. Ellenberger, *Existence*. New York, Basic Books, 1958.

242. LAING, R. D.: *The Divided Self*. Chicago, Quadrangle Books, Inc., 1961.

243. OPLER, M. K.: *op. cit.*, 1956a.

244. OPLER, M. K.: *op. cit.*, 1959b.

245. OPLER, M. K.: *op. cit.*, 1942.

246. BIERER, J.: *Therapeutic Social Clubs* (edited by J. Bierer). London, H. K. Lewis & Co., 1949.

BIERER, J.: Past, present and future. *International Journal of Social Psychiatry*, 6:165–173, 1960.

247. OPLER, M. K.: *op. cit.*, 1959b.

248. OPLER, M. K.: *op. cit.*, 1958a.

249. OPLER, M. K.: *op. cit.*, 1956a.

250. OPLER, M. K.: *op. cit.*, 1959a.

251. OPLER, M. K.: *op. cit.*, 1959b.

252. OPLER, M. K.: The contribution of social psychiatry to preventive psychiatry. *Dis. of the Nerv. System*, Monograph Supplement, 20, No. 5:22–29, May 1959c.

418

253. BLEULER, EUGEN: *Dementia Praecox, or the Group of Schizophrenias.* New York, International Universities Press, 1950.
254. OPLER, M. K.: *op. cit.,* 1956a.
255. DIETHELM, OSKAR: *Etiology of Chronic Alcoholism.* Springfield, Ill., Charles C Thomas, 1955.
256. STAINBROOK, EDWARD: *op. cit.,* 1952.
257. SINGER, JEROME L., and OPLER, MARVIN K.: Contrasting patterns of fantasy and motility in Irish and Italian schizophrenics. *Journal of Abnormal and Social Psychology,* 53:42–47, 1956; Ethnic differences in behavior and psychopathology. *International Journal of Social Psychiatry,* 2:11–23, 1956.
258. STANTON, ALFRED H., and SCHWARTZ, MORRIS S.: *op. cit.,* 1954.
259. FROMM-REICHMANN, FRIEDA: *op. cit.,* 1950.
260. OPLER, MARVIN K.: *op. cit.,* 1955a.
261. HOLLINGSHEAD, A. B. and REDLICH, F. C.: *Social Class and Mental Illness.* New York, Wiley, 1958; OPLER, M. K.: *op. cit.,* 1956a.
262. OPLER, M. K.: *op. cit.,* 1958a.
263. OPLER, M. K.: Anthropological aspects of psychiatry. In *Progress in Psychotherapy,* Eds., J. H. Masserman and J. L. Moreno. New York, Grune & Stratton, 1959d; Cultural evolution and the psychology of peoples. In *Essays in the Science of Culture,* Eds., R. Carneiro and G. E. Dole. New York, Crowell, 1960.
264. OPLER, M. K.: *op. cit.,* 1959b.
265. HOLLINGSHEAD, A. B., and REDLICH, F. C.: *op. cit.,* 1958; SROLE, L.; LANGLER, T. S.; MICHAEL, S.; OPLER, M. K.; and RENNIE, T. A. C.: *op. cit.,* 1962.
266. FIELD, M. J.: *The Search for Security.* Evanston, Northwestern University Press, 1960.
267. JEWELL, D. P.: A case of a "psychotic Navajo Indian male." In *Sociological Studies of Health and Sickness,* Ed., D. Apple. New York, McGraw-Hill, 1960.
268. HOHMANN, G. H.: A stoic faces stress. In *Clinical Studies in Culture Conflict,* Ed., G. Seward. New York, Ronald, 1958.
269. OPLER, M. K.: *op. cit.,* 1955a.
270. OPLER, M. K.: *op. cit.,* 1959b.
271. OPLER, M. K.: *op. cit.,* 1942.
272. OPLER, M. K.: Cf. *op. cit.,* 1956b; and *op. cit.,* 1942.
273. OPLER, M. K.: *op. cit.,* 1960.
274. FIELD, M. J., *op. cit.,* 1960.
275. BOHANNAN, PAUL D.: Review of M. J. Field's *The Search for Security. Amer. Anthropologist,* 63:435, 1961.
276. FIELD, M. J.: *op. cit.,* 1960, p. 449.
277. *Accra Daily Graphic:* May 19, 1961, p. 22.
278. FIELD, M. J.: *op. cit.,* 1960, p. 358.

279. FORSTER, E. F. B.: Psychiatry in a changing world. *Amer. J. of Psychotherapy.* In press.

280. FIELD, M. J.: *op. cit.,* 1960, p. 149.

281. *Ibid.,* p. 105.

282. LYSTAD, ROBERT A.: Marriage and kinship among the Ashanti and the Agni. A study of differential acculturation. In *Continuity and Change in African Cultures,* Eds., William R. Bascom and Melville J. Herskovits. Chicago, University of Chicago Press, 1959.

283. LOUDON, J. B.: Zulu. In *Culture and Mental Health, op. cit.,* 1959b.

284. FIELD, M. J., *op. cit.,* 1960, p. 444.

285. *Ibid.,* p. 318.

286. MALINOWSKI, B.: *Dynamics of Culture Change.* London and New York, Oxford University Press, 1945.

287. LAMBO, T. ADEOYE: *Journal of Mental Science,* 101(423), April 1955.

288. LEAVELL, H. R., and CLARK, E. G.: *Preventive Medicine.* New York, McGraw-Hill, 1958.

289. See OPLER, M. K.: Ethnic differences in behavior and health practice, in *The Family: A Focal Point in Health Education,* I. Galdston, ed. New York, International Universities Press, 1961.

290. NOYES, ARTHUR P., and KOLB, LAWRENCE C.: *Modern Clinical Psychiatry.* Philadelphia, Pa., W. B. Saunders, 1958, p. 471.

291. ENGEL, GEORGE: *Psychological Development in Health and Disease.* Philadelphia, Pa., W. B. Saunders, 1962, p. 391.

292. FREUD, SIGMUND: *The Problem of Anxiety.* New York, W. W. Norton, 1936.

293. ZBOROWSKI, M., and HERZOG, E.: *Life Is With People.* New York, International Universities Press, 1952.

294. RAYCHAUDHURY, A. K.: A case of diabetes mellitus: A study in psychosomatic medicine, *Psychosomatic Medicine,* 20:33–40, 1958.

295. DUNBAR, F.: *Psychiatry in the Medical Specialties.* New York, McGraw-Hill, 1959, p. 172.

296. BRUCH, H.: Physiologic and psychologic interrelationships in diabetes of children, *Psychosomatic Medicine,* 12:200–210, 1949.

297. BARR, D. P.: Health and obesity, *New England Journal of Medicine,* 23:967, 1953.

298. OPLER, M. K., History of the family as a social and cultural institution, in *The Family in Contemporary Society.* I. Galdston, ed. New York, International Universities Press, 1958c, pp. 33–36.

299. ROSEN, H., and LIDZ, T.: Emotional factors in the precipitation of recurrent diabetes acidosis, *Psychosomatic Medicine,* 11:211, 1949.

300. MIRSKY, I. A.: Emotional factors in patients with diabetes mellitus, *Bulletin of Menninger Clinic,* 12:187, 1948.

301. HINKLE, L. E., and WOLF, S.: Studies in diabetes mellitus: changes in glucose, ketone, and water metabolism during stress, in *Life Stress*

and Bodily Disease, H. G. Wolff, ed., Vol. 29, Association for Research in Nervous and Mental Disease, Williams and Wilkins, 1950, pp. 338–389.

302. SEFTEL, H., and SCHULTZ, E.: Diabetes mellitus in the urbanized Johannesburg African," *South African Medical Journal,* 35:66–71, 1961.

303. See OPLER, M. K.: *op. cit.,* 1959b.

Index

426

Heart disease, 287
Heidegger, Martin, 275
Helvétius, Claude Adrien, 243
Henderson, D. K., 120
Henry, G. W., 155–56
Henry, Jules, 10, 81, 85–86, 91
Hermaphrodites, 257–58
Herzog, E., 337
High blood pressure. *See* Hypertension
Hilliboe and Larimore, 268, 331
Hindus, 78, 338
Hinkle and Wolf, 340
"History and Science in Anthropology" (Kroeber), 244–45
Hoch, Paul, 46
Hogben, Lancelot, 12, 239
Hohmann, G. H., 307
Hokkaido. *See* Imu illness
Holland, the Dutch, 17, 69, 103, 283
Hollingshead, A. B., 43, 94, 278
Holmberg, Allan R., 32, 263, 336
Holmes, William H., 240
Holtzman, Philip, 191
Homicide, homicidal acts, 124, 131, 134, 135
Homosexuality, 121, 122, 126, 152, 154, 155–56, 249–64, 292ff; in case history, 386ff; Kinsey and, 152
Hoover Commission, 98
Hopi Indians, 9, 24
Horney, Karen, 20, 31–33, 35, 146, 155, 189
Hospitals, xii, 43ff, 48–49, 205–6, 214, 278
Housing, 268. *See also* Population density; Slums; Urban areas
Hsu, Francis, 193, 304
Human Animal, The (LaBarre), 201–2
"Human nature," 244
Hungarians, 34–35, 99, 267, 269, 289
Hunting and gathering societies, 184–85, 252
Huston, L., 95
Hutterites, 42–43, 65
Huxley, Thomas, 233

Hyde, R. W., 33, 35, 41, 42, 102, 163, 164, 287, 288
Hyperglycemia, 334–35, 336
Hypertension (high blood pressure), 82, 83, 199–200, 267, 268, 269, 287
Hypochondria, 294ff. *See also* Psychosomatic diseases
Hysterias, 49, 81, 106, 107, 144, 271; Arctic, 17; "French," 70, 86

Id, 144, 188, 251
Identification, 53, 60, 144, 275. *See also* Sex
Ifaluk, 271
Impotence, 124
Impounded People, 360n
Imu illness, 17, 23, 133
"In Defense of Culture-Personality Studies" (Eaton), 67
Incest, 37, 183, 186, 259. *See also* Oedipus theory
Incidence of psychiatric disorders, 40–63
Income, 268
India (Indians), 17, 69, 128, 137, 142, 144, 337–38
Indians, American, 140–41, 240; and homosexuality, 252–53; Plains, 23, 71, 132, 200
Indians of North America (Driver), 252–53
Individual and His Culture, The (Kardiner), 174
Infancy, 59. *See also* Children; Families and kinship
Inside Story: Psychiatry and Everyday Life, The (Redlich and Bingham), 105
Intergenerational conflict, 60, 91–92, 97, 338–39; in Ghana, 321–23
International Journal of Social Psychiatry, 272, 273
Interpersonal Theory of Psychiatry (Sullivan), 7–8
Inventions, 246–47
Involutional disorders, 30–31, 107